Common Sense Dictionary

for First Responders

Common Sense Dictionary

for First Responders

Frank L. Fire

Fire Engineering

PennWell

DISCLAIMER

The recommendations, advice, descriptions, and the methods in this book are presented solely for educational purposes. The author and publisher assume no liability whatsoever for any loss or damage that results from the use of any of the material in this book. Use of the material in this book is solely at the risk of the user.

PennWell Corporation
1421 South Sheridan Road
Tulsa, Oklahoma 74112-6600 USA
800.752.9764
+1.918.831.9421
sales@pennwell.com
www.FireEngineering Books.com
www.pennwellbooks.com
www.pennwell.com

Director: Mary McGee
Managing Editor: Jerry Naylis
Production/Operations Manager: Traci Huntsman
Production Editor: Tony Quinn
Book Designer: Robin Remaley
Cover Designer: Sheila Brock

Library of Congress Cataloging-in-Publication Data

Fire, Frank L., 1937-
Common sense dictionary for first responders / Frank L. Fire.
p. cm.
ISBN-13: 978-1-59370-099-7 (softcover)
ISBN-10: 1-59370-099-7 (softcover)
1. Emergency management--United States--Dictionaries. 2. First aid in illness and injury--Dictionaries. 3. Hazardous substances--Dictionaries. I. Title.
HV551.3.F565 2006
363.003--dc22

2006029119

Printed in the United States of America

1 2 3 4 5 10 09 08 07 06

This book is dedicated to my grandchildren:

Kurt Fire
Mark Fire
Jennifer Fire
Nicholas Fire
Amanda Fire
Emily Fire
Aidan Fire

Contents

INTRODUCTION

It is appropriate for a dictionary for emergency responders to begin with definitions. Although everyone knows what a dictionary is, a simple definition is as follows: a reference book that contains words listed in alphabetical order and gives explanations of their meanings. Although dictionaries usually provide additional information about grammar, pronunciation, and etymology, *Common Sense Dictionary for First Responders* will not provide that information. Instead, it is presented as a reference book that gives the meanings of, and often other information about, terms relating to particular subjects or fields, arranged alphabetically.

An emergency responder may be defined as any person whose duty it is to respond to an emergency situation. A first responder is an individual who arrives first at the scene of a fire, a hazardous materials incident, or an emergency of any kind, with the responsibility to act. There are many federal, state, and local regulations that further define an emergency responder and/or first responder. These regulations often list the training and education one must possess before he or she may be classified as any type of responder.

This dictionary contains selected words and their meanings that will be important to first responders to fires and/or hazardous materials incidents, environmentalists, and safety engineers. It will also be helpful to anyone else who may, because of profession or interest, come into contact with an environment made dangerous by the presence of hazardous chemicals. No attempt has been made to include every word in the English language that has something to do with such a complex subject, since such an undertaking would require a work much larger than this one. Nor has an attempt been made to include every word that every first responder learns in his or her training. The emphasis here is on specialized words that will describe certain hazards and conditions that are dangerous to the responder or an ordinary citizen.

The words selected are those that provide a basic understanding of the dangers faced by individual and teams of emergency responders, and further study and training will lead them to individual dictionaries and glossaries specific to each science involved. In some cases, a word or title will be obsolete due to the changing of a law, or the disappearance or merger of a governmental agency. Since the word or title may still appear in the literature, its definition will still be included.

Where multiple definitions of a word or term are given, the order in which they are numbered is not necessarily important. Each discipline (firefighting, hazardous materials response, or environmental occupations, etc.) may have a slightly different or pertinent definition.

Chemical warfare agents are listed under their chemical name, the military designation, and their agent designation. For example, sarin is listed as methylphosphonofluoridic acid and isopropyl ester in the dictionary section. It is also listed as GB in the abbreviations and acronyms section, and it is described as a chemical nerve agent in both sections.

Definitions of words and a listing of abbreviations are provided for the following subjects:

electricity
emergency medical services
environment
firefighting
general chemistry (as it relates to hazardous materials)
general science
hazardous materials
material safety data sheet (MSDS)
plastics
protective clothing
radioactivity
shipping regulations
transportation

There are more than 4,200 terms defined. Section II includes general abbreviations and acronyms.

Definition of Terms

A

abandoned well. A well where use has been permanently discontinued or which is in such a state that it cannot be used for its intended purpose.

abatement. The action of reducing the degree or intensity of an incident, or to eliminate it entirely.

abatement debris. Waste from remediation activities.

A/B/C/D sides. Terminology used by responding fire departments at a building fire to identify the sides of buildings. *A* is the front of the building, and sides *B*, *C*, and *D* follow clockwise around the building.

ABC extinguisher. A fire extinguisher that can be used on fires involving ordinary combustibles, flammable liquids, and energized electrical equipment. May also be called a *multipurpose extinguisher*.

Abel tester. A device used to test for the flash points of kerosene and other liquids having flash points of 120°F and lower.

abrasion resistance. Resistance to surface wear.

absolute. Any chemical that is free from any other material, except for up to 1% water.

absolute alcohol. Alcohol that is free from any other material, except for up to 1% water. The term usually refers to ethyl alcohol.

absolute zero. The temperature at which all molecular motion ceases; –459.6°F (0°R) or –273.16°C (0 K).

absorb. When one material penetrates into the structure of another substance.

absorbed dose. The amount of a substance that penetrates an exposed organism's absorption barriers (e.g., skin, lung tissue, and gastrointestinal tract) through physical or biological processes. May also be called the **internal dose**.

absorbent. Any material that allows another substance to penetrate into its inner physical structure, thus allowing it to be "captured" and moved.

absorption. 1. The penetration of one substance into the physical structure of another substance. 2. The uptake of water, other fluids, or dissolved chemicals by a cell or an organism. *Contrast with* **adsorption**.

absorption barrier. Any of the exchange sites of the body that permit uptake of various substances at different rates (e.g., skin, lung tissue, and gastrointestinal-tract wall).

ABS resins. A group of terpolymers of acrylonitrile, butadiene, and styrene.

accelerant. A substance used to accelerate, intensify, or speed up the spread of a fire.

accelerator. A compound that will speed up the vulcanization process.

acceptable daily intake (ADI). The amount of a chemical a person can be exposed to on a daily basis over an extended period of time (usually a lifetime) without suffering deleterious effects.

accident site. The location of an unexpected occurrence, failure, or loss, either at a plant or along a transportation route, resulting in a release of hazardous materials.

acclimatization. The physiological and behavioral adjustments of an organism to changes in its environment.

acetal resins. Unbranched polyoxymethylene. Also called *polyformaldehyde.*

acetaminophen. A crystalline painkiller and fever reducer ($C_8H_9NO_2$).

acetate. A salt of acetic acid, with a metal ion replacing the acid's hydrogen.

acetylcholine. A chemical involved in the transmission of nerve impulses, secreted from nerve fiber ends.

acetylcholinesterase. 1. An enzyme present in blood that participates in the breakdown of acetylcholine. 2. An enzyme that will suppress the stimulation of nerve endings by acetylcholine.

acetylsalicylic acid. The chemical name for aspirin.

acid. A chemical compound containing one or more hydrogen ions that will liberate hydrogen gas on contact with certain metals, has a pH of less than 7.0, and may be very active chemically.

acid aerosol. Acidic liquid or solid particles small enough to become airborne. High concentrations can irritate the lungs and have been associated with respiratory diseases like asthma.

acid deposition. 1. Any form of wet precipitation having a pH of 5.6 or less. 2. A complex chemical and atmospheric phenomenon that occurs when emissions of sulfur and nitrogen compounds and other substances are transformed by chemical processes in the atmosphere and deposited on Earth in either wet or dry form. The wet forms, popularly called *acid rain,* can fall to Earth as rain, snow, or fog. The dry forms are acidic gases or particulates.

acid gas. A gas that forms an acid when it dissolves in water.

acidic. 1. Having the properties of an acid. 2. The condition of water or soil that contains a sufficient amount of acid substances to lower the pH below 7.0.

acid ionization constant. The equilibrium constant describing the degree of dissociation of an acid.

acid mine drainage. Drainage of water from areas that have been mined for coal or other mineral ores; usually acidic.

acid neutralizing capacity. The measure of the ability of a base (e.g., water or soil) to resist changes in pH.

acid of sugar. Archaic name for oxalic acid.

acidosis. A condition of the blood and tissues caused by decreased alkalinity. Symptoms are a sickly sweet breath, headache, nausea, vomiting, and visual disturbances.

acid rain. *See* **acid deposition**.

acid suit. A totally encapsulating suit with supplied air that will offer resistance to corrosive materials and atmospheres.

ackey. Archaic name for nitric acid.

acrid. A bitter, harsh, and sharp taste or smell.

acrylate elastomers. A family of synthetic elastomers based on polyethylene acrylate copolymerized with a monomer that allows crosslinking.

acrylic resins. Polymers prepared from monomers such as acrylic acid and some of its derivatives.

acrylonitrile. A monomer with the structure CH_2=CHCN. Highly toxic.

acrylonitrile-butadiene-styrene resins. A group of tough thermoplastic materials known as *ABS plastics.*

actinides. 1. The 14 elements in the bottom row of the inner transition elements of the periodic table of the elements (actinium, Ac, atomic number 89, and the elements that follow, with atomic numbers through 103). 2. The actinide series is a subseries of the transition metals. 3. The row of elements below the periodic table, from thorium to lawrencium.

actinium. A solid, silvery white, metallic, radioactive element, symbol Ac, with atomic number 89, and atomic weight 227. It is used as a source of alpha particles.

action levels. 1. Regulatory levels recommended by EPA for enforcement by FDA and USDA when pesticide residues occur in food or feed commodities for reasons other than the direct application of the pesticide. 2. In the Superfund program, the existence of a contaminant concentration in the environment high enough to warrant action or trigger a response under the Superfund Amendments and Reauthorization Act of 1986 (SARA) and the National Oil and Hazardous Substances Contingency Plan. 3. The term is also used in other regulatory programs.

activated carbon (activated charcoal). 1. A form of carbon treated to become highly adsorbent so it can be used to remove odors and other objectionable substances or properties from liquids or gases. 2. In waste treatment, it is used to remove dissolved organic matter from waste drinking water.

activated sludge. The product that results when primary effluent is mixed with bacteria-laden sludge and then agitated and aerated, thus speeding the breakdown of organic matter in raw sewage undergoing secondary waste treatment.

activation energy. The minimum energy required to start a chemical reaction.

activator. A chemical added to a substance to increase its activity.

active ingredient. 1. The chemical that, through its action, will accomplish what the product is manufactured to do. 2. In any pesticide product, the component that kills, or otherwise controls, target pests. Pesticides are regulated primarily on the basis of active ingredients.

activity. 1. The speed with which an element will seek out ways to satisfy the octet rule. 2. Generally refers to the speed and number of other chemicals with which a chemical will react.

acute effect. An adverse effect on a human or animal body, with severe symptoms that develop rapidly and may subside after the exposure stops.

acute exposure. 1. A single exposure to a toxic substance that may result in severe biological harm or death. 2. Acute exposures are usually characterized as lasting no longer than a day, as compared to longer, continuing exposure over a period of time. 3. One dose or multiple doses of short duration spanning less than or equal to 24 hours.

acute lethality. The death of test animals immediately or within 14 days after a single dose of, or exposure to, a toxic substance.

acute toxicity. 1. The ability of a substance to cause severe biological harm or death soon after a single exposure or dose. 2. Any adverse effect resulting from a single short-term exposure to a toxic substance. 3. Any poisonous effect produced within a short period of time following an exposure, usually within 24 to 96 hours.

adamsite. A chemical vomiting agent (diphenylaminearsine); agent DM.

adaptation. Changes in an organism's physiological structure, function, or habits that allow it to survive in new surroundings.

added risk. *See* **additional risk**.

additional risk (AR). 1. The calculated difference in risk of a particular condition between those who are exposed and those who are not. 2. An absolute measure of the excess risk attributed to exposure. Also called *added risk, attributable risk,* or *risk difference.*

additive. 1. Any material mixed with a plastic or resin to modify its properties. 2. Any chemical added to the active ingredient that will somehow modify its activity or effectiveness.

additive effect. The combined effect of two chemicals equals the sum of the agents acting alone.

add-on control device. An air pollution control device, such as carbon absorber or incinerator, that reduces the pollution in an exhaust gas. The control device usually does not affect the process being controlled and thus is "add-on" technology, as opposed to a scheme to control pollution through altering the basic process itself.

adequately wet. Asbestos-containing material that is sufficiently mixed or penetrated with liquid to prevent the release of particulates.

adhesive. Any substance capable of bonding other materials together.

administered dose. The amount of a substance given to a test subject (human or animal) to determine dose-response relationships. Also may be called the **potential dose**.

administrative control. A series of policies and practices written before work begins to minimize exposure to chemical and physical hazards.

administrative order. A legal document signed by EPA directing an individual, business, or other entity to take corrective action or refrain from an activity. It describes the violations and actions to be taken and can be enforced in court.

administrative order on consent. A legal agreement signed by EPA and an individual, business, or other entity through which the violator agrees to pay for correction of violations, take the required corrective or cleanup actions, or refrain from an activity. It describes the actions to be taken, may be subject to a comment period, applies to civil actions, and can be enforced in court.

Administrative Procedures Act. A law that specifies procedures and requirements related to the promulgation of regulations.

administrative record. All documents that EPA considered or relied on in selecting the response action at a Superfund site, culminating in the record of decision for remedial action; or, an action memorandum for removal actions.

adsorb. To condense or hold molecules of another substance on the surface.

adsorbent. Any material that has the ability to condense or hold molecules of another substance on its surface.

adsorption. 1. Removal of a pollutant from air or water by collecting the pollutant on the surface of a solid material. 2. The adherence of one substance to the outer surface of another substance. *Contrast with* **absorption**.

adulterants. Chemical impurities or substances that by law do not belong in a food, pesticide, or other controlled material.

adulterated. 1. Any pesticide whose strength or purity falls below the quality stated on its label. 2. A food, feed, or product that contains illegal pesticide residues.

advanced life support (ALS). A level of emergency medical care typified by paramedics capable of delivering advanced skills performed by emergency medical services (EMS) practitioners.

advanced treatment. A level of wastewater treatment more stringent than secondary treatment; requires an 85% reduction in conventional pollutant concentration or a significant reduction in nonconventional pollutants. Also may be called **tertiary treatment**.

advanced wastewater treatment. Any treatment of sewage that goes beyond the secondary or biological water treatment stage and includes the removal of nutrients such as phosphorus and nitrogen and a high percentage of suspended solids.

adverse effect. A biochemical change, functional impairment, or pathologic lesion that affects the performance of the whole organism, or reduces an organism's ability to respond to an additional environmental challenge.

adverse effects data. The Federal Insecticide, Fungicide, and Rodenticide Act (FIFRA) requires a pesticide registrant to submit data to EPA on any studies or other information regarding unreasonable adverse effects of a pesticide at any time after its registration.

advisory. A nonregulatory document that communicates risk information to those who may have to make risk management decisions.

aerated lagoon. A holding or treatment pond, or both, that speeds up the natural process of biological decomposition of organic waste by stimulating the growth and activity of bacteria that degrade organic waste.

aeration. 1. A process that promotes biological degradation of organic matter in water. 2. A method of purification of liquids. 3. A process by which air is introduced into a liquid, either by bubbling the air through it or by spraying the liquid into the air at normal pressures.

aeration tank. A chamber used to inject air into water.

aerobic. Life or processes that require, or are not destroyed by, the presence of oxygen.

aerobic treatment. Process by which microbes decompose complex organic compounds in the presence of oxygen.

aerosol. 1. A finely divided material suspended in air or other gaseous environment. 2. Small droplets or particles suspended in the atmosphere, typically containing sulfur, that are usually emitted naturally (e.g., in volcanic eruptions) or as the result of activities such as burning fossil fuels. 3. A colloid in which solid particles or liquid droplets are suspended in a gas. Smoke is an example of a solid aerosol; fog is an example of a liquid aerosol. 4. The pressurized gas used to propel substances out of a container. 5. A fine suspension of liquid particles in air.

affected landfill. Under the Clean Air Act, landfills that meet criteria for capacity, age, and emissions rates set by the EPA. These landfills are required to collect and combust their gas emissions.

affected public. 1. The people who live and/or work near a hazardous waste site. 2. The human population adversely impacted following exposure to a toxic pollutant in food, water, air, or soil.

aflatoxin. A poisonous chemical released in certain agricultural crops by a mold fungus, particularly peanuts. May also occur in animal feed.

afterburner. In incinerator technology, a burner located so that the combustion gases are made to pass through its flame in order to remove smoke and odors.

agent. Any physical, chemical, or biological substance that can be harmful to an organism.

Agent Orange. A toxic herbicide and defoliant, containing 2,4,5-trichlorophenoxyacetic acid (2,4,5-T) and 2-4 dichlorophenoxyacetic acid (2,4-D) with trace amounts of dioxin.

age tank. A tank used to store a chemical solution of known concentration for feed to a chemical feeder. May also be called a *day tank*.

aging. The effect of exposure of articles to the environment for an extended period of time. If the environment is an artificial one for test purposes, or the test is designed to provide exposure to the article faster than would occur in the environment in which it is to perform, the aging is said to be *artificial* or *accelerated*.

agricultural pollution. Farming wastes, including: runoff and leaching of pesticides and fertilizers; erosion and dust from plowing; improper disposal of animal manure and carcasses; and crop residues and debris.

agroecosystem. Land used for crops, pasture, and livestock; the adjacent uncultivated land that supports other vegetation and wildlife; and the associated atmosphere, including the underlying soils, groundwater, and drainage networks.

AHERA designated person (ADP). A person designated by a local education agency to ensure that the Asbestos Hazard Emergency Response Act of 1986 (AHERA) requirements for asbestos management and abatement are properly implemented.

air. A mixture of gases that varies throughout the atmosphere. Dry air at sea level usually contains 78% nitrogen, 20.95% oxygen, and 0.93% argon. The other 0.12% is made up of carbon dioxide, helium, hydrogen, krypton, methane, neon, nitrous oxide, ozone, and xenon.

air binding. Situation where air enters the filter media and harms both the filtration and backwash processes.

airborne particulates. Total suspended particulate matter found in the atmosphere as solid particles or liquid droplets. Sources of airborne particulates include: dust, emissions from industrial processes, combustion products from the burning of wood and coal, combustion products associated with motor vehicle or nonroad engine exhausts, and reactions to gases in the atmosphere.

airborne release. Release of any pollutant into the air.

air changes per hour (ACH). The movement of a volume of air in a given period of time.

air cleaning. Indoor air quality control strategy to remove various airborne particulates and/or gases from the air. Most common methods are particulate filtration, electrostatic precipitation, and gas sorption.

air contaminant. Any particulate matter, gas, or combination thereof, other than water vapor. *See* **air pollutant**.

air curtain. A method of containing oil spills. Air bubbling through a perforated pipe causes an upward water flow that slows the spread of oil. It can also be used to stop fish from entering polluted water.

air exchange rate. The rate at which outside air replaces indoor air in a given space.

air gap. Open vertical gap or empty space that separates and protects a drinking water supply from another water system in a treatment plant or other location.

air handling unit. Equipment that includes a fan or blower, heating and/or cooling coils, regulator controls, condensate drain pans, and air filters.

air inlet. *See* **vapor valve**.

air mass. A large volume of air with certain meteorological or polluted characteristics—e.g., a heat inversion or smog—while in one location. The characteristics can change as the air mass moves away.

air monitoring. *See* **monitoring**.

air/oil table. The surface between the vadose zone and ambient oil. The pressure of oil in the porous medium is equal to atmospheric pressure.

air padding. Pumping dry air into a container to assist with the withdrawal of liquid or to force a liquefied gas such as chlorine out of the container.

air permeability. Permeability of soil with respect to air. Important to the design of soil-gas surveys. Measured in Darcies or centimeters per second.

air plenum. Any space used to convey air in a building, furnace, or structure. The space above a suspended ceiling is often used as an air plenum.

air pollutant. Any substance in air that could, in high enough concentration, harm man, other animals, vegetation, or material.

air pollution. The presence of contaminants or pollutant substances in the air that interferes with human health or welfare, or produces other harmful environmental effects.

air pollution control device. A mechanism or piece of equipment that cleans emissions generated by a source by removing pollutants that would otherwise be released into the atmosphere.

air pollution episode. A period of abnormally high concentration of air pollutants, often due to low winds and temperature inversion, that can cause illness and death. Also called *emergency episode.*

air purification respirator (APR). A device worn to filter particulates and contaminants from the air. Also called an *air purifying respirator*.

air quality criteria. The levels of pollution and lengths of exposure above which adverse health and welfare effects may occur.

air quality index (AQI). The EPA's 1999 update of the pollutant standards index to include standards for ozone and PM2.5. *See also* **pollutant standards index**.

air quality standards. The level of pollutants prescribed by regulations that are not to be exceeded during a given time in a defined area.

air reactive. A substance that will self-react and/or ignite when exposed to air.

air sparging. Injecting air or oxygen into an aquifer to strip or flush volatile contaminants as the air bubbles up through the groundwater and is captured by a vapor extraction system.

air stripping. 1. A method of removing volatile organic compounds (VOCs) from contaminated water by forcing an airstream through the water and causing the compounds to evaporate. 2. The process by which a material is pumped through an air chamber or sprayed into the open air at high pressure to remove contaminants.

air toxics. Any air pollutant for which a National Ambient Air Quality Standard (NAAQS) does not exist.

air valve. *See* **vapor valve**.

alachlor. A herbicide, marketed under the trade name Lasso, used mainly to control weeds in corn and soybean fields.

Alar. Trade name for daminozide, a pesticide that makes apples redder, firmer, and less likely to drop off trees before growers are ready to pick them. It is also used to a lesser extent on peanuts, tart cherries, concord grapes, and other fruits.

alchemy. The unscientific predecessor of chemistry. Alchemists spent their lives trying to convert base metals like lead into gold.

alcohol. A hydrocarbon derivative having the general formula R-OH, where the R- is the hydrocarbon backbone and the -OH is the hydroxyl radical.

alcohol foam/alcohol resistant foam. 1. A firefighting foam that is resistant to "polar" chemicals such as ketones and esters that may break down other types of foam. 2. A type of foam developed to suppress ignitable vapors of polar solvents (those miscible in water).

aldehyde. A hydrocarbon derivative having the general formula R-CHO, where the R- is the hydrocarbon backbone and the -CHO is the aldehyde radical.

aldicarb. An insecticide sold under the trade name Temik. It is made from ethyl isocyanate.

algae. Simple rootless plants that grow in sunlit waters in proportion to the amount of available nutrients and are food for fish and small aquatic animals.

algal blooms. Sudden spurts of algal growth, which can affect water quality adversely and indicate potentially hazardous changes in local water chemistry.

algicide. A substance or chemical used specifically to kill or control algae.

alicyclic. Organic compounds whose carbon atoms are arranged in a closed ring but do not contain the hexagonal benzene ring and are therefore not aromatic compounds.

aliphatic. Organic compounds such as hydrocarbons characterized by straight-chain or branched-chain arrangement of the carbon atoms. There are three groups of aliphatic hydrocarbons: alkanes (paraffins), alkenes (olefins), and alkynes (acetylenes).

aliquot. A measured portion of a sample taken for analysis.

alkali. Any substance that has a pH greater than 7.0 (neutral). The chemicals known as alkalis are corrosive. The hydroxides are also referred to as *bases.*

alkali metal. A member of group I on the periodic table of the elements. The alkali metals are lithium, sodium, potassium, rubidium, cesium, and francium.

alkaline. 1. The condition of water or soil that contains a sufficient amount of alkali substance to raise the pH above 7.0. 2. The property of being an alkali. 3. Being caustic in nature. 4. The chemical opposite of acidic. 5. Having a pH greater than 7.0. 6. Any substance that is basic (rather than acidic) in water solutions. 7. Usually pertains to hydroxides.

alkaline earth metal. A member of group II on the periodic table of the elements. The alkaline earth metals are beryllium, magnesium, calcium, strontium, barium, and radium.

alkalinity. 1. The capacity of bases to neutralize acids. 2. The property of being alkaline.

alkaloids. Chemical compounds containing nitrogen, found in plants, that are highly toxic. At certain concentrations, they are effective as drugs or medicines.

alkanes. The analogous family of saturated hydrocarbons that has the general formula C_nH_{2n+2}. The first 10 straight-chain alkanes are methane, ethane, propane, butane, pentane, hexane, heptane, octane, nonane, and decane.

alkenes. 1. The analogous family of unsaturated hydrocarbons that has the general formula C_nH_{2n}. The first nine straight-chain alkenes are ethene, propene, butene, pentene, hexene, heptene, octene, nonene, and decene. 2. All alkenes have one double bond between carbon atoms.

alkyd resins. Polyester resins made with a fatty acid modifier. The most important surface coating resins.

alkyl. A hydrocarbon radical or backbone derived from the alkanes by removing one hydrogen from the molecule (e.g., methane → methyl, ethane → ethyl, propane → propyl, etc.).

alkylated. The introduction of an alkyl radical onto an organic molecule.

alkyl radical. In a general formula, R- is the first alkyl radical in the formula, R'- may represent the same radical, or it may represent a different alkyl radical. If a third alkyl radical appears, it would be designated R"-.

alkynes. The analogous family of saturated hydrocarbons that has the general formula C_nH_{2n-2}. The simplest alkyne is acetylene (C_2H_2), and all alkynes have one triple bond between carbon atoms.

allergen. A substance that causes an allergic reaction in individuals sensitive to it.

allergic reaction. Abnormal physiological response to a chemical stimuli by a sensitive person.

allergic respiratory reaction. One or more of the following symptoms: labored breathing, coughing, or gasping caused by inhaling a particular substance.

allergic skin reaction. One or more of the following symptoms: reddening, swelling, and/or itching of the skin following contact with a substance to which a person has become sensitized due to previous skin contact or natural body conditions.

allergy. A condition in which a person has been sensitized to a substance, subsequently reacting adversely to further exposure.

allotrope. One of two or more possible forms of an element.

alloy. 1. A physical mixture, usually of metals, created by melting the metals together. 2. Alloys are mixtures, and not chemical compounds. 3. Alloys may also be mixtures of polymers and polymer compounds.

alluvial. 1. Relating to sediments deposited by flowing water 2. The sand or other sediment deposited by flowing water.

allyl resins. Plastics made by the polymerization of monomers containing the allyl group (CH_2=CH–CH_2-).

alpha particle. 1. A specific particle ejected from a radioactive atom. It has low penetrating power and short range. Alpha particles will generally fail to penetrate the skin. However, alpha-emitting atoms can cause health effects if introduced into the lungs or wounds. 2. The nucleus of an atom of helium (two protons and two neutrons). 3. A helium ion (He^{+2}). 4. Also denoted as *α-particle.*

alpha radiation. *See* **alpha ray.**

alpha ray. A stream of alpha particles. Alpha rays rapidly dissipate their energy as they pass through materials and are far less penetrating than beta particles and gamma rays. Also called *alpha radiation.*

alternate method. Any method of sampling and analyzing for an air or water pollutant that is not a reference or equivalent method but is acceptable to EPA as adequate for compliance monitoring.

alternative compliance. A policy that allows facilities to choose among methods for achieving emission reduction or risk reduction instead of following specified standards.

alternative fuels. Substitutes for traditional liquid, oil-derived motor vehicle fuels like gasoline and diesel. Includes mixtures of alcohol-based fuels with gasoline, methanol, ethanol, compressed natural gas, hydrogen, and others.

alternative preservatives. Wood preservatives other than CCA, ACZA, penta, and creosote.

alternative remedial contract strategy contractors. Government contractors that provide project management and technical services to support remedial response activities at National Priorities List (NPL) sites.

alum. 1. Originally potassium aluminum sulfate, $KAl(SO_4)_2 \cdot 12H_2O$. 2. The term now includes salts in which sodium or ammonium substitute for potassium.

alumina. Aluminum oxide.

aluminum. A light, silvery white, solid, metallic element, symbol Al, with atomic number 13, and atomic weight 26.98. It corrodes rapidly to form a very thin layer of aluminum oxide on its surface, and then is resistant to further corrosion.

alveoli. Small air spaces deep in the lungs where oxygen enters the blood.

amatol. A mixture of ammonium nitrate (NH_4NO_3) and TNT (trinitrotoluene) used in bombs and artillery shells.

ambient air. 1. Any unconfined portion of the atmosphere. 2. Open air. 3. Surrounding air.

ambient air quality standards. *See* **criteria pollutants** and **National Ambient Air Quality Standards.**

ambient measurement. A measurement of the concentration of a substance or pollutant within the immediate surroundings of an organism or point.

ambient medium. Material surrounding or contacting an organism.

ambient temperature. Temperature of the surrounding air or other medium.

American Conference of Governmental Industrial Hygienists (ACGIH). An organization of professional personnel in governmental agencies or educational institutions that sets limits on worker exposure to hazardous substances. It publishes threshold limit value–time-weighted average (TLV-TWA) and short-term exposure limit (STEL) information.

American Society for Testing and Materials (ASTM). A voluntary, consensus organization that publishes test methods for numerous materials.

American Wood Preservers Institute (AWPI). The association representing the treated wood industry, whose members include wood treaters, preservative manufacturers, and supporting members supplying goods and services.

americium. A white, solid, metallic, radioactive element, symbol Am, with atomic number 95, and atomic weight 243. Used as a source of alpha particles.

amide. A hydrocarbon derivative containing the amide group ($-CONH_2$).

amine. A hydrocarbon (or ammonia) derivative having the general formula $R-NH_2$, where the R- is the hydrocarbon backbone and the $-NH_2$ is the amine radical.

amino plastics. Polymers containing the -NH or $-NH_2$ group. They are based on reactions of formaldehyde with melamine or urea.

amiton. One of the second-generation nerve agents similar to VX-gas, estimated to be 10 times more toxic than sarin.

ammeter. A device that measures electrical current.

ammoniacal copper zinc arsenate (ACZA). 1. An inorganic arsenic compound. 2. A waterborne wood preservative with uses similar to those of chromated copper arsenate (CCA), a wood preservative.

ammonium. A complex cation (NH_4^{+1}).

amorphous. 1. Noncrystalline. 2. Having no formal structure.

ampere. A measure of electrical current used to describe the number of electrons moving through a wire in 1 second (1 coulomb per second); amp. or A.

amperometric titration. A way of measuring concentrations of certain substances in water using an electric current that flows during a chemical reaction.

amphiprotic. *See* **amphoteric.**

amphoteric. A substance having both acid and base characteristics. It is now more commonly called *amphiprotic.*

amyl. A pentyl radical or substituent ($-C_5H_{11}$).

amylene. A pentene, C_5H_{11}, usually 1-pentene or 2-pentene. Isoamylene is one of the isomers of 2-methyl-2-butene.

amyl hydrate. An amyl (i.e., pentyl) alcohol.

anaerobic. 1. A life or process that occurs in, or is not destroyed by, the absence of oxygen. 2. In the absence of oxygen.

anaerobic decomposition. A change in the chemical composition of organic matter caused by microorganisms in an oxygen-free environment.

analog. A compound in one analogous series that has a property in common with a compound in another analogous series; for example, methyl chloride is an analog of methyl fluoride.

analogous. Similar or alike in a way that allows analogies to be made. An analogous series of chemical compounds all belong to the same "family," and the similarities allow certain conclusions to be drawn.

analogous series. A series of compounds that have differences of the same type between compounds. That is, in an analogous series of hydrocarbon compounds, each compound is different from the one succeeding it by one more carbon atom in the chain.

anecdotal data. Data based on the description of individual cases rather than controlled studies.

anesthetic. A substance that renders a human or animal drowsy, and in large doses or exposures can produce unconsciousness and death.

angstrom. A measure of length that is 1/10,000,000,000 of a meter (10^{-10} m) or 1/10th of a nanometer; Å.

anhydride. A chemical or other substance with all water removed.

anhydrous. A chemical term meaning "no water present."

animal dander. Tiny scales of animal skin; a common indoor air pollutant.

animal studies. Investigations using animals as surrogates for humans with the expectation that the results are pertinent to humans.

anion. A negatively charged ion.

anisotropy. In hydrology, the conditions under which one or more hydraulic properties of an aquifer vary from a reference point.

annular space. The space between two concentric tubes or casings, or between the casing and the borehole wall. Also called an *annulus*.

annulus. *See* **annular space**.

anode. 1. The positive electrode of a catalytic cell. 2. When an electric current is passed through an ionic solution, the negatively charged ions (anions) will migrate to the anode. 3. The electrode at which oxidation occurs.

anodize. To coat a metal with a protective film by electrolysis.

anoxia. Condition of cells whereby a deficiency of oxygen causes permanent damage.

antagonism. Interference or inhibition of the effect of one chemical by the action of another.

Antarctic "ozone hole." Refers to the seasonal depletion of ozone in the upper atmosphere above a large area of Antarctica. *See also* **ozone hole**.

anthrax. Derived from the bacterium *Bacillus anthracis*, it is an acute bacterial infection of the skin, lungs, or gastrointestinal (GI) tract. Can be transmitted via direct contact (with infected animals), inhalation, or ingestion. Symptoms include (depending on contraction method): sores, blisters, respiratory distress, fever, shock, intense stomach pain, bowel obstruction, dehydration, diarrhea, fever, blood poisoning, and death.

anthropogenic. Man-made.

antibody. 1. A biological molecule (protein) that specifically recognizes a foreign substance (antigen) as a means of natural defense. 2. Proteins used commonly in diagnostic tests.

antichlor. Sodium thiosulfate.

anti-degradation clause. Part of federal air quality and water quality requirements prohibiting deterioration where pollution levels are above the legal limit.

antidote. A remedy that will counteract the effects of a poison.

antigen. 1. A substance that generates or stimulates a specific antibody immune response. 2. A substance that is specifically bound or attracted to a given antibody molecule.

antimatter. Species of subatomic particles that have the same mass and spin as normal particles but have opposite electrical charges from their normal matter counterparts. When a particle of matter collides with a particle of antimatter, both particles are destroyed, and their masses are converted to photons of equivalent energy. Also called an *antiparticle.*

antimicrobial. An agent that kills microbes.

antioxidant. 1. Compounds that slow the oxidation processes. 2. Antioxidants will slow or prevent the oxidation processes that degrade foods, fuels, rubber, plastic, and other materials by scavenging destructive free radicals from the food. 3. A chemical additive that has the ability to minimize the effects of oxygen on a substance.

antiozonant. Compounds that reverse or prevent severe oxidation by ozone.

antimony. A solid, silver-white, toxic element, symbol Sb, with atomic number 51, and atomic weight 121.75. Used to harden lead.

antiparticle. *See* **antimatter**.

antistatic agent. A chemical additive designed to prevent the accumulation of electrostatic charges on the surface of the article. The chemical may be sprayed on the surface, or it may be incorporated within the plastic compound. The antistatic agent may be a mixture, a chemical compound, another polymer, metal flakes or fibers, or any other conductive material.

apparatus. A truck or group of trucks of any variety used in the fire service.

appearance. The manner in which a substance appears (including color, size, and consistency) at normal room temperature and normal atmospheric conditions.

appliance. Any variety of tools or devices carried on an apparatus that connect hoses or stream devices together.

applicable or relevant and appropriate requirement (ARAR). Any state or federal statute that pertains to protection of human life and the environment in addressing specific conditions or use of a particular cleanup technology at a Superfund site.

applied dose. In exposure assessment, the amount of a substance in contact with the primary absorption boundaries of an organism (e.g., skin, lung tissue, and/or gastrointestinal tract) and available for absorption.

approach suit. Personal protective equipment used with SCBA that allows response personnel to operate in high-temperature atmospheres for short periods of time. This suit will not withstand direct flame.

aqua ammonia. Aqueous solution of ammonium hydroxide.

aqua fortis. Nitric acid, HNO_3; literally "strong water."

aqua regia. 1. Literally "water of the king," a mixture of concentrated nitric and hydrochloric acids capable of dissolving the so-called royal metal, gold. 2. Also called *aqua regis* or *nitrohydrochloric acid.*

aqua vitae. Literally "water of life." Concentrated aqueous ethanol, C_2H_5OH.

aqueous. Pertaining to water or a substance dissolved in water.

aqueous solubility. The maximum concentration of a chemical that will dissolve in pure water at a reference temperature.

aquifer. An underground geological formation, or group of formations, containing water. Aquifers are sources of groundwater for wells and springs.

aquifer test. A test to determine hydraulic properties of an aquifer.

aquitard. Geological formation that may contain groundwater but is not capable of transmitting significant quantities of it under normal hydraulic gradients. May function as a confining bed.

aramid. Generic name for a class of highly aromatic polyamide fibers that are flame resistant. The aramid best known to firefighters is Nomex.

architectural coatings. Coverings such as paint and roof tar that are used on exteriors of buildings.

area of command. A system established to oversee the management of multiple incidents [with multiple incident command systems (ICS)] or to oversee management of a very large incident that has multiple ICS assigned to it.

area of review. In the Underground Injection Control (UIC) Program, the area surrounding an injection well that is reviewed during the permitting process to determine if flow between aquifers will be induced by the injection operation.

area source. Any source of air pollution that is released over a relatively small area but which cannot be classified as a point source.

argentum. Latin for "silver," hence the symbol, Ag.

argon. A nonflammable, gaseous, nonmetallic element, symbol Ar, with atomic number 18, and atomic weight 39.95. It is a member of group VIII on the periodic table of the elements (the inert or "noble" gases).

aromatic. 1. A type of hydrocarbon, such as benzene or toluene, with a specific type of ring structure. 2. Pertaining to benzene-based organic compounds. 3. *Contrast with* **aliphatic** compounds, which have straight or branched chains. 4. The simplest aromatic compound is benzene.

arrhythmia. An irregular heartbeat.

arsenate. A salt of arsenic acid; AsO_4^{-3}.

arsenic. A gray, solid, nonmetallic, toxic element, symbol As, with atomic number 33, and atomic weight 74.9.

arsenicals. Pesticides containing arsenic.

arsenic trichloride. Chemical choking agent.

arsenite. A salt of arsenious acid; AsO_3^{-3}.

arsine. A chemical blood agent; agent SA.

arson. The crime of deliberately burning property for malicious purposes.

artesian aquifer. Water held under pressure in porous rock or soil confined by impermeable geological formations.

artesian well. Well supplied by an aquifer that contains water under pressure.

aryl group. 1. The radical remaining after a hydrogen atom is removed from an aromatic system. 2. A molecular fragment or group attached to a molecule by an atom that is on an aromatic ring.

asbestos. A naturally occurring mineral fiber that can pollute air or water and cause cancer or asbestosis when inhaled.

asbestos abatement. Procedures to control fiber release from asbestos-containing materials in a building, including removal, encapsulation, repair, enclosure, encasement, and operations and maintenance programs.

asbestos assessment. In the asbestos-in-schools program, the evaluation of the physical condition and potential for damage of all friable asbestos containing materials and thermal insulation systems.

asbestos-containing waste materials (ACWM). Mill tailings or any waste that contains commercial asbestos and is generated by a source covered by the Clean Air Act asbestos National Emissions Standards for Hazardous Air Pollutants (NESHAP).

asbestosis. A disease associated with inhalation of asbestos fibers. The disease makes breathing progressively more difficult and can be fatal.

asbestos program manager. A building owner or designated representative who supervises all aspects of the facility asbestos management and control program.

A-scale sound level. A measurement of sound approximating the sensitivity of the human ear, used to note the intensity or annoyance level of sounds.

ash. The powered mineral (inorganic) residue produced by the complete combustion of a material.

aspartame. A trademarked nonnutritive artificial sweetener that is a combination of aspartic acid and L-phenylalanine.

asphalt. A dark brown to black, solid to semisolid, cementitious material usually used in paving. It is a mixture of paraffinic and aromatic hydrocarbons and heterocyclic compounds.

asphyxia. The state caused by a lack of oxygen and interference with oxygenation of the blood. Can lead to unconsciousness and death.

asphyxiant. 1. A substance, either a gas or a vapor, that interferes with the respiratory process. 2. A gas that is essentially nontoxic, but can cause unconsciousness or death (suffocation) by lowering the concentration of oxygen in the air or by totally replacing the oxygen in breathing air.

asphyxiation. Unconsciousness or death caused by the lack of oxygen.

aspiration hazard. A danger produced by drawing a substance into the lungs. The resulting symptoms range from mild irritation to death.

aspirin. Acetylsalicylic acid; an analgesic and anti-inflammatory.

assay. A test for a specific chemical, microbe, or effect. An analytical test used to measure the amount or presence of a specific substance.

assay zone. The portion of a treated wood product to which the minimum quantity standards apply.

assessment endpoint. In ecological risk assessment, an explicit expression of the environmental value to be protected. Includes both an ecological entity and the specific attributes thereof.

assimilation. The ability of a body of water to purify itself of pollutants.

assimilative capacity. The capacity of a natural body of water to receive wastewaters or toxic materials without deleterious effects and without damage to aquatic life or humans who consume the water.

Association of Boards of Certification (ABC). An international organization representing boards that certify the operators of waterworks and wastewater facilities.

astatine. A highly unstable, solid, nonmetallic, radioactive element, symbol At, with atomic number 85, and atomic weight 211. It is the heaviest of the halogens. Can be made by the bombardment of bismuth.

asymmetrical. Referring to a particular arrangement of elements within a chemical molecule.

atactic. A polymer molecule that has substituted groups arranged randomly above and below the backbone chain. *Contrast with* **isotactic**.

-ate. 1. The ending of the name of a salt that contains oxygen. 2. The ending of the name of a salt, the metal or radical of which is in its highest oxidation state.

atmosphere. 1. A unit of pressure. One atmosphere is the pressure that will support a column of mercury 760 mm (29.92 inches of water) high. One atmosphere is 101,325 pascals and 1.01325 bar. 2. The absolute total of all the gases surrounding the Earth.

atom. 1. The smallest piece of an element that cannot be divided or broken up by chemical means. 2. The smallest part of an element that can still be identified as the element.

atomic mass. *See* **atomic weight**.

atomic mass unit (AMU). 1. The unit of weight used to state atomic or molecular weights of atoms or molecules. The proton and the neutron both have atomic weights of 1 AMU.

atomic number. The number of protons in the nucleus of an atom. All atoms of the same element have the same number of protons in their nuclei, and each atomic number stands for one and only one element; designated as *Z*.

atomic orbital. The region or volume in space around the nucleus in which the probability of finding electrons is highest.

atomic weight. The total amount of protons and neutrons in the nucleus. A fractional atomic weight is due to the averaging of the weights of all the isotopes of the element. Also known as atomic mass; designated as *A*.

atropine. 1. An antidote for nerve agent poisoning by binding to acetylcholine receptors, it inhibits the action of acetylcholine at muscle receptors. 2. An alkaloid used as an antidote for cholinesterase-inhibiting compounds, organophosphorus insecticides, and nerve gases.

attainment area. An area considered to have air quality as good as or better than the national ambient air quality standards as defined in the Clean Air Act. An area may be an attainment area for one pollutant and a nonattainment area for others.

attenuation. 1. The process by which a compound is reduced in concentration over time through absorption, adsorption, degradation, dilution, and/or transformation. 2. The decrease with distance of sight caused by attenuation of light by particulate pollution.

atto-. Prefix used in the SI system meaning "multiply by 10-18" (10^{-18}); designated as *a*.

attractant. A chemical or agent that lures insects or other pests by stimulating their sense of smell.

attributable risk. *See* **additional risk.**

attrition. Wearing or grinding down of a substance by friction.

aurum. Latin for "gold," hence the symbol, Au.

autoignition temperature. The minimum temperature to which a material must be raised before combustion will occur. No external ignition source is required for ignition. Also called **ignition temperature**.

Automated Resource for Chemical Hazard Incident Evaluation (ARCHIE). A DOS-based software program for use in hazard analysis.

availability session. Informal meeting at a public location where interested citizens can talk with EPA and state officials on a one-to-one basis.

available chlorine. A measure of the amount of chlorine available in chlorinated lime, hypochlorite compounds, and other materials used as a source of chlorine when compared with that of liquid or gaseous chlorines.

average daily dose (ADD). Dose rate averaged over a pathway-specific period of exposure expressed as a daily dose on a per-unit-bodyweight basis. The ADD is usually expressed in terms of mg/kg-day or other mass-time units.

Avogadro's number. The number of atoms present in 12 grams of the carbon-12 isotope (1 mole of ^{12}C); 6.023 x 10^{23}. Designated as N.

avoided cost. The cost a utility would incur to generate the next increment of electric capacity using its own resources.

awareness level. First responders at the awareness level are those persons who, in the course of their normal duties, may be the first on the scene of an emergency involving hazardous materials. First responders at the awareness level are expected to recognize the presence of hazardous materials, protect themselves, call for trained personnel, and secure the area (NFPA 472).

azide. A compound with the general formula $R(N_3)_x$, where R may be a metal, hydrogen, a halogen, ammonium, a complex radical, or any of a large group of other radicals.

azo-. The prefix indicating the presence of the -N=N- radical.

azotic acid. *See* **nitric acid**.

B

bacillus. A form of bacteria having a rod-like shape.

Bacillus anthracis. 1. A biological agent. 2. A toxin; bacterial or viral organism that can cause casualties when released. *See* **anthrax**.

backdraft. The term given to a type of explosion caused by the sudden influx of air into a mixture of gases that has been heated to above the ignition temperature of at least one of its components, in a confined space.

backfit. *See* **retrofit**.

backflow. A reverse flow condition created by a difference in water pressures that causes water to flow back into the distribution pipes of a drinking water supply from any source other than the intended one. Also called *back siphonage*.

background level. 1. The concentration of a substance in an environmental medium (air, water, or soil) that occurs naturally or is not the result of human activities. 2. In exposure assessment, the concentration of a substance in a defined control area, during a fixed period of time before, during, or after a data-gathering operation. 3. Chemical substances that exist in either of the following:

1. Naturally occurring levels, or ambient concentrations of substances present in the environment, without human influence.
2. Anthropogenic levels, or concentrations of substances present in the environment due to man-made, nonsite sources.

background radiation. The radiation in the natural environment, including cosmic rays and radiation from the naturally radioactive elements, both outside and inside the bodies of humans and animals. It is also called *natural radiation*. Man-made sources of radioactivity contribute to total background radiation levels.

background samples. *See* **prevalent level samples**.

back pressure. A pressure that can cause water to backflow into the water supply when a user's wastewater system is at a higher pressure than the public system.

back siphonage. *See* **backflow**.

backwashing. Reversing the flow of water back through the filter media to remove entrapped solids.

backyard composting. Composting yard and kitchen wastes in one's yard through controlled decomposition of organic matter by bacteria and fungi into a humus-like product.

bacteria. 1. Microscopic living organisms that can aid in nitrogen fixation and pollution control in sewage, oil spills, or other pollutants. Harmful bacteria in soil, water, or air can cause human, animal, and plant health problems. 2. The singular form is *bacterium*.

bactericide. Any material that will kill bacteria.

baffle. 1. A partial wall to control the movement of a liquid in a tank, especially useful in the transportation of liquids. 2. A device placed in flowing water or slurry systems to cause more uniform flow velocities to absorb energy and to divert, guide, or agitate liquids.

baffle chamber. A chamber in an incinerator designed to cause settling of fly ash and coarse particulate matter.

baghouse filter. Large fabric bag, similar to a vacuum cleaner bag, used to eliminate intermediate and large particles.

bailer. A pipe with a valve at the lower end, used to remove slurry from the bottom or side of a well as it is being drilled, or to collect groundwater samples from wells or open boreholes. 2. A tube of varying length.

Bakelite. A trade name for a series of thermoplastic and thermosetting plastics.

baking powder. Usually sodium carbonate.

baking soda. Sodium bicarbonate.

baling. Compacting solid waste into blocks to reduce volume and simplify handling.

ballistic separator. A machine that sorts organic from inorganic matter for composting.

balloon frame. A building with studs running two or more stories without fire stops.

banana oil. Amyl acetate.

Banbury. An intensive mixing device using counterrotating, sigma-shaped mixing blades inside a closed chamber. Used to masticate, flux, and thoroughly mix plastic and rubber compounds.

band application. The spreading of chemicals over, or next to, each row of plants in a field.

banking. A system for recording qualified air emission reductions for later use in bubble, offset, or netting transactions.

bar. Unit of pressure; 1 bar = 105 pascals = 1.01325 atmospheres.

barbiturate. A derivative of barbituric acid that depresses the central nervous system, which will eventually produce sedation.

barite. Barium sulfate, $BaSO_4$. Also called *barytes*.

barium. 1. A soft, silver-white, solid metallic element, symbol Ba, with atomic number 56, and atomic weight 137.3. 2. Barium belongs to the group of metals known as **alkaline earth metals**.

barn. A measurement of area equal to 10^{-24} cm^2.

barometric pressure. Essentially the weight, at any given point in the atmosphere, of the gases directly above that point.

barrel sampler. Open-ended steel tube used to collect soil samples.

barrier coating. A layer of a material that obstructs or prevents passage of something through a surface that is to be protected.

barrier plastic. A term used to describe a plastic compound that, when processed into an article, will not allow the passage of products through itself. The barrier is intended to stop gases, aromas, and flavors from passing in either direction.

bar screen. In wastewater treatment, a device used to remove large solids.

basal application. In pesticides, the application of a chemical on plant stems or tree trunks just above the soil line.

base. 1. A chemical compound that contains the hydroxide ion (OH^{-1}), is the chemical opposite of an inorganic acid, is active chemically, and has a pH greater than 7.0. When it reacts with an acid, it forms a salt and water. Some of the bases are as corrosive as strong acid. 2. Central location where primary logistics for an incident are coordinated and administered. Incident command post may also be located there.

basic life support (BLS). A level of emergency medical care typified by an emergency medical technician (EMT), capable of delivering basic emergency interventions performed by emergency medical services (EMS) practitioners trained and credentialed to do so.

basic solution. A solution of a substance in water that has a pH greater than 7.0.

battery acid. Sulfuric acid.

bayonet (firefighting). *See* **puncture nozzle**.

bean sheet. Common term for a pesticide data package record.

becquerel. The SI unit of radioactivity. One disintegration per second; 37 billion becquerels (Bq) = 1 curie.

bed load. Sediment particles resting on or near the channel bottom that are pushed or rolled along by the flow of water.

BEN. EPA's computer model for analyzing a violator's economic gain from not complying with the law.

benchmark concentration (BMC). *See* **benchmark dose**.

benchmark dose (BMD). A statistical lower confidence limit on the dose that produces a predetermined change in response rate of an adverse effect. Also called *benchmark concentration.*

benchmark response (BMR). An adverse effect, used to define a benchmark dose from which a reference dose (RfD) or reference concentration (RfC) can be developed.

bench-scale tests. Laboratory testing of potential cleanup technologies. *See also* **treatability studies**.

benign tumor. A tumor that does not spread to a secondary localization, but may impair normal biological function through obstruction or may progress to malignancy later.

benthic. Having to do with the bottom of a body of water such as an ocean, lake, or river.

benthos. An organism that feeds on the sediment at the bottom of a water body such as an ocean, lake, or river.

bentonite. A colloidal clay, expansible when moist, commonly used to provide a tight seal around a well casing.

benzene ring. The six-sided, closed molecular structure with a carbon atom at each apex, typical of benzene and all its substituted compounds.

benzine. Ligroin or petroleum ether; sometimes benzene, C_6H_6.

benzol. Benzene, C_6H_6.

berkelium. A solid, synthetic, radioactive, metallic element, symbol Bk, with atomic number 97, and atomic weight 247. Made by bombarding americium-241.

beryllium. A solid, gray-white, light, metallic element, symbol Be, with atomic number 4, and atomic weight 9.01. Hazardous to human health when inhaled as an airborne pollutant.

best available control measures (BACM). A term used to refer to the most effective measures (according to EPA guidance) for controlling small or dispersed particulates and other emissions from sources such as roadway dust, soot and ash from woodstoves, and open burning of rush, timber, grasslands, or trash.

best available control technology (BACT). An emission limitation based on the maximum degree of emission reduction (considering energy, environmental, and economic impacts) achievable through application of production processes and available methods, systems, and techniques. BACT does not permit emissions in excess of those allowed under any applicable Clean Air Act provisions. Use of the BACT concept is allowable on a case-by-case basis for major new or modified emissions sources in attainment areas and applies to each regulated pollutant.

best demonstrated available technology (BDAT). As identified by EPA, the most effective commercially available means of treating specific types of hazardous waste. The BDATs may change with advances in treatment technologies.

best management practice (BMP). Methods that have been determined to be the most effective practical means of preventing or reducing pollution from nonpoint sources.

beta particle. 1. A charged particle emitted from the nucleus of some atoms as part of those atoms' radioactive decay. 2. Moderate penetrating power and a range of up to a few meters in air. Beta particles will penetrate only a fraction of an inch of skin tissue but can cause burns and are harmful to living tissues. May be stopped by a thin sheet of metal. 3. Positively charged beta particles are called *positrons* and negatively charged beta particles are called *electrons.* 4. Also denoted as β-*particle.*

beta ray. Electrons emitted by an unstable nucleus. In some cases, beta radiation consists of positrons ("anti-electrons," which are identical to electrons but carry a +1 charge).

bi-. A prefix used in chemical nomenclature meaning "two." *See also* **di-**.

bimetal. Beverage containers with steel bodies and aluminum tops; handled differently from pure aluminum in recycling.

binary. An alternate word meaning "two."

binary compound. 1. A compound made up of two elements. 2. A compound that contains the atoms or ions of two elements. It may contain more than one atom or ion of an element, but only two elements may be represented in the compound.

binary munitions. A two-part shell that allows the two chemicals necessary in the final stage of sarin synthesis to begin the chemical reaction shortly before its explosion.

binder. The portion of a plastics compound that holds the active ingredients together. Usually, it is the compound before the additives are added.

bioaccumulants. Substances that are very slowly metabolized or excreted that increase in concentration in living organisms as they breathe contaminated air, drink contaminated water, or eat contaminated food.

bioassay. A test developed to determine the relative strength of a substance by comparing its effect on a test organism with that of a standard preparation similarly given to the test organism.

bioavailabiliity. Degree of ability to be absorbed and ready to interact in organism metabolism.

biochemical oxygen demand (BOD). The amount of oxygen determined to be consumed in the biological processes that break down organic matter in water. The greater the BOD, the greater the degree of pollution.

bioconcentration. The accumulation of a chemical in tissues of a fish or other organism to levels greater than in the surrounding medium.

biodegradable. Substance that is capable of being decomposed under natural conditions.

biodegradation. Decomposition of a substance by bacterial action.

biodiversity. 1. The variety and variability among living organisms and the ecological complexes in which they occur. 2. The number of different items and their relative frequencies. Biodiversity encompasses different ecosystems, species, and genes.

biohazard. Organisms that have a pathogenic effect on life and the environment and can exist in normal ambient environments as disease-causing germs and viruses.

biological agents. Living organisms that can cause disease, sickness, and mortality in humans.

biological contaminants. Living organisms or derivates that can cause harmful health effects when inhaled, swallowed, or otherwise taken into the body.

biological control. The use of animals and organisms that eat or otherwise kill or outcompete pests.

biological exposure index (BEI). A measure of the amount of material absorbed by a body. Either the material or its metabolic products in tissue, fluids, or exhaled air can be measured.

biological integrity. The ability to support and maintain balanced, integrated functionality in the natural habitat of a given region.

biologically based dose-response model. A predictive tool used to estimate potential human health risks by describing and quantifying the key steps in the cellular, tissue, and organismal responses as a result of chemical exposure.

biologically effective dose. The amount of a deposited or absorbed compound reaching the cells or target sites where adverse effect occurs, or where the chemical interacts with a membrane.

biological magnification. The process whereby certain substances such as pesticides or heavy metals move up the food chain and are eaten by aquatic organisms such as fish, which in turn are eaten by large birds, animals, or humans, and then become concentrated in tissues or internal organs.

biological measurement. A measurement taken in a biological medium.

biological medium. One of the major components of an organism; e.g., blood, fatty tissue, lymph nodes, or breath, in which chemicals can be stored or transformed.

biological oxidation. Decomposition of complex organic materials by micro-organisms that occurs in self-purification of water bodies and in activated sludge wastewater treatment.

biological oxygen demand (BOD). An indirect measure of the concentration of biologically degradable material present in organic wastes.

biologicals. Vaccines, cultures, and other preparations made from living organisms and their products, intended for use in diagnosing, immunizing, or treating humans or animals, or in related research.

biological stressors. Organisms accidentally or intentionally introduced into habitats in which they do not evolve naturally.

biological treatment. A treatment technology that uses bacteria to consume organic waste.

biological weapon. A weapon that disperses biological agents.

biomass. 1. All of the living material in a given area. 2. Often refers to vegetation.

biome. Entire community of living organisms in a single major ecological area.

biomonitoring. 1. Introduction of living organisms to test the suitability of effluents for discharge into receiving waters and to test the quality of such waters downstream from the discharge. 2. The analysis of blood, urine, and tissues to measure chemical exposure in humans.

bioremediation. 1. Use of living organisms to clean up oil spills or remove other pollutants from soil, water, or wastewater. 2. Use of organisms such as nonharmful insects to remove agricultural pests or counteract diseases of trees, plants, and garden soil.

biosensor. An analytical mechanism consisting of a biological recognition element in contact with an electrochemical, optical, thermal, or acoustic signal transducer. Together they permit analyses of chemical properties or quantities.

biosphere. The portion of Earth and its atmosphere that can support life.

biostabilizer. A device that converts solid waste into compost by grinding and aeration.

biota. The animal and plant life of a given region.

biotechnology. Techniques that use living organisms or parts of organisms to produce a variety of products to improve plants or animals, or to develop microorganisms to remove toxins from bodies of water or to act as pesticides.

biotic community. A naturally occurring assemblage of plants and animals that live in the same environment and are mutually sustaining and interdependent.

biotransformation. The conversion of a substance into other compounds by organisms.

bis(chloromethyl) ether. A chemical choking agent.

bismuth. A heavy, solid, reddish-white, metallic element, symbol Bi, with atomic number 83, and atomic weight 208.98.

bitumen. Solid to semisolid mixture of hydrocarbons that exists naturally or as a residue from certain petroleum distillation methods.

bivalent. Having a valance of two.

blackbody temperature. The temperature of a perfect radiator (ASTM E 648).

blackwater. Water that contains animal, human, or food waste.

blanc fixe. Barium sulfate.

blasting agent. 1. A substance made up of a mixture of materials, none of which is classified as an explosive, but operates by exploding. 2. After testing in accordance with Sec. 13.114a (49 CFR), it must be so insensitive that there is very little probability of it exploding accidentally or transitioning from burning to detonation.

bleaching powder. 1. Calcium oxychloride, $CaOCl_2$. 2. Produced by passing chlorine gas over dry calcium hydroxide. 3. After absorbing moisture, it becomes a mixture of calcium chloride ($CaCl_2$) and calcium hypochlorite [$Ca(OCl)_2$].

bleeding. 1. The undesirable movement of materials from plastic compounds to the surface of the finished article. 2. Also called *migration*.

blister agents. 1. Substances that cause blistering of the skin. 2. Exposure is through liquid or vapor contact with any exposed tissue (i.e., eyes, skin, or lungs). 3. Mustard (H), distilled mustard (HD), nitrogen mustard (HN), and lewisite (L) are blister agents. 4. Symptoms include red eyes, skin irritation, burning of skin, blisters, upper respiratory damage, cough, and hoarseness.

blood agents. 1. Substances that injure a person by interfering with the exchange of oxygen and carbon dioxide between blood and tissues. 2. Hydrogen cyanide (AC) and cyanogen chloride (CK) are blood agents. 3. Symptoms include respiratory distress, headache, unresponsiveness, seizures, and coma.

blood asphyxiant. A substance that will render the red blood cells incapable of carrying oxygen by attaching itself to the red blood cell.

blood products. Any product derived from human blood, including, but not limited to, blood plasma, platelets, red or white corpuscles, and derived licensed products such as interferon.

blood-to-air partition coefficient. A ratio of a chemical's concentration between blood and air when at equilibrium.

bloom. 1. A proliferation of algae and/or higher aquatic plants in a body of water. 2. In plastics, colors carried to the surface by incompatible liquids in the compound.

blowing agent. 1. A substance that produces a uniform amount of gas when heated to a specific temperature or contacted by a specific chemical. 2. In plastics, the gas will produce cells that turn a solid material into a foam.

blow molding. A process by which a hot plastic tube or parison is made to take shape by being forced against the inside of a mold by a blast of air from inside the tube.

blown film. Plastic film produced by extruding film, passing it around a mandrel, and expanding it to the desired dimensions by forcing air against it from within the mandrel.

blue verdigris. Copper(II) acetate, $Cu(C_2H_3O_2)_2 \cdot H_2O$.

blue vitriol. An archaic name for copper sulfate, $CuSO_4{\cdot}5H_2O$.

BOD_5. The amount of dissolved oxygen consumed in five days by biological processes that break down organic matter.

body burden. The amount of a chemical stored in the body at a given time, especially a potential toxin in the body as the result of exposure.

bog. A type of wetland that accumulates appreciable peat deposits.

bohrium. A solid, metallic element, symbol Bh , with atomic number 107, and atomic weight 262. Formerly called *nielsbohrium.*

boiler. 1. A vessel designed to transfer heat produced by combustion or electric resistance to water. 2. Boilers may provide hot water and/or steam.

boiling liquid expanding vapor explosion (BLEVE). The explosion associated with the sudden failure of a container whose contents are a flammable liquefied compressed gas. Typically a BLEVE is due to flame impingement that causes an increased pressure inside the vessel and a weakening of the vessel material. Upon rupture, the pressure inside the vessel is immediately reduced to atmospheric pressure, and the contents of the vessel instantly boil and vaporize. The vapors of the material occupy several hundred times the space that the liquid had required. This produces a quickly expanding vapor cloud that can be ignited, causing a massive explosion and fireball.

boiling point. The minimum temperature at which the vapor pressure of a liquid just equals atmospheric pressure.

boilover. The overflow of crude oil from its container when the heat wave of burning oil reaches the water level in the tank. The heat energy causes water to flash to steam, causing a violent expulsion of the material as a froth.

bond. In chemistry, the covalent bond, which holds covalent compounds together by the sharing of a pair of electrons.

bond energy. The energy required to break the bonds in 1 g-mole of a compound.

bone ash. Crude calcium phosphate.

boom. 1. A floating device used to contain oil on a body of water. 2. A piece of equipment used to apply pesticides from a tractor or truck.

borax. Sodium tetraborate.

borehole. Hole made with drilling equipment.

boride. A binary compound containing boron and a metal.

boron. A solid, yellow-brown, nonmetallic element, symbol B, with atomic number 5, and atomic weight 10.81.

botanical pesticide. 1. A pesticide with an active ingredient that is a plant-produced chemical, such as nicotine or strychnine. 2. Also called a *plant-derived pesticide.*

bottom ash. 1. The nonairborne combustion residue from burning pulverized coal in a boiler. 2. The material that falls to the bottom of the boiler and is removed mechanically. A concentration of non-combustible materials, which may include toxics.

botulinum toxin. Botulinum toxin is most often found in improperly prepared foods. *Clostridium botulinum* is highly toxic. Once infected, untreated victims may stand little chance of survival. Symptoms include drooping eyelids, dry mouth, dry throat, difficulty talking and swallowing, impaired vision, difficulty breathing, and death from asphyxia.

bounding estimate. An estimate of exposure, dose, or risk that is higher than that incurred by people in the population with the currently highest exposure, dose, or risk.

Boyle's law. 1. The pressure of a gas is inversely proportional to its volume at a given temperature. 2. The volume of a confined gas at a constant temperature varies inversely with its pressure.

brackish. Mixed fresh and salt water.

branched. The molecular structure characterized by the presence of side chains attached to the main chain. *Contrast with* **linear**.

branching. 1. A configuration in which a carbon atom attaches itself to another carbon atom that has two or three other carbon atoms attached to it, forming a *branch,* or side chain. 2. When the carbon attaches to another carbon that has a chain consisting only of carbons attached to either one or two atoms, a straight chain is formed, rather than a branched chain.

brass. A copper-zinc alloy.

breach. The physical action of breaking or damaging a container.

breakpoint chlorination. Addition of chlorine to water until the chlorine demand has been satisfied.

breakthrough. A crack or break in a filter bed that allows the passage of floc or particulate matter through a filter.

breathing apparatus support. A mobile unit designed and constructed for the purpose of providing a specified level of breathing air support capacity and personnel capable of refilling self-contained breathing apparatus (SCBA) at remote incident locations (compressor systems or cascade). *See also* **self-contained breathing apparatus** and **firefighting gear.**

breathing zone. Area of air in which an organism inhales.

brimstone. Sulfur.

brine mud. Waste material, often associated with well drilling or mining, composed of mineral salts or other inorganic compounds.

brisance. The explosive power of an explosive or a material that explodes.

British anti-lewisite. The common name for dimercaprol, which is used to treat inhalation or ingestion of certain toxic metal compounds.

British thermal unit. The unit of heat energy equal to the amount of heat required to raise the temperature of 1 lb of water by 1°F at sea level.

broadcast application. The spreading of pesticides over an entire area.

bromate. An anion (BrO_3^{-1}) derived from bromic acid ($HBrO_3$). Bromates are often oxidizers.

bromide. A compound containing the Br^{-1} ion or the -Br radical.

brominate. 1. The act of chemically adding bromine to a molecule. 2. A chemical reaction in which bromine becomes attached to a molecule of some other material.

bromine. A dark red, liquid, nonmetallic element, symbol Br, with atomic number 35, and atomic weight 79.9. It is a member of the halogen family. A chemical choking agent.

bromite. An anion (BrO_2^{-1}) derived from bromous acid ($HBrO_2$). Bromites are usually oxidizers.

bromo-. A prefix denoting the presence of bromine in the compound.

bromobenzylcyanide. A riot control chemical; agent CA.

bronze. A copper-tin alloy.

brownfields. Abandoned, idled, or under-used industrial and commercial facilities or sites where expansion or redevelopment is complicated by real or perceived environmental contamination.

brucella. Parasitic organisms capable of invading any animal tissue and causing infections in the genital organs, mammary glands, and intestinal tracts. Can be used as a biological warfare agent. Symptoms include prolonged fever, headaches, profuse sweating, chills, muscle and joint pain, and fatigue.

bubble. A system under which existing emissions sources can propose alternate means to comply with a set of emissions limitations. Under the bubble concept, sources can control more than required at one emission point where control costs are relatively low in return for a comparable relaxation of controls at a second emission point where costs are higher.

bubble policy. *See* **emissions trading**.

buddy system. A work practice in which workers team up in pairs during work activities.

buffer. A solution or liquid with a chemical makeup such that it minimizes changes in pH when acids or bases are added to it.

buffer strips. Strips of grass or other erosion-resisting vegetation between or below cultivated strips or fields.

building code. A list of rules, usually adopted by city ordinance, to regulate the safe construction of buildings in a community. There are several national building codes that are widely adopted in the United States.

building envelope. 1. The exterior surface of a building's construction, including the walls, windows, floors, roof, and floor. 2. Also called a *building shell.*

building shell. *See* **building envelope**.

building-related illness. Diagnosable illness whose cause and symptoms can be directly attributed to a specific pollutant source within a building.

bulk sample. A small portion (usually thumbnail size) of a suspected asbestos-containing building material collected by an asbestos inspector for laboratory analysis to determine asbestos content.

bulky waste. Large items of waste materials, such as appliances, furniture, large auto parts, trees, and stumps.

bung. The cap or plug that fits into the holes in a drum.

bunker gear. An entire set of firefighter's protective clothing that includes helmet, coat, pants, boots, and gloves. *See also* **turnout gear** and **full turnouts**.

burial ground. A disposal site for radioactive waste materials that uses earth or water as a shield. Also called a *graveyard.*

burn. 1. To undergo combustion (ASTM E176). 2. As used in the plastics processing industry, the pyrolysis or degradation of a batch of material in the processing equipment. It is said that the batch "burned" or "burned up." 3. A chemical or thermal burn. The former may be caused by corrosive substances and the latter by liquefied cryogenic gases, hot molten substances, or flames.

burn degree. The degree of burn traditionally classified according to the depth of tissue damage that is produced. Also called *degree of burn.*

- *first-degree burn.* The mildest type of burn, limited to the most superficial layers of skin and characterized by redness and pain. Sunburn is an example.
- *second-degree burn.* A penetration of the skin causing damage to both the epidermis and the underlying dermis. A second-degree burn looks mottled or red, swollen, and somewhat wet. These burns are characterized by blister formation.
- *third-degree burn.* Damage or destruction of the full thickness of the skin, from the epidermis down to the subcutaneous fat, and sometimes underlying muscle as well. The skin appears charred, leathery, or pearly gray. Third-degree burns are insensitive to painful stimuli because of destruction of the nerve endings for pain in the dermis.

- *fourth-degree burn.* A burn similar to the characteristics of the third-degree burn. When muscle or bone is involved, the burn is sometimes categorized as fourth-, fifth-, or sixth-degree burn.

burning behavior. The manner in which a material acts when it is subjected to a specific ignition source, as in a fire test.

burning velocity. Speed of a planar (two-dimensional) flame front, normal to its surface and relative to the unburned (gaseous and fuel) oxidizer mixture (ASTM E 176).

burnt lime. Calcium oxide, CaO.

burnt ochre. Ferric oxide.

butadiene, 1,3-. $CH_2=CH-CH=CH_2$. The monomer of polybutadiene.

butyl. The radical $-C_4H_9$, formed by removing one hydrogen from butane, C_4H_{10}. It has four isomers.

butyl rubber. A synthetic rubber made by the copolymerization of isobutylene with isoprene.

buyback center. Facility where individuals or groups bring recyclables in return for payment.

by-product. Material, other than the principal product, generated as a consequence of an industrial process or as a breakdown product in a living system.

C

cadmium. A soft, blue-white, solid, metallic element, symbol Cd, with atomic number 48, and atomic weight 112.4.

cadmium oxide. A chemical choking agent.

calcium. A soft, silver-white, solid, metallic element, symbol Ca, with atomic number 20, and atomic weight 40.08. A member of the alkaline earth metals.

calendering. The forming of a plastic into film or sheet by forcing the plastic through a series of rolls called a calender.

californium. A man-made, radioactive, solid, metallic element, symbol Cf, with atomic number 98, and atomic weight 251. Made by bombarding curium or americium with neutrons.

calorie. The amount of energy required to raise 1 gram (g) of water 1° Celsius (1°C) at 1 atmosphere (atm) of pressure. The calorie referred to in connection with food is the kilogram calorie (kc), also called a *kilocalorie*, which is 1,000 times larger than a calorie (c).

calorimeter. A device used to determine the amount of heat released or absorbed in a chemical reaction.

CAMEO. Acronym for Computer-Aided Management of Emergency Operations, developed by the National Oceanic and Atmospheric Administration.

cancellation. Refers to Section 6 (b) of the Federal Insecticide, Fungicide, and Rodenticide Act (FIFRA), which authorizes cancellation of a pesticide registration if unreasonable adverse effects to the environment and public health develop when a product is used according to widespread and commonly recognized practice, or if its labeling or other material required to be submitted does not comply with FIFRA provisions.

cancer. A disease of heritable, somatic mutations affecting cell growth and differentiation, characterized by an abnormal, uncontrolled growth of cells.

cap. A layer of clay, or other impermeable material installed over the top of a closed landfill to prevent entry of rainwater and minimize leachate.

capacity assurance plan. A statewide plan that supports a state's ability to manage the hazardous waste generated within its boundaries over a 20-year period.

capillarity. A property of surface tension that draws water upwards.

capillary action. Movement of water through very small spaces due to molecular forces called capillary forces.

capillary fringe. 1. The porous material just above the water table that may hold water by capillarity in the smaller void spaces. 2. The zone above the water table within which the porous medium is saturated by water under less than atmospheric pressure.

caprolactam. The monomer of polycaprolactam, or nylon-6.

capture efficiency. The fraction of organic vapors generated by a process that is directed to an abatement or recovery device.

carbide. A binary compound of carbon and another element, usually metals. Silver, mercury, and copper carbides are explosive.

carbohydrate. An organic compound containing only carbon, hydrogen, and oxygen, with the hydrogen to oxygen ratio at two to one.

carbolic acid. An older name for phenol (C_6H_5OH).

carbon. A solid metallic element, symbol C, with atomic number 6, and atomic weight 12.01; the basis of organic chemistry.

carbon absorber. An add-on control device that uses activated carbon to absorb volatile organic compounds from a gas stream.

carbon adsorption. A treatment system that removes contaminants from groundwater or surface water by forcing it through tanks containing activated carbon treated to attract the contaminants.

carbonate. An ionic compound containing the CO_3^{-2} ion. The organic compounds are esters.

carbon dioxide. A colorless, odorless gas produced by fossil fuel combustion, or any carbon-containing material; CO_2.

carbonic acid. Archaic name for carbon dioxide dissolved in water; H_2CO_3.

carbon monoxide. A colorless, odorless, poisonous gas produced by incomplete fossil fuel combustion, or any carbon-containing material; CO.

carbon tetrachloride. Compound consisting of one carbon atom and four chlorine atoms (CCl_4), once widely used as a industrial raw material, as a solvent, and in the production of CFCs. Its use as a solvent ended when it was discovered to be carcinogenic.

carbonyl. The functional group with the structural formula of a carbon with a double bond to an oxygen. It is present in both aldehydes and ketones.

carboxyhemoglobin. Hemoglobin in which the iron is bound to carbon monoxide instead of oxygen.

carboxylic acid. A hydrocarbon derivative having the general formula R-COOH, where R- is the hydrocarbon backbone and -COOH is the carboxyl radical.

carboy. A glass or plastic bottle enclosed in a wooden crate.

carburetted hydrogen. An archaic name for methane, CH_4.

carcinogen. Any substance that can cause or aggravate cancer. A chemical is considered to be a carcinogen if one of the following applies:

1. It has been evaluated by the International Agency for Research on Cancer (IARC) and found to be a carcinogen or potential carcinogen.
2. It is listed as a carcinogen or potential carcinogen in the latest edition of the *Annual Report on Carcinogens* published by the National Toxicology Program (NTP).
3. It is regulated by OSHA as a carcinogen.

carcinogenesis. The origin or production of a benign or malignant tumor.

carcinogenic. The ability or tendency to cause cancer.

cardiopulmonary resuscitation (CPR). 1. An emergency procedure used to maintain and restore breathing and blood circulation. 2. A combination of artificial resuscitation and closed-chest cardiac (heart) compression.

Caro's acid. Persulfuric acid (H_2SO_5).

carrier. 1. The inert liquid or solid material in a pesticide product that serves as a delivery vehicle for the active ingredient. 2. Any material or system that can facilitate the movement of a pollutant into the body or cells.

carrying capacity. 1. In recreation management, the amount of use a recreation area can sustain without loss of quality. 2. In wildlife management, the maximum number of animals an area can support during a given period.

case-control study. An epidemiologic study contrasting those with the disease of interest (cases) to those without the disease (controls).

case study. A brief fact sheet providing risk, cost, and performance information on alternative methods and other pollution prevention ideas, compliance initiatives, and voluntary efforts.

cask. A thick-walled container (usually lead) used to transport radioactive material. Also called a *coffin*.

CAS registration number. A number assigned by the Chemical Abstracts Service of the American Chemical Society to uniquely identify a chemical.

casting. Forming of shapes by pouring a liquid plastic into a mold or onto a moving belt or other surface.

catalyst. A substance that speeds up or slows down a chemical reaction. The catalyst does not enter into and is not consumed by the chemical reaction.

catalytic converter. An air pollution abatement device that removes pollutants from motor vehicle exhaust, either by oxidizing them into carbon dioxide and water or reducing them to nitrogen.

catalytic incinerator. A control device that oxidizes volatile organic compounds (VOCs) by using a catalyst to promote the combustion process.

cat cracker. A catalytic cracking unit used in refining oil.

categorical exclusion. A class of actions that either individually or cumulatively would not have a significant effect on the human environment and therefore would not require preparation of an environmental assessment or environmental impact statement under the National Environmental Policy Act (NEPA).

categorical pretreatment standard. A technology-based effluent limitation for an industrial facility discharging into a municipal sewer system.

catenation. The bonding together of atoms of the same element into chains or rings.

cathode. 1. The negative electrode of a catalytic cell. 2. When an electric current is passed through an ionic solution, the positively charged ions (cations) will migrate to the cathode. 3. The electrode where reduction occurs.

cathode ray. A negatively charged beam that emanates from the cathode of a discharge tube. Cathode rays are streams of electrons.

cathodic protection. A technique to prevent corrosion of a metal surface by making it the cathode of an electrochemical cell.

cation. A positively charged ion.

caustic. 1. Any strongly alkaline substance that has a corrosive effect on tissue. 2. Usually refers to bases such as lithium hydroxide, sodium hydroxide, and potassium hydroxide; may include hydroxides of calcium, beryllium, and magnesium.

caustic lime. Calcium hydroxide.

caustic potash. Potassium hydroxide.

caustic soda. Sodium hydroxide.

caustic vegetable alkali. Archaic term for potassium hydroxide.

cavitation. 1. The formation and collapse of gas pockets or bubbles on the blade of an impeller or the gate of a valve. 2. Collapse of these pockets or bubbles drives water with such force that it can cause pitting of the gate or valve surface.

ceiling (C). The maximum allowable exposure limit for an airborne substance, not to be exceeded during the work shift.

ceiling limit. Set by the ACGIH as a limit above which no surpassing of the concentration of regulated substance is permitted, not even briefly. *See also* **threshold limit value-ceiling**.

cell asphyxiant. A substance that, upon entering the body, inhibits the normal function of cells, particularly the dumping of carbon dioxide to make room for oxygen.

cellophane. Regenerated cellulose.

cells. 1. The smallest structural part of living matter capable of functioning as an independent unit. 2. In solid waste disposal, holes where waste is dumped, compacted, and covered with layers of dirt on a daily basis.

cellular plastic. A plastic that has been processed to contain many empty cells throughout its mass. Also referred to as *foamed plastic.*

cellulose. 1. A naturally occurring, carbohydrate-high polymer. 2. The principal constituent in all plant material. 3. The most abundant organic material in the world. (Wood is approximately 50% cellulose, while cotton is almost pure cellulose.)

cellulose acetate. A thermoplastic acetic acid ester of cellulose.

cellulose acetate butyrate. A thermoplastic acetic and butyric acid ester of cellulose.

cellulose nitrate. 1. A thermoplastic nitric acid ester of cellulose. 2. Also known as *pyroxylin, guncotton,* and *nitrocellulose,* it has a high risk for rapid burning and explosion.

cellulose propionate. A thermoplastic propionic acid ester of cellulose.

cellulose triacetate. A thermoplastic acetic triester of cellulose.

cellulosic plastics. Thermoplastics made by replacing the hydroxide groups of natural cellulose with acidic groups. Includes cellulose acetate, cellulose acetate propionate, cellulose acetate butyrate, cellulose nitrate, cellulose propionate, and cellulose triacetate. Also called *cellulosics.*

Celsius scale. Temperatures on this scale are denoted by °C, where the normal freezing point of water is 0°C and the normal boiling point of water is 100°C. Also called *centigrade scale.*

cementitious. Densely packed and non-fibrous, friable materials.

centi-. The prefix that means "one hundredth of," or 10^{-2}; c.

centigrade scale. *See* **Celsius scale**.

centimeter. One hundredth of a meter, or 0.3937 inch; 1 in. = 2.54 cm.

centipoise. 1. One hundredth of a poise. 2. Poise is the unit of viscosity in the centimeter-gram-second (cgs) metric system.

centistoke. One hundredth of a stoke, the unit of kinematic viscosity.

central collection point. 1. Location where a generator of regulated medical waste consolidates wastes originally generated at various locations in its facility. 2. Community hazardous waste collections, and/or industrial and other waste management systems.

central nervous system (CNS). In humans, the brain and spinal cord, as opposed to the peripheral nerves found in the extremities.

centrifugal collector. A mechanical system using centrifugal force to remove aerosols from a gas stream or to remove water from sludge.

ceramics. A group of products produced by the effect of heat, principally on silicates.

CERCLA hazardous substance. A Superfund hazardous substance listed in Table 302.4 of 40 CFR Part 302.4, and Section 101(14) of CERCLA, which subjects facilities to CERCLA and Title III release notification.

cerium. A gray, solid, metallic element, symbol Ce, with atomic number 58, and atomic weight 140.12. It is the most abundant element of the rare earth group.

cesium. A soft, silver-white, solid, metallic element, symbol Cs, with atomic number 55, and atomic weight 132.9. It is an alkali metal, a powerful oxidizer, and the most reactive of all the elements.

cetane number. The corresponding number for diesel fuel as octane is to gasoline.

cgs. An older metric system of units that uses centimeters, grams, and seconds as base units.

chain. 1. The way carbon atoms react with each other, producing covalent bonds between them, resembling a chain with carbon atoms existing as the links. 2. A unit of linear measurement equal to 66 feet.

chain length. 1. The number of repeating monomer units in a polymer molecule. 2. The degree of polymerization.

chain of command. A hierarchy of management positions ranked in order of authority.

chain reaction. A reaction that, once initiated, sustains itself and expands.

chalk. Calcium carbonate.

channelization. Straightening and deepening streams so water will move faster.

char. Carbonaceous material formed by pyrolysis or incomplete combustion (ASTM E 176).

characteristic. Any one of the four categories used in defining hazardous waste: ignitability, corrosivity, reactivity, and toxicity.

characterization of ecological effects. The part of an ecological risk assessment that evaluates the ability of a stressor to cause adverse effects under given circumstances.

characterization of exposure. The part of an ecological risk assessment that evaluates the interaction of a stressor with one or more ecological entities.

Charles' Law. 1. A gas will expand or contract in direct proportion to an increase or decrease in its temperature. 2. If the gas is confined so it cannot expand, its pressure will increase or decrease in direct proportion to temperature.

checking. The separation of wood that normally occurs across or through the annual rings, usually as a result of seasoning.

check-valve tubing pump. A water sampling tool also referred to as a water pump.

chelating agent. Any chemical compound capable of forming multiple chemical bonds to a metal ion.

chemical asphyxiant. A substance that will reduce the body's ability to transport, absorb, or utilize oxygen. *See also* **respiratory asphyxiant** and **simple asphyxiant.**

chemical/biological (C/B) protective ensemble. A compliant vapor-protective ensemble that is also certified as being compliant with the additional requirements for protection against C/B warfare agents such as vapors, gases, liquids, and particulate; National Fire Protection Association (NFPA) Standard #1991.

chemical bond. A strong attraction between two or more atoms. Bonds hold atoms in molecules and crystals together. There are many types of chemical bonds, but all involve electrons that are either shared or transferred between the bonded atoms.

chemical cartridge. A filtering device that is attached to an air-purifying respirator.

chemical compound. 1. A chemical combination of two or more atoms, either from the same elements or from different elements, that is electrically neutral. 2. A distinct and pure substance formed by the union of two or more elements in definite proportion by weight.

chemical element. A fundamental substance made up of one kind of atom.

chemical emergency. *See* **emergency, chemical**.

chemical equation. A method of depicting a chemical reaction by using symbols.

chemical foam. A foam formed when an alkaline solution and an acid solution unite to produce carbon dioxide combined with a foaming agent that traps the gas in bubbles.

chemical formula. A shorthand using chemical symbols to show which elements are present and their quantity. *See also* **molecular formula** and **structural formula**.

Chemical Hazards Response Information System (CHRIS). A series of reference manuals used to provide emergency response information regarding chemical release emergencies. Developed by the U.S. Coast Guard (USCG).

chemical hygiene officer (CHO). A person or employee who is qualified by training or experience to provide technical guidance in the development and implementation of the provisions of a chemical hygiene plan (CHP).

chemical hygiene plan. A set of policies and procedures implemented to protect laboratory workers from injury by exposure to chemicals, as required by the OSHA Laboratory Standard (29 CFR 1910.1450).

chemically pure (CP). A purified element or compound. No detectable impurities.

chemical name. The proper scientific name of a chemical. Since there are several systems for naming chemical compounds, a chemical may have more than one chemical name.

chemical oxygen demand (COD). A measure of the oxygen required to oxidize all compounds, both organic and inorganic, in water.

chemical plant. Any chemical industry facility including manufacturing plants, distribution facilities, warehouses, and transportation systems.

chemical pneumonitis. An inflammation of the lungs caused by accumulation of fluids due to a chemical irritation.

chemical property. A description of how matter reacts chemically with other substances. Chemical properties include flammability, corrosiveness, oxidation state, and reactivity.

chemical protection equipment (CPE). Protective clothing and respiratory protection for chemicals that may be encountered at a hazardous materials incident.

chemical protective clothing material. Any material or combination of materials used in an item of clothing for the purpose of isolating parts of the wearer's body from contact with a hazardous chemical (NFPA #1991, 1–3).

chemical protective suit. Single or multipiece garment constructed of chemical protective clothing materials designed and configured to protect the wearer's torso, head, arms, legs, hands, and feet (NFPA #1991, 1–3).

chemical reaction. 1. A chemical change that occurs when two or more substances are brought together and energy is either absorbed or liberated. Includes combustion, condensation, hydrolysis, ionization, oxidation, photosynthesis, polymerization, pyrolysis, and reduction. 2. A chemical change that occurs when one substance is acted upon by a form of energy.

chemical reactivity. The speed and ease with which a substance enters into chemical reactions.

Chemical Referral Center (CRC). A service of CHEMTREC connecting members of the public to chemical producers for answers to health and safety questions.

chemical resistance. The ability of a material to resist chemical reaction by other chemicals.

chemical stressors. Chemicals released to the environment through industrial waste, auto emissions, pesticides, and other human activity.

chemical symbol. The chemical shorthand used for the full name of an element. It is always one or two letters. If one letter, it is always a capital letter. If two letters, the first is always capitalized and the second is always lower cased.

Chemical Transportation Emergency Center (CHEMTREC). A public service of the American Chemistry Council [formerly the Chemical Manufacturers Association (CMA)]. It is located in Washington D.C. and is available 24 hours a day at: (800) 424-9300.

chemical treatment. Any one of a variety of reactions that use chemicals or a variety of chemical processes to treat other materials, including wastes.

chemical warfare agent. A chemical substance (such as a nerve agent, blister agent, blood agent, choking agent, or irritating agent) used to kill, seriously injure, or incapacitate people through its physiological effects (excluding riot control agents, herbicides, smoke, and flame (NATO).

chemiluminescence. Light generated by a chemical reaction.

chemistry. The science of matter, energy, and reactions.

CHEMNET. A program established by the CMA to provide mutual aid information and programs to organizations desiring such information.

chemosterilant. A chemical that controls pests by preventing reproduction.

CHEMTREC. The industry-sponsored Chemical Transportation Emergency Center; provides information and/or emergency assistance to emergency responders.

chief. The title for persons responsible for command of functional divisions or sections, such as administration, finance, inspections, logistics, manpower, operations, and planning.

child resistant packaging (CRP). Packaging, required by FIFRA regulations, that protects children or adults from injury or illness resulting from accidental contact with or ingestion of residential pesticides that meet or exceed specific toxicity levels. 2. Also used for the protective packaging of medicines.

Chile niter. Sodium nitrate ($NaNO_3$). Also called **Chile saltpeter**.

Chile saltpeter. Sodium nitrate ($NaNO_3$). Also called **Chile niter.**

chiller. A device that cools gases or liquids.

chilling effect. 1. The greenhouse effect. 2. The lowering of the Earth's temperature because of increased particles or gases in the air blocking the Sun's rays.

chlorate. 1. Any compound containing the chlorate ion (ClO_3^{-1}). 2. A compound derived from chloric acid ($HClO_3$). 3. Usually a strong oxidizing agent.

CHLOREP. The Chlorine Emergency Plan, established by the Chlorine Institute, which enables the nearest producer of chlorine to respond to an incident involving chlorine. (Contact is made through CHEMTREC.)

chloride. Any binary compound containing the chloride ion (Cl^{-1}) or the chloride radical (-Cl).

chlorinate. 1. The act of adding chlorine to a molecule. 2. A chemical reaction in which chlorine becomes attached to a molecule of some other material.

chlorinated. A chemical compound that has had chlorine incorporated into it.

chlorinated hydrocarbons. 1. Chemicals containing only carbon, hydrogen, and chlorine. 2. Any chlorinated organic compounds, including chlorinated solvents such as dichloromethane, trichloromethylene, and chloroform.

chlorinated lime. *See* **bleaching powder**.

chlorinated polyether. The polymer of chlorinated oxetane.

chlorinated solvent. An organic solvent containing chlorine atoms.

chlorination. 1. The chemical addition of chlorine to a compound. 2. The application of chlorine to drinking water, sewage, or industrial waste to disinfect or to oxidize undesirable compounds.

chlorinator. A device that adds chlorine, in gas or liquid form, to water or sewage to kill infectious bacteria.

chlorine. A greenish-yellow, toxic, corrosive, gaseous, nonmetallic element, symbol Cl, with atomic number 17, and atomic weight 35.453. It is a member of the halogen family and is a powerful oxidizer. A chemical choking agent.

chlorine-contact chamber. That part of a water treatment plant where effluent is disinfected by chlorine.

chlorine kit. A standardized kit custom manufactured to provide safety equipment to control or stop leaks in chlorine cylinders, tanks, and transportation tank cars.

chlorine trifluoride. A chemical choking agent, ClF_3.

chlorite. 1. Any compound containing the chlorite ion (ClO_2^{-1}). 2. A compound derived from chlorous acid ($HClO_2$). 3. Usually an oxidizing agent.

chloro-. A prefix denoting an organic compound containing chlorine substituted for a hydrogen atom.

chloroacetophenone. A riot control chemical (C_8H_7ClO); agent CN.

chlorofluorocarbons (CFCs). 1. A family of inert, nontoxic, and easily liquefiable compounds used as solvents and aerosol propellants or in refrigeration and air conditioning. 2. CFCs are relatively inert, and they slowly disperse into the upper atmosphere, where their chlorine components may destroy the protective ozone layer.

chlorophenoxy. A class of herbicides that may be found in domestic water supplies and cause adverse health effects.

chloropicrin. A riot control, chemical choking agent (CCl_3NO_2); agent PS.

chlorosis. Discoloration of normally green plant parts caused by pollution, disease, or lack of nutrients.

choking agent. A chemical substance that causes physical injury to the lungs, through inhalation. Membranes may swell and lungs become filled with liquid (pulmonary edema), causing death. Symptoms include irritation to eyes, nose, and/or throat, respiratory distress, nausea and vomiting, and a burning sensation on exposed skin. Included (with agent designation) are:

- arsenic trichloride (no military designation)
- bis(chloromethyl) ether (no military designation)
- bromine (no military designation)
- cadmium oxide (no military designation)
- chlorine (agent CL)
- chlorine trifluoride (no military designation)
- chloropicrin (agent PS)
- cyanide
- diphosgene (agent DP)

disulfur decafluoride (no military designation)

nickel carbonyl (no military designation)

nitrogen oxide (NO)

perchloromethyl mercaptan (no military designation)

perfluoroisobutylene (PHIB)

phosgene (CG)

red phosphorous (RP)

selenium oxide fume (no military designation)

sulfur trioxide-chlorosulfonic acid (FS)

Teflon and perfluoroisobutylene (PHIB)

titanium tetrachloride (FM)

zinc oxide (HC)

choline. One of the products from the hydrolysis of acetylcholine.

cholinesterase. An enzyme found in animals that regulates nerve impulses by the inhibition of acetylcholine.

chromate. A complex ion containing chromium and oxygen $(CrO_4)^{-2}$, where chromium has a valency of six. It is usually an oxidizing agent.

chromated copper arsenate (CCA). An inorganic arsenical. The most prevalent of the waterborne wood preservatives, commonly used to prevent attack by termites and decay, both indoors and outdoors.

chromatography. A method for separating mixtures based on differences in the speed at which they migrate over or through a stationary phase.

chromic acid. Chromium(VI) oxide, CrO_3, or its formal hydrate, H_2CrO_4.

chromium. A bluish-white, solid, metallic element, symbol Cr, with atomic number 24, and atomic weight 51.996. Commonly used in metal plating and in alloys.

chromophore. Chemical functional groups with characteristic optical absorptions.

chronic effect. Any adverse effect on a human or animal in which symptoms recur frequently or develop slowly over a long period of time.

chronic exposure. Multiple exposures occurring over an extended period of time or over a significant fraction of an animal's or a human's lifetime.

chronic study. A toxicity study designed to measure the (toxic) effects of chronic exposure to a chemical.

chronic toxicity. The capacity of a substance to cause long-term poisonous health effects in humans, animals, fish, and other organisms.

cinnabar. Mercury(II) sulfide (HgS), a red pigment. *See also* **vermillion**.

circle of influence. The circular outer edge of a depression produced in the water table by the pumping of water from a well.

cis-. Refers to a particular arrangement of elements within a chemical molecule, having two atoms or groups of atoms on the same side of a double bond between two carbon atoms.

cistern. Small tank or storage facility used to store water for a home or farm; often used to store rain water.

claimant. A person submitting a claim of trade secrecy to EPA in connection with a chemical otherwise required to be disclosed in a report or other filing made under Title III.

clarification. Clearing action that occurs during wastewater treatment when solids settle out, often aided by centrifugal action and chemically induced coagulation in wastewater.

clarifier. A tank in which solids settle to the bottom and are subsequently removed as sludge.

class A fire. A fire involving class A materials, such as wood, plastics, cloth, paper, and paper products.

class A materials. Wood, paper, plastics, and cloth.

class B fire. A fire involving class B materials, such as flammable and combustible liquids.

class B materials. Flammable and combustible liquids.

class C fire. A fire involving charged electrical equipment and wires.

class C materials. Charged electrical equipment and wires.

class D fire. A fire involving metals.

class D materials. Metals, including chips and powders.

class I area. Under the Clean Air Act, a class I area is one in which visibility is protected more stringently than under the national ambient air quality standards. It includes national parks, wilderness areas, monuments, and other areas of special national and cultural significance.

class I substance. One of several groups of chemicals with an ozone depletion potential of 0.2 or higher, including CFCs, halons, carbon tetrachloride, and methyl chloroform (listed in the Clean Air Act); and hydrobromofluorocarbons (HBFCs) and ethyl bromide (added by EPA regulations). *See also* **global warming potential**.

class II substance. A substance with an ozone depletion potential of less than 0.2. All hydrofluorocarbons (HCFCs) are currently included in this classification. (*See* **global warming potential**.)

clay soil. Soil material containing more than 40% clay, less than 45% sand, and less than 40% silt.

Clean Air Act (CAA). A set of national standards for ambient air quality that defines the principal types and levels of pollution that should not be exceeded. This law requires states to develop state implementation plans for achieving the ambient air standards in each air quality control region in the state.

clean coal technology. Any technology not in widespread use prior to the Clean Air Act Amendments of 1990.

clean distillate. A creosote preservative introduced in 1985. Clean distillate products, such as utility poles, exhibit clean, dry surfaces with little or no surface residue.

Cleaner Technologies Substitutes Assessment. A document that systematically evaluates the relative risk, performance, and cost trade-offs of technological alternatives.

clean fuels. Includes blends or substitutes for gasoline fuels, including compressed natural gas, methanol, ethanol, and liquefied petroleum gas.

cleanup. Actions taken to deal with a release or threat of release of a hazardous substance that could affect humans and/or the environment. Often used interchangeably with the terms **remedial action**, **removal action**, **response action**, or **corrective action**.

Clean Water Act (CWA). Federal legislation to protect the nation's water and set state water quality standards for interstate navigable waters as the basis for pollution control and enforcement.

clear-cutting. Harvesting all the trees in one area at one time.

clear well. A reservoir for storing filtered water of sufficient quantity to prevent the need to vary the filtration rate with variations in demand.

climate change. Sometimes used to refer to all forms of climatic inconsistency, but because the Earth's climate is never static, the term is more properly used to imply a significant change from one climatic condition to another. Also called *global climate change*.

cloning. In biotechnology, obtaining a group of genetically identical cells from a single cell; making identical copies of a gene.

closed-loop recycling. Reclaiming or reusing wastewater for nonpotable purposes in an enclosed process.

closure. The procedure a landfill operator must follow when a landfill reaches its legal capacity for solids, ceasing acceptance of solid waste and placing a cap on the landfill site.

cloud. A visible mass of condensed water floating in the air.

coagulation. Clumping of particles in wastewater to settle out impurities, often induced by chemicals such as lime, alum, and iron salts.

coal cleaning technology. A precombustion process by which coal is physically or chemically treated to remove some of its sulfur to reduce sulfur dioxide emissions.

coal gasification. The conversion of coal to a gaseous product by one of several available technologies.

coastal zone. Lands and waters adjacent to the coast that exert an influence on the uses of the sea and its ecology; its uses and ecology also are affected by the sea.

cobalt. A silvery white, solid, metallic element, symbol Co, with atomic number 27, and atomic weight 58.93.

cocarcinogen. An agent, when administered with a carcinogen, that enhances the activity of the carcinogen.

Code of Federal Regulations (CFR). Document that codifies all rules of the executive departments and agencies of the federal government. It is divided into 50 volumes, known as titles. Title 40 of the CFR (referenced as 40 CFR) lists all environmental regulations. Title 49 (49 CFR) lists rules set forth by the Department of Transportation (DOT) governing the transportation of hazardous materials within the continental United States.

coefficient of haze (COH). A measurement of visibility interference in the atmosphere.

coefficient of permeability. *See* **hydraulic conductivity**.

coextrusion. 1. The process by which two or more layers of an extruded product are produced simultaneously. 2. Two (or more) extruders are used and the two (or more) extrudates are laid on each other while still hot.

cofire. Burning of two different fuels in the same combustion unit.

cogeneration. The consecutive generation of useful thermal and electric energy from the same fuel source.

coke. An impure form of carbon obtained by destructive distillation of coal or petroleum.

coke oven. An industrial process that converts coal into coke, one of the basic materials used in blast furnaces for the conversion of iron ore into iron.

cold temperature CO standard. A standard for automobile emissions of carbon monoxide emissions to be met at a low temperature (i.e., 20°F). Conventional automobile catalytic converters are not efficient in cold weather until they warm up.

cold zone. A clearly marked and controlled area where the command post and support functions that are necessary to control the incident are located. This is also referred to as the *clean zone*, *green zone*, or *support zone* in other documents (EPA standard operating safety guidelines, OSHA 29 CFR 1910.120, and NFPA 472). *See also* **support zone** and **safe zone**.

coliform index. A rating of the purity of water based on a count of fecal bacteria.

coliform organism. Microorganisms found in the intestinal tract of humans and animals. Their presence in water indicates fecal pollution and potentially adverse contamination by pathogens.

collector. Public or private hauler that collects nonhazardous waste and recyclable materials from residential, commercial, institutional, and industrial sources.

collector sewers. Pipes used to collect and carry wastewater from individual sources to an interceptor sewer that will carry it to a treatment facility.

colloidal dispersion. Not a true solution or suspension. The particles have a size between 1 and 100 nanometers (nm).

colloids. Very small, finely divided insoluble solids that remain dispersed in a liquid for a long time due to their small size and electrical charge.

combined sewer overflows. Discharge of a mixture of storm water and domestic waste when the flow capacity of a sewer system is exceeded during rainstorms.

combined sewers. A sewer system that carries both sewage and stormwater runoff.

combustible. Capable of combustion.

combustible liquid. A liquid with a flash point of 100°F or higher.

combustibility. 1. The ease with which a material burns. 2. May be determined by properties such as flash point, ignition temperature, and flammable range. 3. May be synonymous with **flammability**.

combustion. 1. Burning, or rapid oxidation, accompanied by release of energy in the form of heat and light. 2. In waste disposal, it refers to the controlled burning of waste, in which heat chemically alters organic compounds, converting the waste into stable inorganic products such as carbon dioxide and water. 3. *See also* **fire**.

combustion chamber. The actual compartment where waste is burned in an incinerator.

combustion product. Substance produced during the burning or oxidation of a material. Airborne effluent from a material undergoing combustion. May also include pyrosylates (ASTM E 800).

command-and-control regulations. Specific requirements prescribing how to comply with specific standards defining acceptable levels of pollution.

command post. Facility located at a safe distance upwind from an accident site, where the on-scene coordinator, responders, and technical representatives make response decisions, deploy manpower and equipment, maintain liaison with news media, and handle communications.

comment period. Time provided for the public to review and comment on a proposed EPA action or rulemaking after publication in the Federal Register.

commercial waste. All solid waste emanating from business establishments such as stores, markets, office buildings, restaurants, shopping centers, and theaters.

commercial waste management facility. A treatment, storage, disposal, or transfer facility that accepts waste from a variety of sources, as compared to a private facility that normally manages a limited waste stream generated by its own operations.

commingled recyclables. Mixed recyclables that are collected together.

comminuter. A machine that shreds or pulverizes solids to make waste treatment easier.

comminution. Mechanical shredding or pulverizing of waste. Used in both solid waste management and wastewater treatment.

common name. 1. The name originally given to a chemical compound upon its discovery, prior to the adoption of an organized system of assigning proper names. 2. Any designation or identification such as code name, code number, trade name, brand name, or generic name used to identify a chemical other than by its proper chemical name.

Common Sense Initiative. Voluntary program to simplify environmental regulation to achieve cleaner, cheaper, smarter results, starting with six major industry sectors.

community. In ecology, an assemblage of populations of different species within a specified location in space and time.

Community Awareness and Emergency Response (CAER). A program adopted by the Chemical Manufacturers Association (CMA), designed to provide the public with information on chemicals manufactured, used, or stored in the community, and to integrate facility emergency response plans with community emergency response plans.

community relations. The EPA effort to establish two-way communication with the public to create understanding of EPA programs and related actions, to ensure public input into decision-making processes related to affected communities, and to make certain that the agency is aware of and responsive to public concerns.

community water system. A public water system that serves at least 15 service connections used by year-round residents or regularly serves at least 25 year-round residents.

comonomer. A monomer copolymerized with another monomer, to form a copolymer. The copolymer will have many of the properties of each polymer.

compact fluorescent lamp (CFL). Small fluorescent lamps used as more efficient alternatives to incandescent lighting. Also called *PL, Twin-Tube*, or *BIAX lamps*.

compaction. Reduction of the bulk of solid waste by rolling and tamping.

comparative risk assessment. Process that generally uses the judgment of experts to predict effects and set priorities among a wide range of environmental problems.

compatibility. The ability of two materials to be brought together without reacting.

compatibility group. Letters identify explosives that are deemed to be compatible. Class 1 materials are considered to be "compatible" if they can be transported together without significantly increasing either the probability of an incident or, for a given quantity, the magnitude of the effects of such an incident. Letter designations include:

- A. Substances that are expected to mass detonate very soon after fire reaches them.
- B. Articles that are expected to mass detonate very soon after fire reaches them.
- C. Substances or articles that may be readily ignited and burn violently without necessarily exploding.
- D. Substances or articles that may mass detonate (with blast and/or fragment hazard) when exposed to fire.
- E. Articles that may mass detonate in a fire.
- F. Articles that may mass detonate in a fire.
- G. Substances and articles that may mass explode and give off smoke or toxic gases.
- H. Articles that in a fire may eject hazardous projectiles and dense white smoke.
- J. Articles that may mass explode.
- K. Articles that in a fire may eject hazardous projectiles and toxic gases.
- L. Substances and articles that present a special risk and could be activated by exposure to air or water.
- N. Articles that contain only extremely insensitive detonating substances and demonstrate a negligible probability of accidental ignition or propagation.
- S. Packaged substances or articles that, if accidentally initiated, produce effects that are usually confined to the immediate vicinity.

complete combustion. A combustion reaction that converts all of the fuel's carbon, hydrogen, sulfur, and nitrogen into carbon dioxide, water, sulfur dioxide, and molecular nitrogen (N_2), respectively.

complete treatment. A method of treating water that consists of the addition of coagulant chemicals, flash mixing, coagulation-flocculation, sedimentation, and filtration. Also called **conventional filtration**.

complex ion. A charged particle that started as two or more atoms, bound together chemically, which collectively gained or lost one or more electrons.

compliance coal. Any coal that emits less than 1.2 pounds of sulfur dioxide per million British thermal units (Btus) when burned. Also known as *low sulfur coal*.

compliance coating. A coating with a volatile organic compound content that does not exceed that allowed by regulation.

compliance cycle. A nine-year calendar-year cycle (the first of which began on January 1, 1993) during which public water systems must monitor. Each cycle consists of three compliance periods of three years each.

compliance monitoring. Collection and evaluation of data, including self-monitoring reports and verification to show whether pollutant concentrations and loads contained in permitted discharges are in compliance with the limits and conditions specified in the permit.

compliance schedule. A negotiated agreement between a pollution source and a government agency that specifies dates and procedures by which a source will reduce emissions and, thereby, comply with a regulation.

composite sample. A series of water samples taken over a given period of time and weighted by flow rate.

compost. The relatively stable humus material that is produced from a composting process in which bacteria in soil mixed with garbage and degradable trash break down the mixture into organic fertilizer.

composting. The controlled biological decomposition of organic material in the presence of air to form a humus-like material.

composting facility. 1. An off-site facility where the organic component of municipal solid waste is decomposed under controlled conditions. 2. An aerobic process in which organic materials are ground or shredded and then decomposed to humus in windrow piles or in mechanical digesters, drums, or similar enclosures.

compound. 1. As in a chemical compound, a chemical combination of two or more atoms, either from the same element or from different elements, that is electrically neutral. 2. In plastics, a mixture of resin and the necessary additives to give the resin the required properties of the finished part.

Comprehensive Environmental Response, Compensation, and Liability Act (CERCLA). Enacted in 1980 and known as CERCLA or Superfund, it addresses hazardous substance releases into the environment and the cleanup of inactive hazardous waste sites. It also requires those who release hazardous substances, as defined by the EPA, above certain levels (reportable quantities) to notify the National Response Center (NRC).

compressed gas. A gas that is under pressure, either still in the gaseous state or liquefied. It will have an absolute pressure greater than 40 psi at 21.1°C.

Compressed Gas Association. A nonprofit technical association representing about 300 businesses, including most of the world's leading producers of compressed, liquefied, and cryogenic gases.

compressed natural gas (CNG). One of the cleanest motor vehicle fuels because of low hydrocarbon emissions. As a fuel, it produces very little ozone. However, vehicles fueled with CNG do emit a significant quantity of nitrogen oxides.

compression molding. The process by which a compound or a sheet of thermoplastic is placed in a molding cavity while heat is applied to the mold and pressure is applied to the sheet by part of the mold moving against the sheet.

Computer-Aided Management of Emergency Operations (CAMEO). Computer database storage retrieval of preplanning data for on-scene response use in hazmat incidents.

concentrate. 1. An additive that is a plastics compound containing many more times the active ingredient required by the final article. This concentrate is then added to a "natural" compound at a predetermined rate in the processing equipment to achieve the desired final result. The concentrate can contain colorants, antioxidants, flame retardants, or any other active ingredient. 2. Also called a *masterbatch*.

concentration. 1. The amount of one material mixed or dissolved in another expressed as a percentage. 2. In an acid, the amount of the anhydrous acid dissolver in water. 3. The relative amount of a substance mixed with another substance. For example, 10 ppm of nitrogen dioxide in air or 1 mg/L of calcium in water.

condensate. 1. Water created by cooling steam or water vapor. 2. A liquid formed when warm landfill gas cools as it travels through a collection system.

condensate return system. System that returns the heated water condensing within steam piping to the boiler and thus saves energy.

condensation. 1. The process by which a gas or vapor passes into the liquid phase. 2. A type of chemical reaction by which water is formed and separated from the other products of the reaction.

condensation point. The temperature at which a gas or vapor changes into a liquid by cooling.

condensed states. The solid and liquid states of matter.

conditionally exempt (CE) generators. Persons or enterprises that produce less than 220 pounds of hazardous waste per month. *Contrast with* **small quantity generator**.

conditional registration. Under special circumstances, the FIFRA permits registration of pesticide products that is conditional upon the submission of additional data.

conditions to avoid. Conditions encountered during handling or storage that could cause a substance to become unstable and react.

conductance. 1. A rapid method of estimating the dissolved solids content of water supply by determining the capacity of a water sample to carry an electrical current. 2. The ability of a substance to conduct electrical current. *See also* **conductivity**.

conduction. Transfer of heat through a medium.

conductivity. A measure of the ability of a solution to carry an electrical current.

conductor. A material through which electrons travel freely. The best electrical conductors are metals.

cone of depression. A depression in the water table that develops around a pumped well.

cone of influence. The depression, roughly conical in shape, produced in a water table by the pumping of water from a well.

cone penterometer testing (CPT). A direct push system used to measure lithology based on soil penetration resistance.

confidential business information (CBI). Material that contains trade secrets or commercial or financial information that has been claimed as confidential by its source.

confidential statement of formula (CSF). A list of the ingredients in a new pesticide or chemical formulation. The list is submitted at the time for application for registration or change in formulation.

confined aquifer. An aquifer in which groundwater is confined under pressure that is significantly greater than atmospheric pressure.

confined space. Any area that has limited openings for entry and exit that would make escape difficult in an emergency, has a lack of ventilation, contains known and potential hazards, and is neither intended nor designated for continuous human occupancy.

confinement. Actions taken to keep a material in a defined or local area after it is released.

conflagration. A large, uncontrollable fire covering a considerable area and crossing natural fire barriers such as streets and streams.

confluent growth. A continuous bacterial growth covering all or part of the filtration area of a membrane filter in which the bacteria colonies are not discrete.

confounder. A condition or variable that is both a risk factor for disease and associated with an exposure of interest. Also called a *confounding factor*.

confounding factor. *See* **confounder.**

conjugated double bonds. A structure in which there are double covalent bonds between two carbon atoms that are separated from each other by one single bond between two carbon atoms (-C=C-C=C-).

consent decree. A legal document, approved by a judge, that formalizes an agreement reached between EPA and potentially responsible parties (PRPs) through which PRPs will conduct all or part of a cleanup action at a Superfund site; cease or correct actions or processes that are polluting the environment; or otherwise comply with EPA-initiated regulatory enforcement actions to resolve the contamination at the Superfund site involved.

conservation. 1. Preserving and renewing, when possible, human and natural resources. 2. The use, protection, and improvement of natural resources according to principles that will ensure their highest economic or social benefits.

conservation easement. Easement restricting a landowner to land uses that are compatible with long-term conservation and environmental values.

consignee. 1. The person or company to whom a shipment is being made. 2. The buyer of the product or a warehouse or other enterprise that will hold the shipment until it is ready to be used.

consignor. The person named in the bill of lading as the one from whom the goods have been received for shipment.

consist. 1. A rail shipping paper similar to a cargo manifest. 2. A list of the cars in the train, in order, or a list of those cars carrying hazardous materials and their locations on the train.

constituent(s) of concern. Specific chemicals that are identified for evaluation in the site assessment process.

construction and demolition waste. Waste building materials, dredging materials, tree stumps, and rubble resulting from construction, remodeling, repair, and demolition of homes, commercial buildings, and other structures and pavements.

construction ban. If, under the Clean Air Act, EPA disapproves an area's planning requirements for correcting nonattainment, EPA can ban the construction or modification of any major stationary source of the pollutant for which the area is in nonattainment.

consumer information sheets (CIS). EPA-approved guidelines for handling treated wood generally available to the consumer at retail outlets where treated lumber is sold and from AWPI and the wood-treating industry.

consumptive water use. Water removed from available supplies without return to a water resources system.

contact pesticide. A chemical that kills pests by touch, instead of by ingestion.

container. Anything that holds material, including storage tanks, pipelines, packaging drums, and carboys, etc.

contaminant. Any physical, chemical, biological, or radiological substance or matter that has an adverse effect on air, water, or soil.

contamination. 1. Introduction into water, air, and soil of microorganisms, chemicals, toxic substances, wastes, or wastewater in a concentration that makes the medium unfit for its next intended use. 2. Also applies to surfaces of objects, buildings, and various household and agricultural use products. 3. Deposition of radioactive material in any place where it is not desired, particularly where its presence can be harmful. 4. A release of hazardous material from its source to people, animals, the environment, or equipment.

contamination reduction corridor (CRC). *See* **warm zone**.

contamination reduction zone (CRZ). *See* **warm zone**.

contamination source inventory. An inventory of contaminant sources within delineated state water quality protection areas.

contingency plan. A document setting out organized, planned, and coordinated courses of action to be followed in case of a fire, explosion, or other accident that releases toxic chemicals, hazardous waste, or radioactive materials that threaten human health or the environment.

continuous discharge. A routine release to the environment that occurs without interruption, except for infrequent shutdowns for maintenance and process changes, etc.

continuous sample. A flow of water, waste, or other material from a particular place in a plant to the location where samples are collected for testing.

contour strip farming. A kind of contour farming in which row crops are planted in strips, between alternating strips of close-growing, erosion-resistant forage crops.

contract labs. Laboratories under contract to EPA that analyze samples taken from waste, soil, air, and water or carry out research projects.

control group. A group used as the baseline for comparison in epidemiologic studies or laboratory studies. Also called a **reference group**.

controlled area. An area where entry, activities, and exit are controlled to help ensure radiation protection and to prevent the spread of contamination.

controlled reaction. A chemical reaction under precise temperature and pressure conditions maintained within safe limits to produce a desired product or process.

control technique guidelines (CTG). EPA documents designed to assist state and local pollution authorities to achieve and maintain air quality standards for certain sources through reasonably available control technologies (RACT).

control zone. A designated area at a hazardous materials incident, based on safety and the degree of hazard. Many terms are used to describe control zones; however, these zones are defined as the *hot, exclusion, or restricted zone*; the *warm, contamination reduction,* or *limited access zone*; and the *cold, support,* or *clean zone* (EPA standard operating safety guidelines, OSHA 29 CFR 1910.120, and NFPA 472).

convection. Transfer of heat with a medium.

convection column. *See* **thermal column**.

conventional filtration. *See* **complete treatment**.

conventional pollutant. A pollutants listed by regulation. These may be in the form of organic waste, sediment, acid, bacteria, viruses, nutrients, oil and grease, or heat.

conventional site assessment. Assessment in which most of the sample analysis and interpretation of data are completed off-site.

conventional system. A systems that has been traditionally used to collect municipal wastewater in gravity sewers and convey it to a central primary or secondary treatment plant prior to discharge to surface waters.

conversion. *See* **process (plastics)**.

conversion process. *See* **process (plastics)**.

conveyance loss. Water loss in pipes, channels, conduits, or ditches by leakage or evaporation.

cooling electricity use. Amount of electricity used to meet a building cooling load.

cooling tower. 1. A structure that helps remove heat from water used as a coolant. 2. A mechanism that dissipates the heat from water-cooled systems by spraying the water through streams of rapidly moving air.

coordinate bond. A covalent bond in which a pair of electrons is donated by only one of the atoms that it joins.

copolymer. 1. A rubber or plastic material made by the copolymerization of two monomers, such as styrene and butadiene to make styrene-butadiene rubber. Three monomers, such as those in acrylonitrile-butadiene-styrene (ABS) make a **terpolymer**, even though the three monomers were not polymerized together.

copper. A reddish-brown, solid, metallic element, symbol Cu, with atomic number 29, and atomic weight 63.546. It is ductile and therefore can be drawn into wire. It is a very good conductor of electricity.

copperas. Ferrous sulfate.

copper naphthenate. An organic unrestricted-use wood preservative that protects against wood-destroying organisms. Uses include the pressure treatment of utility poles, lumber, timbers, pilings, and laminated beams. Also recommended for brush, spray, or dip treatments for end cuts and cutoffs of pressure-treated wood products.

cordite. A smokeless explosive that is made by mixing nitrocellulose, nitroglycerine, and a small amount of additive.

core. The uranium-containing heart of a nuclear reactor, where energy is released.

core program cooperative agreement. An assistance agreement whereby EPA supports states or tribal governments with funds to help defray the cost of certain expenses that are not item specific, such as administrative and training activities.

corrective action. EPA can require treatment, storage, and disposal facilities (TSDF) handling hazardous waste to undertake corrective actions to clean up spills resulting from failure to follow hazardous waste management procedures or other mistakes.

corridor. An enclosed space connecting a room or compartment with an exit. The corridor may include normal extensions, such as lobbies and other enlarged spaces (ASTM E 648).

corrosion. The process by which a metal is progressively destroyed, usually caused by a chemical reaction such as that occurring between water and the pipes, chemicals touching a metal surface, or contact between two dissimilar metals.

corrosive. 1. A chemical agent that reacts with the surface of a material, causing it to deteriorate or wear away. 2. A chemical that causes visible destruction of, or irreversible alterations in, living tissue by chemical action at the site of contact. 3. Any material that will attack and injure or destroy, by chemical action, any living tissue with which it comes into contact.

corrosiveness. The ability to attack and damage or destroy materials by chemical action.

cosmic rays. High-energy radiation that originates outside the Earth's atmosphere.

cost-benefit analysis. A quantitative evaluation of the costs that would have incurred by implementing a particular program versus the overall benefits to society of the proposed action.

cost-effective alternative. An alternative control or corrective method identified after analysis as being the best available in terms of reliability, performance, and cost.

cost recovery. A legal process by which potentially responsible parties who contributed to contamination at a Superfund site can be required to reimburse the Trust Fund for money spent during any cleanup actions by the federal government.

cost sharing. A publicly financed program through which society, as a beneficiary of environmental protection, shares part of the cost of pollution control with those who must actually install the controls.

coulomb. 1. An SI unit of electric charge, equal to the amount of charge delivered by a current of 1 ampere (amp) running for 1 second. 2. One mole of electrons has a charge of about 96,487 coulombs (C).

covalent. A type of chemical bonding characterized by the sharing of one or more pairs of electrons between the bonded atoms. The resulting chemical compound is called a covalent compound.

covalent bond. The sharing of a pair of electrons between two atoms. It represents stored energy, which is released when the bond is broken.

covalent compound. A compound containing atoms bonded together by covalent bonds.

covered facility. A facility subject to a reporting requirement of Title III. It has four different meanings in Title III, depending on the section of the act.

covered substance. A hazardous chemical that subjects a facility to the requirements of Title III.

cover material. Soil used to cover compacted solid waste in a sanitary landfill.

cracking. The breaking of covalent bonds, usually between carbon atoms.

cradle-to-grave system. A procedure in which hazardous materials are identified and followed as they are produced, treated, transported, and disposed of by a series of permanent, linkable, descriptive documents (e.g., manifests). Also called **manifest system**.

creep. The tendency of a material to deform (permanently) under prolonged stress or pressure.

creosote. 1. A distillate of coal tar. An oil most commonly used to preserve railroad ties, utility poles, pilings, bridges, guard posts, and marine applications. 2. A tar deposited inside a chimney when resinous wood is burned.

criteria. Descriptive factors taken into account by EPA in setting standards for various pollutants.

criteria pollutant. 1. A pollutant known to be hazardous to human health as specified by the 1970 amendments to the Clean Air Act. EPA, required to set national ambient air quality standards, identified and set standards to protect human health and welfare for six pollutants: ozone, carbon monoxide, total suspended particulates, sulfur dioxide, lead, and nitrogen oxide. 2. The term *criteria pollutants* derives from the requirement that EPA must describe the characteristics and potential health and welfare effects of these pollutants. It is on the basis of these criteria that standards are set or revised.

critical concentration. An ambient chemical concentration expressed in units of micrograms per cubic meter and used in the operational derivation of the inhalation of the reference concentration. This concentration will be the no-observed-adverse-effect level (NOAEL) human equivalent concentration (HEC) adjusted from principal study data.

critical effect. The first adverse effect, or its known precursor, that occurs as a dose rate increases.

critical mass. The minimum mass of a particular fissionable radioactive material in a given volume required to sustain a nuclear chain reaction.

critical pressure. 1. The pressure of a gas at its critical temperature. 2. The pressure required to liquefy a gas at its critical temperature.

critical radiant flux. The level of incident radiant heat energy on the floor covering system at the most distant flameout point. It is reported as watts per square centimeter (W/cm^2) or Btus per square foot (Btu/ft^2) (ASTM E 648).

critical study. The study that contributes most significantly to the qualitative and quantitative assessment of risk. Also called *principal study*.

critical temperature. 1. The maximum temperature at which a gas may remain in the liquid phase. 2. The temperature above which it is impossible for a gas to be liquefied or remain a liquid.

crop consumptive use. The amount of water transpired during plant growth plus that which evaporated from the soil surface and foliage in the crop area.

crop rotation. Planting a succession of different crops on the same land area as opposed to planting the same crop time after time.

cross contamination. The movement of underground contaminants from one level or area to another due to invasive subsurface activities.

cross connection. Any actual or potential connection between a drinking water system and an unapproved water supply or other source of contamination.

cross-linking. The chemical reaction where chemical bonds are set up between polymer chains. The process occurs mostly in thermoset resins or by cross-blending fillers and other additives with a thermoplastic resin, which will cause the conversion to a thermosetting resin.

crown fire. The movement of fire through the crowns of trees or shrubs, more or less independently of the surface fire. Also called *crowning*.

crowning. *See* **crown fire**.

crumb rubber. Ground rubber fragments the size of sand or silt used in rubber or plastic products, or processed further into reclaimed rubber or asphalt products.

cryogen. Synonym for a cryogenic material. A substance, usually a gas, that is produced and/or is used at temperatures of –150°F and below.

cryogenic gas. A gas with a boiling point of –150°F or lower.

cryogenic liquid. A refrigerated, liquefied gas, with a boiling point colder than –150°C (–238°F) at atmospheric pressure. Also called *refrigerated liquid*.

cryogenics. The study of the behavior of matter at temperatures of –150°F and below.

cryptosporidium. A protozoan microbe associated with the disease cryptosporidiosis in humans.

crystal. A solid that has a regular shape bound by plane surfaces (facets) that intersect at characteristic angles.

crystallinity. Denotes uniformity and compactness of the molecular chains, forming a crystal-like structure. *Contrast with* **amorphous.**

cubic centimeter. 1. Metric measurement of volume equal to 1 mL. 2. One cubic centimeter (cc) equals 0.061 $in.^3$. 3. One cubic inch equals 16.4 cc. 4. One quart equals approximately 946 cc.

cubic feet per minute (cfm). A measure of the volume of a substance flowing through air within a fixed period of time. With regard to indoor air, refers to the amount of air, in cubic feet, that is exchanged with outdoor air in 1 min; i.e., the air exchange rate.

cullet. Crushed glass.

cultural eutrophication. Increasing rate at which water bodies "die" by pollution from human activities.

cultures and stocks. 1. Infectious agents and associated biologicals, including cultures from medical and pathological laboratories. 2. Waste from the production of biologicals. 3. Discarded live and attenuated vaccines and culture dishes and devices used to transfer, inoculate, and mix cultures.

cumulative ecological risk assessment. Consideration of the total ecological risk from multiple stressors to a given eco-zone.

cumulative exposure. The sum of exposures of an organism to a pollutant over a period of time.

cumulative working level months (CWLM). The sum of lifetime exposure to radon working levels expressed in total working level months.

cuprum. Latin for "copper," hence the symbol, Cu.

curbside collection. Method of collecting recyclable materials at homes, community districts, or businesses.

curb stop. A water service shutoff valve located in a water service pipe near the curb and between the water main and the building.

cure. 1. The process by which the chemical properties of a material are changed due to a chemical reaction. 2. Usually refers to the chemical reaction involving a thermosetting resin, where the polymerization is called *curing* or *setting up*.

curie. A unit of activity, which is defined as the number of nuclei in a sample that disintegrate every second (3.7^{10}). Curies (Ci) are used to define the rate of decay of a radioactive material.

curium. A silvery white, radioactive, solid, metallic element, symbol Cm, with atomic number 96, and atomic weight 244. Artificially produced from plutonium.

cutaneous. Relates to the skin.

cutaneous hazard. A chemical that affects the dermal layer of the body.

cutie-pie. An instrument used to measure radiation levels.

cuttings. Spoils left by conventional drilling with hollow stem auger or rotary drilling equipment.

cyanate. The cyanate ion (CNO^{-1}), or a salt or ester of cyanic acid (HCNO). Always toxic.

cyanide. Any compound containing the cyanide ion (CN^{-1}) or the cyanide radical (-CN). Always toxic. Organic compounds containing the cyanide radical may be called nitriles.

cyano-. A prefix indicating the presence of the cyanide radical (-CN). Always toxic.

cyanogen. A chemical blood agent.

cyanogen chloride. A chemical blood agent, CNCl; agent CK.

cyclic. An organic compound structure characterized by the presence of one or more closed rings. The number of rings present is designated by the prefixes *mono-*, *bi-*, *tri-*, or *poly-*.

cyclical. A molecular structure that forms a closed ring, instead of being open-ended. 2. The structure of certain molecules where there is no end to the carbon chain. The molecule is a closed structure resembling a ring; what would be the "last" carbon in the chain is bonded to the "first" carbon in the chain. There are cyclical compounds in which the closed structure contains the atoms of other elements in addition to carbon.

cyclohexyl sarin. A chemical nerve gas; agent GF.

cyclone collector. A device that uses centrifugal force to remove large particles from polluted air.

cyclonite. High explosive, more powerful than TNT; agent RDX.

cyclosarin. Also known as sarin, a chemical nerve gas; agent GF.

D

Dalton's law. *See* **partial pressure, law of.**

dangerous goods. Another term for hazardous materials.

dangerous goods by road (ADR). Accord European Relatif au Transport International des Marchandises Dangereuses par Route (European regulations).

dangerous when wet. A class of hazardous materials that when exposed to water allows a chemical reaction to take place and often produces flammable or poisonous gases, heat, and a caustic solution.

dash method. 1. A method of showing the configuration of an atom's unpaired electrons by drawing a dash for every unpaired electron. 2. The dash, when used around the symbol of one element, is not a covalent bond, but an unpaired electron.

data call-in. A part of the Office of Pesticide Programs' (OPP) process of developing key required test data, especially on the long-term, chronic effects of existing pesticides, in advance of scheduled registration standard reviews.

data quality objectives (DQOs). Qualitative and quantitative statements of the overall level of uncertainty that a decision maker will accept in results or decisions based on environmental data.

day tank. Another name for *deaerating tank*.

dead end. The end of a water main that is not connected to other parts of the distribution system.

decant. To draw off the upper layer of liquid after the heaviest material (a solid or another liquid) has settled.

decay. The process by which radioactive materials give off particles. 2. Decomposition of wood by wood-destroying fungi.

decay products. Degraded radioactive materials, often referred to as *daughters* or *progeny*. Radon decay products of most concern from a public health standpoint are polonium-214 and polonium-218.

dechlor. Sodium thiophosphate.

dechlorination. Removal of chlorine from a substance.

decibel (dB). 1. A unit of relative loudness, voltage, or current equal to the common logarithm of the ratio of two readings. 2. A unit of measurement to detect noise levels.

decomposition. 1. The breakdown of a chemical compound by heat, decay, chemical reaction, electrolysis, or other process. 2. The breakdown of matter by bacteria and fungi, changing the chemical makeup and physical appearance of materials.

decomposition products. Products of a chemical or thermal breakdown of a substance.

decomposition temperature. The temperature at which a chemical substance breaks down into two or more substances.

decontamination. 1. Removal of harmful substances such as noxious chemicals, harmful bacteria or other organisms, or radioactive material from exposed individuals, rooms, and furnishings in buildings, or the exterior environment. 2. The reduction or removal of contaminating radioactive material from a structure, area, object, or person.

decontamination area. An area located on the upwind edge of the hot zone used to decontaminate personnel and equipment. All personnel coming out of the hot zone must undergo decontamination. *See also* **hot zone**.

decontamination line. A line set up with stations for decontamination procedures between the exclusion zone and the support zone.

decyl. The radical ($-C_{10}H_{21}$) formed when one hydrogen is removed from decane ($C_{10}H_{22}$).

deep-well injection. Deposition of raw or treated, filtered hazardous waste by pumping it into deep wells, where it is contained in the pores of permeable subsurface rock.

defatting. The process whereby the solvent action of the material dissolves the fat from human skin.

defensive mode. The strategy of firefighting whereby the fire department's resources are dedicated to protecting exposures and limiting risk to firefighters when the fire has progressed to the point that an offensive attack will accomplish nothing. The goal is to simply confine the fire to the building or area of origin. No aggressive interior firefighting operations take place in the defensive mode. All fire streams are operated onto the fire from the outside. This strategy is employed when a fire has advanced to the point where attack operations are judged too dangerous, and/or the fire is beyond the capabilities of on-scene resources.

defibrillation. The use of direct current electric shock to terminate ventricular fibrillation and restore effective cardiac function.

deflagrate. To burn very rapidly.

deflagration. 1. The very rapid combustion of a material, usually a low explosive. 2. A property of class B explosives. 3. Some references say deflagration is an explosion that operates by a shock wave moving at subsonic speed. 4. Compare with **detonation**.

deflocculating agent. A material added to a suspension to prevent settling of solids.

defluoridation. The removal of excess fluoride in drinking water to prevent the staining of teeth.

defoliant. A herbicide that removes leaves from trees and growing plants.

degasification. A water treatment that removes dissolved gases from the water.

degradation. 1. A deleterious change in the chemical structure, physical properties, or appearance of a plastic (ASTM D883). 2. The breakdown of a chemical compound.

degree-day. 1. A rough measure used to estimate the amount of heating required in a given area, defined as the difference between the mean daily temperature and 65°F. 2. Degree-days are also calculated to estimate cooling requirements.

degree of flammability. *See* **flammability, degree of**.

dehydration. The removal or loss of water.

deionizing. A method of purifying water by removing soluble salts.

delegated state. A state that has received authority to administer an environmental regulatory program in lieu of a federal counterpart.

deliquescent. The property by which a substance absorbs moisture from the air (or other substances) in such quantities that it dissolves in that moisture.

delist. Use of the petition process to have a facility's toxic designation rescinded.

deluge. In firefighting, the delivery of water in flooding amounts.

demand regulator. A device that reduces tank pressure to provide air to the mask when the wearer inhales.

demineralization. A treatment process that removes dissolved minerals from water.

denaturant. A substance added to ethanol to render it unfit for human consumption.

denatured alcohol. Referring to ethanol (ethyl alcohol) to which another liquid has been added to render it unfit for human consumption.

denier. An older unit of fineness of fibers where 1 denier equals 1 gram (g) of fiber stretched to 9,000 meters (m). If the 9,000 m of fiber weighs 2 g, then the denier is 2, and so on.

denitrification. The biological reduction of nitrate to nitrogen gas by denitrifying bacteria in soil.

dense nonaqueous phase liquid (DNAPL). Nonaqueous phase liquids, such as chlorinated hydrocarbon solvents or petroleum fractions with a specific gravity greater than 1.0, that sink through the water column until they reach a confining layer.

density. 1. A measure of how heavy a specific volume of a solid, liquid, or gas is in comparison to water. 2. Weight per unit volume, usually expressed in grams per cubic centimeter (g/cc or g/cm^3) or pounds per cubic foot (lb/ft^3).

deoxyribonucleic acid (DNA). A complex sugar-protein polymer that contains the genetic code of every enzyme in the cell.

Department of Transportation (DOT). An agency, either federal or state, that regulates shipments and transfer of hazardous materials.

Department of Transportation specification. Tank car specification consisting of a class designation followed by identifying letters and numbers. The second set of numerals, where present, indicates tank test pressure in pounds per square inch, followed by the type of tank material and lining or thermal protection that may be present. In all classes except classes 103, 104, and 113, the two-number series is separated by an "A," which has no special significance.

depletion curve. In hydraulics, a graphical representation of water depletion from storage-stream channels, surface soil, and groundwater.

depolymerization. 1. The breakdown, usually by heat, of a polymer into simpler molecules. 2. The process whereby a polymer reverts to its monomer, or a lower molecular weight polymer, usually occurring upon the polymer's exposure to high temperature.

depressurization. A condition that occurs when the air pressure inside a structure is lower than the air pressure outdoors.

derivative. In organic chemistry, a compound made from a hydrocarbon by substituting another atom or group of atoms for one of the hydrogen atoms in the compound.

dermal. Pertaining to the skin.

dermal absorption. Process by which a chemical penetrates the skin and enters the body. Also called *dermal penetration.*

dermal exposure. Contact between a chemical and the skin.

dermal penetration. *See* **dermal absorption.**

dermal toxicity. The ability of a pesticide or toxic chemical to poison people or animals by contact with the skin.

dermatitis. An inflammation, redness, or irritation of the skin.

desalination. 1. The removal of salts from ocean or brackish water by using various technologies. 2. Removal of salts from soil by artificial means, usually leaching. Also called *desalinization.*

desalinization. *See* **desalination.**

desiccant. A chemical agent that absorbs moisture. Some desiccants are capable of drying out plants or insects, causing death.

design capacity. The average daily flow that a treatment plant or other facility is designed to accommodate.

design value. The monitored reading used by EPA to determine an area's air quality status.

designated pollutant. An air pollutant that is neither a criteria nor hazardous pollutant, as described in the Clean Air Act, but for which new source performance standards exist.

designated uses. Those water uses identified in state water quality standards that must be achieved and maintained as required under the Clean Water Act.

designer bugs. Popular term for microbes developed through biotechnology that can degrade specific toxic chemicals at their source in toxic waste dumps or in groundwater.

desorption. The process of removing a material from the surface of another material on which it is adsorbed.

destination facility. The facility to which regulated medical waste is shipped for treatment and destruction, incineration, and/or disposal.

destratification. Vertical mixing within a lake or reservoir to totally or partially eliminate separate layers of temperature, plant, or animal life.

destroyed medical waste. Regulated medical waste that has been ruined, torn apart, or mutilated through thermal treatment, melting, shredding, grinding, tearing, or breaking, so that it is no longer generally recognized as medical waste.

destruction and removal efficiency (DRE). A percentage that represents the number of molecules of a compound removed or destroyed in an incinerator relative to the number of molecules entering the system.

destruction facility. A facility that destroys regulated medical waste.

desulfurization. Removal of sulfur from fossil fuels to reduce pollution.

detectable leak rate. The smallest leak (from a storage tank), expressed in terms of gallons per hour or liters per hour, that a test can reliably discern with a certain probability of detection or false alarm.

detection criterion. A predetermined rule to ascertain whether a tank is leaking or not.

detection limit. The lowest concentration of a chemical that can reliably be distinguished from a zero concentration.

detector. A device that is sensitive to radiation and can produce a response signal suitable for measurement or analysis. A radiation detection instrument.

detention time. 1. The theoretical calculated time required for a small amount of water to pass through a tank at a given rate of flow. 2. The actual time that a small amount of water is in a settling basin, flocculating basin, or rapid-mix chamber. 3. In storage reservoirs, the length of time water will be held before being used.

detergent. 1. Synthetic washing agent that helps to remove dirt and oil. 2. A soaplike emulsifier that contains a sulfate (SO_3^{-2}) or a phosphate (PO_4^{-3}) group instead of a carboxylate (-C-O-O) group.

detonate. To explode.

detonation. 1. The extremely rapid combustion of a material such as a high explosive. 2. An explosion accompanied by a shock wave moving at supersonic speed. 3. A property of class A explosives. 4. Compare with **deflagration**.

deuterium. Radioactive isotope of hydrogen with an atomic weight of 2; symbol D.

developmental toxicity. Adverse effects on the developing organism that may result from exposure prior to conception (either parent), during prenatal development, or postnatally until the time of sexual maturation.

development effects. Adverse effects such as altered growth, structural abnormality, functional deficiency, or death observed in a developing organism.

dewater. 1. Remove or separate a portion of the water in a sludge or slurry to dry the sludge so it can be handled and disposed of. 2. Remove or drain the water from a tank or trench.

dew point. The temperature at which air, by cooling, becomes saturated with water vapor, which then condenses into liquid water.

di-. A prefix meaning "two." *See also* **bi-**.

diacetylmorphone. Heroin; $C_{17}H_{17}NO(C_2H_3O_2)_2$. Also called *diamorphone.*

diameter index safety system (DISS). Used to avoid erroneous connections of medical gas equipment.

diamond. An allotropic form of carbon.

diatomaceous earth. 1. A chalklike material (fossilized diatoms) used to filter out solid waste in wastewater treatment plants. 2. Used as an active ingredient in some powdered pesticides. Also called *diatomite.*

diatomic. Made up of two atoms, as in a diatomic molecule.

diatomite. *See* **diatomaceous earth**.

Diazinon. A trademarked insecticide.

dibasic. Concerning acids, those having two displaceable hydrogen atoms for each molecule of the acid.

dibenzofurans. A group of organic compounds, some of which are toxic.

dichlorodiphenyltrichloroethane (DDT). Para-dichlorodiphenyltrichloroethane; a chlorinated hydrocarbon disinfectant and insecticide that was used for many years on mosquitoes and body lice. It was banned by the EPA in 1972.

dicofol. A pesticide used on citrus fruits.

differential thermal analysis (DTA). A technique that is used to analyze materials that react or decompose at higher temperatures.

diffused air. A type of aeration that forces oxygen into sewage by pumping air through perforated pipes inside a holding tank.

diffusion. 1. The movement of suspended or dissolved particles (or molecules) from a more concentrated to a less concentrated area. The process tends to distribute the particles or molecules more uniformly. 2. Spontaneous mixing.

diffusion flame. The flame produced by the spontaneous mixture of fuel vapors or gases and air.

digester. 1. In wastewater treatment, a closed tank. 2. In solid waste conversion, a unit in which bacterial action is induced and accelerated in order to break down organic matter and establish the proper carbon to nitrogen ratio.

digestion. The biochemical decomposition of organic matter, resulting in partial gasification, liquefaction, and mineralization of pollutants.

diisocyanate. An organic compound containing two isocyanate (-NCO) groups.

dike. A low wall that can act as a barrier to prevent a spill or leak from spreading. Can be concrete, earth, and other barriers temporarily constructed to hold back the spill or leak.

diluent. Any liquid or solid material used to dilute or carry an active ingredient.

dilute. A solution of low concentration, produced by the addition of water (or another material) to the substance.

dilution. The act of adding water (or other material) to a water soluble material, thereby lowering its concentration.

dilution ratio. The relationship between the volume of water in a stream and the volume of incoming water. It affects the ability of the stream to assimilate waste.

dimension lumber. A size classification of lumber that is from 2 in. up to, but not including, 5 in. thick, and that is 2 in. or more in width.

dimer. 1. A molecule formed from two molecules of a monomer. 2. A chemical compound whose molecule is made up of two molecules of the same chemical composition.

dimercaprol. Used to treat inhalation or ingestion of certain toxic metal compounds. Also called **British anti-lewsite**.

dimethylsulfate. A vesicant or blister agent; $(CH_3)_2SO_4$.

dimictic. Lakes and reservoirs that freeze over and normally go through two stratifications and two mixing cycles a year.

dinocap. A fungicide used primarily by apple growers to control summer diseases.

dinoseb. A herbicide that is also used as a fungicide and insecticide. It was banned by EPA in 1986 because it posed the risk of birth defects and sterility.

dioxin. Any of a family of chlorinated hydrocarbon compounds known chemically as dibenzo-p-dioxins. They are considered dangerous because of their potential toxicity as contaminants in commercial products.

diphenylchloroarsine. A chemical vomiting agent; agent DA.

diphenylcyanoarsine. A chemical vomiting agent; agent DC.

diphosgene. A chemical choking agent; agent PS.

direct discharger. 1. A municipal or industrial facility that introduces pollution through a defined conveyance or system such as outlet pipes. 2. A point source.

direct drive. *See* **direct push**.

direct filtration. A method of treating water that consists of the addition of coagulant chemicals, flash mixing, coagulation, minimal flocculation, and filtration.

direct point. *See* **direct push**.

direct push. The technology used for performing subsurface investigations by driving, pushing, and/or vibrating small-diameter hollow steel rods into the ground. Also known as *direct drive, drive point,* or *push technology*.

direct runoff. Water that flows over the ground surface or through the ground directly into streams, rivers, and lakes.

discharge. 1. Flow of surface water in a stream or canal or the outflow of groundwater from a flowing artesian well, ditch, or spring. 2. May also be the discharge of liquid effluent from a facility or chemical emissions into the air through designated venting mechanisms.

disinfectant. A chemical or physical process that kills pathogenic organisms in water, air, or on surfaces.

disinfectant by-product. 1. A compound formed by the reaction of a disinfectant such as chlorine with organic material in the water supply. 2. A chemical by-product of the disinfection process.

dispatch. To move a resource from one place to another.

dispersant. A chemical agent used to break up concentrations of organic material such as spilled oil.

disperse. To cause to scatter in different directions.

dispersion. 1. The act of dispersing. 2. To cause material to be scattered widely or to dispel from the general area.

displacement savings. Savings realized by displacing purchases of natural gas or electricity from a local utility by using landfill gas for power and heat.

disposables. Consumer products, other items, and packaging used once or a few times and discarded.

disposal. Final placement or destruction of toxic, radioactive, or other wastes, surplus or banned pesticides or other chemicals, polluted soils, and drums containing hazardous materials from removal actions or accidental releases. Disposal may be accomplished through use of approved secure landfills, surface impoundments, land farming, deep-well injection, ocean dumping, or incineration.

disposal facility. A repository for solid waste, such as a landfill or a combustor intended for permanent containment or destruction of waste materials.

dissolved oxygen (DO). The oxygen freely available in water.

dissolved solids. Disintegrated organic and inorganic material in water.

distillate. The vapor collected and condensed from a distillation.

distillation. 1. The separation of a liquid mixture into its components on the basis of differences in boiling points. 2. A method of purifying liquids through boiling, so that the steam or gaseous vapors condense to a pure liquid.

distilled mustard. A chemical vesicant or blister agent; agent HD.

disturbance. Any event or series of events that disrupt an ecosystem, community, or population structure and alter the physical environment.

disulfur decafluoride. A chemical choking agent.

diversion. 1. Use of part of a stream flow as water supply. 2. A dam or dike used to change the flow direction of a liquid.

diversion rate. The percentage of waste materials diverted from traditional disposal, such as by use of a landfill or incineration, to be recycled, composted, or reused.

DMAEDMAPP. Abbreviation for a chemical nerve agent; agent GP.

DMAPDMAPP. Abbreviation for a chemical nerve agent; EA 5414.

DNA hybridization. Use of a segment of DNA, called a DNA probe, to identify its complementary DNA.

Dobson unit (DU). Unit of measurement of ozone in the atmosphere.

domestic application. Pesticide application in and around houses, office buildings, motels, and other living or working areas.

doffing. The act of taking off or removing chemical protective clothing or other gear.

domestic waste. *See* **household waste**.

donning. The act of putting on chemical protective clothing or other gear.

Doppler effect. As a source of waves moves toward an observer, the wavelengths grow shorter, and then longer as the source moves away from the observer.

dosage. *See* **dose.**

dose. 1. The actual quantity of a chemical administered to an organism or to which it is exposed. 2. The amount of a substance that reaches a specific tissue (e.g., the liver). 3. The amount of a substance available for interaction with metabolic processes after crossing the outer boundary of an organism. 4. A general term for the quantity of a chemical taken into the body or radiation or energy absorbed. 5. *See also* **absorbed dose, administered dose, applied dose,** and **potential dose**.

dose equivalent. The product of the absorbed dose from ionizing radiation and factors such as biological differences due to the type of radiation and its distribution in the body.

dose rate. In exposure assessment, dose per time unit (e.g., mg/day), sometimes also called dosage. The dose delivered per unit of time. It is usually expressed as rads per hour or in multiples or submultiples of this unit, such as millirads per hour. The dose rate is commonly used to indicate the level of hazard from a radioactive source.

dose response. Shifts in toxicological responses of an individual or populations that are related to changes in the dose of any given substance.

dose-response assessment. 1. Estimating the potency of a chemical. 2. In exposure assessment, the process of determining the relationship between the dose of a stressor and a specific biological response. 3. Evaluating the quantitative relationship between dose and toxicological responses. 4. A determination of the relationship between the magnitude of an administered, applied, or internal dose and a specific biological response.

dose-response curve. Graphical representation of the relationship between the dose of a stressor and the resulting biological response.

dose-response relationship. The quantitative relationship between the amount of exposure to a substance and the extent of toxic injury or disease produced.

dosimeter. An instrument to measure dosage.

dosimetry. The process or technology of measuring and/or estimating dosage.

DOT. U.S. Department of Transportation.

DOT 103. The classification of an insulated or uninsulated, nonpressure tank car with an expansion dome of 1%. Can be constructed of carbon steel, aluminum, nickel, or alloy steel. A bottom outlet or washout is allowed, depending on specification.

DOT 104. The classification of an insulated, carbon steel, nonpressure tank car with a minimum expansion dome of 2%. Bottom outlet and washout are optional.

DOT 105. The classification of an insulated pressure tank car designed for top loading and unloading. May be constructed of carbon steel or aluminum alloy. No bottom outlet or washout; only one opening in the tank.

DOT 111. The classification of an insulated or uninsulated, nonpressure tank car without an expansion capacity built into the tank. These tanks have varied fittings according to specification. This tank car is the most common one in service.

DOT 112. The classification of an uninsulated carbon steel pressure tank car designed for top loading and unloading. Bottom outlet and washout are prohibited. Thermal protection is designed to meet specific criteria.

DOT 113. The classification of an insulated vacuum tank car for cryogenic service having an inner container and carbon steel outer shell. The insulation system is designed for protection for 30 days, not protection from fire (thermal energy).

DOT 114. The classification similar to the DOT 112 class, except bottom outlets and washouts are allowed.

DOT 115. The classification of a tank car with an inner tank, a layer of polyurethane insulation (supporting the inner tank), and an outer tank constructed of carbon steel. Bottom washout and outlets are optional.

DOT exemption. Authority granted by DOT to deviate from the requirements of 49 CFR 100–199, based on proof that an equivalent level of safety is provided by the deviation. It is applicable to domestic shipments only.

dot method. A method of showing the configuration of an atom's valence electrons. May also be referred to as *electron dot formula* or the *Lewis dot formula*.

DOT reportable quantity (RQ). The quantity of a substance specified in a U.S. Department of Transportation regulation that triggers labeling, packaging, and other requirements related to shipping such substances.

double covalent bond. 1. Two covalent bonds between two atoms. 2. Also called a double bond. 3. Represented in structural formulas as -C=C-.

downgradient. The direction that ground-water flows; similar to "downstream" for surface water.

downstream processors. Industries dependent on crop production.

DP hole. A hole in the ground made with direct push (DP) equipment.

draft. 1. The act of drawing or removing water from a tank or reservoir or any source other than accepting pressurized water from a hydrant or another fire apparatus. 2. The water that is drawn or removed.

draft permit. A preliminary permit drafted and published by EPA, subject to public review and comment before final action on the application.

drainage. Improving the productivity of agricultural land by removing excess water from the soil by such means as ditches or subsurface drainage tiles.

drainage basin. The area of land that drains water, sediment, and dissolved materials to a common outlet at some point along a stream channel.

drainage well. A well drilled to carry excess water off agricultural fields.

dram. A unit of weight equal to 3.888 g. Also called a *drachm*.

drawdown. 1. The drop in the water table or level of water in the ground when water is being pumped from a well. 2. The amount of water used from a tank or reservoir. 3. The drop in the water level of a tank or reservoir.

dredging. The removal of mud from the bottom of water bodies.

drilling fluid. Fluid used to lubricate the bit and convey drill cuttings to the surface with rotary drilling equipment, usually composed of bentonite slurry or muddy water.

drinking water equivalent level. Protective level of exposure related to potentially noncarcinogenic effects of chemicals that are also known to cause cancer.

Drinking Water State Revolving Fund. The fund that provides capitalization grants to states to develop drinking water revolving loan funds to help finance system infrastructure improvements, assure source water protection, enhance operation and management of drinking water systems, and otherwise promote local water system compliance and protection of public health.

drive casing. Heavy-duty steel casing driven along with the sampling tool in cased direct push (DP) systems. Keeps the hole open between sampling runs and is not removed until the last sample has been collected.

drive point profiler. An exposed ground-water direct push (DP) system used to collect multiple depth-discrete groundwater samples.

drop-off. Recyclable materials collection method in which individuals bring recyclable materials to a designated collection site.

drug lab. Usually a clandestine laboratory; an illegal site for the manufacture of drugs or chemicals.

dry chemical. 1. A fire extinguishing agent specially designed for fighting fires involving flammable liquids, pyrophoric substances, and electrical equipment.

2. Common types contain sodium bicarbonate or potassium bicarbonate. 3. May be used on any A, B, or C fire.

dry ice. Solid carbon dioxide (CO_2).

dry powder. The extinguishing agent suitable for use on combustible metal fires.

dual-phase extraction. Active withdrawal of both liquid and gas phases from a well, usually involving the use of a vacuum pump.

dubnium. An extremely rare, man-made, radioactive, solid, metallic element, symbol Db, with atomic number 105, and atomic weight 262.

ductile. Capable of being drawn into wire. Metals are typically ductile materials.

duet rule. A special subset of the octet rule. The duet rule says that for an element to reach stability, it must have two electrons in its only ring.

dump. A site used to dispose of solid waste without environmental controls.

duplicate. A second aliquot or sample that is treated the same as the original sample in order to determine the precision of the analytical method. *See also* **aliquot**.

dust explosion. The ignition of any combustible dust resulting in an explosion.

dustfall jar. An open container used to collect large particles from the air for measurement and analysis.

dyes. Natural or synthetic colorants that are soluble in most solvents, and usually dissolve in the polymer in which they are mixed. *Contrast with* **pigments** and **organic pigments**.

dynamite. A high explosive made from nitroglycerine and an inert filler. There are many dynamite formulations today, varying in sensitivity and brisance. Must be detonated by a blasting cap.

dynamometer. A device used to place a load on an engine and measure its performance.

dyne. The unit of force in the obsolete cgs system of units. A dyne (dyn) is the force required to accelerate a 1 g mass by 1 cm/s^2.

dyspnea. Shortness of breath.

dysprosium. A solid, metallic element, symbol Dy, with atomic number 66, and atomic weight 162.5. A member of the rare earth elements.

dystrophic lake. An acidic, shallow body of water that contains much humus or other organic matter, which contains many plants but few fish.

E

ease of ignition. The ease with which a material or product can be ignited under specified conditions.

easily liquefiable. 1. Pertains to a gas with a relatively high boiling point. 2. Gases may be liquefied by either applying sufficient pressure or by cooling the gas to its boiling point. (A combination of pressure and cooling will liquefy the gas above its boiling point.)

EC_{50}. *See* **effective concentration**.

ecological entity. In ecological risk assessment, a general term referring to a species, a group of species, an ecosystem function or characteristic, or a specific habitat or biome.

ecological exposure. Exposure of a non-human organism to a stressor.

ecological impact. The effect that a man-caused or natural activity has on living organisms and their nonliving (abiotic) environment.

ecological indicator. A characteristic of an ecosystem that is related to, or derived from, a measure of biotic or abiotic variable, which can provide quantitative information on ecological structure and function.

ecological integrity. A living system exhibits integrity if, when subjected to disturbance, it sustains and organizes self-correcting ability to recover toward a biomass end-state that is normal for that system.

ecological risk assessment. The application of a formal framework, analytical process, or model to estimate the effects of human actions(s) on a natural resource and to interpret the significance of those effects in light of the uncertainties identified in each component of the assessment process. Such analysis includes initial hazard identification, exposure and dose-response assessments, and risk characterization.

ecological sustainability. The maintenance of ecosystem components and functions for future generations. Also called *environmental sustainability.*

ecology. The relationship of living things to one another and their environment, or the study of such relationships.

economic poisons. Chemicals used to control pests and to defoliate cash crops such as cotton.

ecosphere. The "bio-envelope" that contains life on the land, in surface waters, and in the air.

ecosystem. The interacting system of a biological community and its nonliving environmental surroundings.

ecosystem structure. Attributes related to the instantaneous physical state of an ecosystem.

ED_{10}. *See* **effective dose.**

edema. The collection of watery fluid in body cavities or connective tissue, usually the lungs. Pulmonary edema is an excessive buildup of water in the lungs.

effective concentration. The effective concentration of gas or smoke that will produce a response in 50% of the test animals within a specified time; EC_{50}. It is a general term and may designate any measured response of the animal.

effective dose. The dose corresponding to a 10% increase in an adverse effect, relative to the control response; ED_{10}.

effluent. Wastewater that flows out of a treatment plant, sewer, or industrial outfall.

effluent guidelines. Technical EPA documents that set effluent limitations for given industries and pollutants.

effluent limitation. Restrictions established by a state or EPA on quantities, rates, and concentrations in wastewater discharges. Also called *effluent standard.*

effluent standard. *See* **effluent limitation**.

einsteinium. A solid, metallic element, symbol Es, with atomic number 99, and atomic weight 254.

ejector. A device used to disperse a chemical solution into water being treated.

elastomer. A material that in its final shape and at room temperature may be stretched to at least twice its length; it will return to its original shape rapidly and with some force.

electric current. The movement of electrons through a material. Electric current is measured in units of amperes (amps).

electricity. The flow of electrons.

electrode. 1. A conductor that gives off or collects electrons in a cell or similar device. 2. An electrically conducting surface that allows electrons to be transferred between reactants in an electrochemical cell.

electrodialysis. A process that uses electrical current applied to permeable membranes to remove minerals from water, such as in desalinization.

electrolysis. Decomposition of compounds in a water solution (or just water itself) by passing an electric current through the solution.

electrolyte. A compound that dissociates into ions when in solution and conducts electricity.

electrolyte imbalance. A chemical imbalance in the body due to the loss of minerals.

electromagnetic geophysical methods. Ways to measure subsurface conductivity via low-frequency electromagnetic induction.

electromagnetic radiation. A traveling wave motion that results from changing electric and magnetic fields (X-rays and gamma rays; ultraviolet waves; visible light; and infrared waves, radar, and radio waves of relatively long wavelengths).

electron. A subatomic particle that has essentially no weight (1/1,837 the mass of a proton, or 10^{-28}g), an electrical charge of −1, and orbits around the nucleus of an atom.

electron dot formula. *See* **dot method**.

electronegativity. A measure of the ability of an atom in a molecule to draw bonding electrons to itself.

electronic configuration. The number and position of the electron(s) orbiting the nucleus of each atom.

electroplating. The electrostatic deposition of metal on plastics and/or other metals.

electrostatic bond. Alternate name for the **ionic bond**.

electrostatic precipitator (ESP). A device that removes particles from a gas stream (smoke) after combustion occurs. The ESP imparts an electrical charge to the particles, causing them to adhere to metal plates inside the precipitator.

electrovalent bond. *See* **ionic bond**.

element. A pure substance that cannot be broken down into simpler substances by chemical means.

elemental. Having the properties of an element.

elemental stability. The atoms of an element seek to reach stability by attaining a full outer ring. A full outer ring has eight electrons in the outer (valence) ring or two electrons in its only ring.

element symbol. An international abbreviation for element names, usually consisting of one letter (capitalized) or two letters (the second letter is always lower cased). Some symbols are abbreviations for ancient names.

eligible costs. The construction costs for wastewater treatment works upon which EPA grants are based.

El Niño. A weather condition caused by the decrease in atmospheric pressure over the eastern Pacific Ocean.

elongation. The increase in length of a material stressed under a certain tension.

EMAP data. Environmental monitoring data collected under the auspices of the Environmental Monitoring and Assessment Program (EMAP). All EMAP data share the common attribute of being of known quality, having been collected in the context of explicit data quality objectives and a consistent quality assurance program.

emergency. An unexpected, sudden, or unplanned event requiring immediate remedial and/or urgent action.

emergency (chemical). A situation created by an accidental release or spill of hazardous chemicals that poses a threat to the safety of workers, residents, the environment, or property.

emergency episode. *See* **air pollution episode**.

emergency exemption. Provision in FIFRA under which EPA can grant temporary exemption to a state or another federal agency to allow the use of a pesticide product not registered for that particular use.

emergency manager (EM). The local official with the broadest general oversight and management of community-wide resources. Acts to support and assist the incident commander (IC).

emergency medical technician (EMT). A certified technician capable of injured victim assessment, triage, stabilization, and transportation at the basic life support (BLS) level.

emergency operating center (EOC). The protected site from which a major incident will be controlled by civil government officials.

emergency operations plan (EOP). The plan each jurisdiction has for handling incidents and emergencies.

emergency planning notification. The notice a facility must make to the state emergency response commission (SERC) when subject to the emergency planning requirements of Title III.

emergency removal action. 1. Steps taken to remove contaminated materials that pose imminent threats to local residents (e.g., removal of leaking drums or the excavation of explosive waste).

emergency response. The response to any occurrence that results, or is likely to result, in a release of a hazardous substance due to an unforeseen event.

Emergency Response Guidebook (ERG). This guidebook, which is produced by the U.S. Department of Transportation, assists responders in making initial decisions upon arriving at the scene of a hazardous materials incident.

emergency response plan. 1. The comprehensive emergency response plan developed by the local emergency planning committee (LEPC). 2. The written descriptions of planned actions and personnel responsibilities for emergency response actions.

emergency response values. Concentrations of chemicals, published by various groups, defining acceptable levels for short-term exposures in emergencies.

emergency support function. Includes all the duties and responsibilities of the staff members of Federal Response Plan participants as enumerated in the Plan.

emergency suspension. Suspension of a pesticide product registration due to an imminent hazard. The action immediately halts distribution, sale, and sometimes actual use of the pesticide involved.

emission. Pollution discharged into the atmosphere from smokestacks and other vents; from surface areas of commercial or industrial facilities; from residential chimneys; and from motor vehicle, locomotive, or aircraft exhausts.

emission cap. A limit designed to prevent projected growth in emissions from existing and future stationary sources from eroding any mandated reductions.

emission factor. The relationship between the amount of pollution produced and the amount of raw material processed.

emission inventory. A listing, by source, of the amount of air pollutants discharged into the atmosphere of a community.

emission standard. The maximum amount of air polluting discharge legally allowed from a single source, mobile or stationary.

emissions trading. The creation of surplus emission reductions at certain stacks, vents, or similar emissions sources, and the use of this surplus to meet or redefine pollution requirements applicable to other emissions sources. Also called *bubble policy*.

emulsified. The condition of two or more immiscible liquids held in suspension together.

emulsifier. 1. A chemical that aids in suspending one liquid in another, usually an organic chemical in an aqueous solution. 2. A surface-active agent.

emulsion. A stable mixture of two or more immiscible liquids held in suspension.

encapsulation. The treatment of asbestos-containing material with a liquid that covers the surface with a protective coating or embeds fibers in an adhesive matrix to prevent their release into the air.

enclosure. Putting an airtight, impermeable, permanent barrier around asbestos-containing materials to prevent the release of asbestos fibers into the air.

endangered species. Animals, birds, fish, plants, or other living organisms threatened with extinction by anthropogenic (man-caused) or natural changes in their environment.

endangerment assessment. A study to determine the nature and extent of contamination at a site on the National Priorities List and the risks posed to public health or the environment.

endemic. Present in a region, community, or group of people.

end-of-the-pipe. Technologies such as scrubbers on smokestacks and catalytic converters on automobile tailpipes that reduce emissions of pollutants after they have formed.

endothermic. A chemical reaction in which heat is absorbed. *Contrast with* **exothermic**, which is a chemical reaction in which heat is liberated by the reaction.

endpoint. An observable or measurable biological event or chemical concentration used as an index of an effect of a chemical exposure.

endrin. A pesticide toxic to freshwater and marine aquatic life that produces adverse health effects in domestic water supplies.

end-use product. A pesticide formulation for field or other end use. The label has instructions for use or application to control pests or regulate plant growth. The term excludes products used to formulate other pesticide products.

end user. Consumer of products for the purpose of recycling. Excludes products for reuse or combustion for energy recovery.

-ene. A suffix related to an open-chain, unsaturated hydrocarbon having one double bond.

energy. The capacity for doing work.

energy management system. A control system capable of monitoring environmental and system loads and adjusting HVAC operations accordingly in order to conserve energy while maintaining comfort.

energy recovery. Obtaining energy from waste through a variety of processes.

enforceable requirements. Conditions or limitations in permits issued under the Clean Water Act Section 402 or 404 that, if violated, could result in the issuance of a compliance order or initiation of a civil or criminal action under federal or applicable state laws.

enforcement. EPA, state, or local legal actions to obtain compliance with environmental laws, rules, regulations, or agreements; and/or to obtain penalties or criminal sanctions for violations.

enforcement decision document (EDD). A document that provides an explanation to the public of EPA's selection of the cleanup alternative at enforcement sites on the National Priorities List. Similar to a **record of decision**.

engineered controls. 1. Methods of managing environmental and health risks by placing a barrier between the contamination and the rest of the site, thus limiting exposure pathways. 2. Substitution, isolation, and ventilation methods used to reduce the level of the contaminant at the source. 3. Also called *engineering controls.*

enrichment. The addition of nutrients (e.g., nitrogen, phosphorus, and carbon compounds) from sewage effluent or agricultural runoff to surface water greatly increases the growth potential for algae and other aquatic plants.

enthalpy. The heat of reaction, either exothermic or endothermic. *See also* **exothermic** and **endothermic**.

entrain. To trap bubbles in water, either mechanically through turbulence or chemically through a reaction.

entry suit. In firefighting, a type of suit that provides protection for brief entry into total flame environment at temperatures as high as 2,000°F.

environment. The sum of all external conditions affecting the life, development, and survival of an organism.

environmental assessment. An environmental analysis prepared pursuant to the National Environmental Policy Act to determine whether a federal action would significantly affect the environment and thus require a more detailed environmental impact statement.

environmental audit. An independent assessment of the current status of a party's compliance with applicable environmental requirements or of a party's environmental compliance policies, practices, and controls.

environmental exposure. Human exposure to pollutants originating from facility emissions.

environmental fate. The destiny of a chemical or biological pollutant after release into the environment.

environmental fate data. Data that characterize a pesticide's fate in the ecosystem, considering factors that foster its degradation, pathways, and resultant products.

environmental impact statement. A document required of federal agencies by the National Environmental Policy Act for major projects or legislative proposals significantly affecting the environment.

environmental medium. A major environmental category that surrounds or contacts humans, animals, plants, and other organisms, and through which chemicals or pollutants move.

Environmental Protection Agency (EPA). A federal agency concerned with environmental air, water, and land quality.

Environmental Response Team (ERT). EPA experts located in Edison, NJ, and Cincinnati, OH, who can provide around-the-clock technical assistance to EPA regional offices and states during all types of hazardous waste site emergencies and spills of hazardous substances.

environmental risk. The potential for adverse effects on living organisms associated with pollution of the environment by effluents, emissions, wastes, or accidental chemical releases, energy use, or the depletion of natural resources. Also called *ecological risk*.

environmental site assessment. The process of determining whether contamination is present on a parcel of real property.

environmental sustainability. Long-term maintenance of ecosystem components and functions for future generations. Also called *ecological sustainability*.

environmental tobacco smoke. Mixture of smoke from the burning end of a cigarette, pipe, or cigar, as well as smoke exhaled by the smoker.

EPA ID number. *See* **identification code**.

epichlorohydrin rubber. A polyether elastomer with very good oil, heat, and ozone resistance, polymerized from the monomer epichlorohydrin.

epidemic. An outbreak of a disease that spreads more quickly than normally would be expected.

epidemiology. Study of the distribution of disease or other health-related states and events in human populations, as related to age, sex, occupation, ethnicity, and economic status.

episode (pollution). An air pollution incident in a given area caused by a concentration of atmospheric pollutants under meteorological conditions that may result in a significant increase in illnesses or deaths.

epoxide. A covalent compound containing the "epoxy" group, which is an oxygen atom connected to two other atoms, usually carbon, in a triangular ring structure.

epoxy resins. Mostly thermosetting polymers based on ethylene oxide and its derivatives.

Epsom salts. Magnesium sulfate; $MgSO_4{\cdot}7H_2O$.

equilibrium. 1. In radiation, the state at which the radioactivity of consecutive elements within a radioactive series is neither increasing nor decreasing. 2. Physical equilibrium occurs when two or more physical states or phases are changing back and forth into each other at the same rate, with no net change in the system. 3. Chemical equilibrium occurs when two or more chemical compounds exist together in specified ratios and are no longer changing back and forth into each other.

equilibrium pressure. The pressure above a liquefied gas in a container. The liquefied gas will evaporate until the pressure above the liquid becomes stable.

equivalent method. Any method of sampling and analyzing for air pollution that has been demonstrated to the EPA administrator's satisfaction to be, under specific conditions, an acceptable alternative to normally used reference methods.

erbium. A solid metallic element, symbol Er, with atomic number 68, and atomic weight 167.26. It is a member of the rare earth elements.

erosion. The wearing away of land surface by wind or water, intensified by land-clearing practices related to farming, residential or industrial development, road building, or logging.

established treatment technologies. Technologies for which cost and performance data are readily available. *Contrast with* **innovative treatment technologies**.

establishment. An economic unit, generally at a single physical location, where business is conducted or where services or industrial operations are performed.

ester. 1. The reaction product of an alcohol and an acid. An organic hydrocarbon derivative with the general formula R-COO-R', where the R- is a hydrocarbon radical or backbone, and the -R' is either the same hydrocarbon radical, or a different one. R may also be a hydrogen atom.

estimated environmental concentration. The estimated pesticide concentration in an ecosystem.

estimated exposure dose (EED). The measured or calculated dose to which humans are likely to be exposed considering all sources and routes of exposure.

estuary. Region of interaction between rivers and near-shore ocean waters, where tidal action and river flow mix fresh and salt water.

ethanol. 1. Proper name for ethyl alcohol, C_2H_5OH. 2. The alcohol in alcoholic beverages. 3. An alternative automotive fuel derived from grain and corn; usually blended with gasoline to form gasohol.

ethene. The proper name for ethylene, C_2H_4.

ether. A hydrocarbon derivative with the general formula R-O-R', where R- is a hydrocarbon backbone or radical, and -R' may be the same or different hydrocarbon backbone. Ethers are subject to slow oxidation in air that will convert some of the ether to an explosive peroxide.

ethyl. The hydrocarbon radical ($-C_2H_5$) formed by removing one hydrogen from ethane, C_2H_6.

ethyl alcohol. Ethanol (C_2H_5OH).

ethyldichloroarsine. A vesicant or blister agent ($C_2H_5AsCl_2$); agent ED.

ethylene dibromide (EDB). A chemical ($C_2H_4Br_2$) used as an agricultural fumigant and in certain industrial processes.

Extremely toxic and found to be a carcinogen in laboratory animals. EDB has been banned for most agricultural uses in the United States.

ethylene vinyl acetate (EVA). A copolymer of ethylene and vinyl acetate that has many of the properties of polyethylene, but has increased flexibility, elongation, and impact resistance.

etiologic agent. An organism or its toxins that contribute to the cause of infection, disease, or other abnormal condition.

etiology. The scientific study of origins or causes of disease.

European Inventory of Existing Commercial Chemical Substances (EINECS). European equivalent of the Toxic Substances Control Act (TSCA).

europium. A steel-gray, solid, metallic element, symbol Eu, with atomic number 63, and atomic weight 151.96. It is a member of the rare earth metals.

eutectic mixture. A mixture of two or more substances with a melting point lower than that for any other mixture of the same substances.

eutrophication. The slow aging process during which a lake, estuary, or bay evolves into a bog or marsh and eventually disappears.

eutrophic lakes. Shallow, murky bodies of water with concentrations of plant nutrients causing excessive production of algae. *Contrast with* **dystrophic lakes**.

evaporation. The process by which a liquid changes into a vapor, always accompanied by an increase in energy of the molecules evaporating. Also known as *vaporization. See also* **vaporization**.

evaporation pond. An area where sewage sludge is dumped and dried.

evaporation rate. The speed at which a liquid converts to a vapor below its boiling point.

evapotranspiration. The loss of water from the soil both by evaporation and by transpiration from the plants growing in the soil.

exceedance. Violation of the pollutant levels permitted by environmental protection standards.

excepted quantities. A shipment of dangerous goods of very small quantities of certain classes allowed in nonspecification packaging without a shipper's declaration.

excess lifetime risk. The additional or extra risk of developing cancer due to exposure to a toxic substance incurred over the lifetime of an individual.

exclusionary ordinance. Zoning that excludes classes of persons or businesses from a particular neighborhood or area.

exclusion zone. 1. The area where the hazard is present. 2. The contaminated area. 3. Also called the **hot zone**.

exempted aquifer. Underground bodies of water defined in the Underground Injection Control Program as aquifers that are potential sources of drinking water, though not being used as such, and thus exempted from regulations barring underground injection activities.

exempt solvent. Specific organic compounds not subject to requirements of regulation because they are deemed by EPA to be of negligible photochemical reactivity.

EX number. The number, preceded by the prefix "EX," which is assigned by the associated administrator for Hazardous Materials Safety to identify an explosive that has been approved.

exothermic. 1. A chemical reaction in which heat is liberated. 2. *Contrast with* **endothermic**, which is a chemical reaction in which heat is absorbed by the reaction.

exotic species. A species that is not indigenous to a region.

expansion ratio. The number of volumes of a gas or vapor produced by the evaporation of one volume of liquid.

experimental use permit. Obtained by manufacturers for testing new pesticides or uses thereof whenever they conduct experimental field studies to support registration on 10 acres or more of land or 1 acre or more of water.

explode. The rapid expansion of a material or container with the release of energy, heat, or pressure.

explosion. 1. The phenomenon characterized by the instantaneous release of heat and pressure caused by the oxidation of fuels or the decomposition of molecules. 2. The sudden and violent release of mechanical, chemical, or nuclear energy from a confined space.

explosion-proof. 1. The covering of all or parts of electrical devices to prevent explosive gases, vapors, dusts, or fumes from reaching an area where an electrical spark or excessive heat may act as an ignition source. 2. Any treatment to prevent explosions.

explosive. 1. (n.) Any pure substance or mixture whose principal purpose is to explode. *Contrast with* its use as an adjective: 2. (adj.) Anything that will explode.

explosive hazard class I. Any substance or article, including a device, that is designed to function by explosion or that, by chemical reaction within itself, is able to function in a similar manner even if not designed to function by explosion. Divisions of explosives include:

- Division 1.1: explosive with mass explosion hazard
- Division 1.2: explosive with projection hazard
- Division 1.3: explosive with fire, minor blast, or minor projection hazard
- Division 1.4: explosive device with minor explosion hazard
- Division 1.5: very insensitive explosives
- Division 1.6: extremely insensitive explosives

explosive limits. 1. The amounts of vapor in the air that form explosive mixtures. 2. Explosive limits are expressed as lower and upper limits and give the range of vapor concentrations in air that will explode if an ignition source is present. 3. Also called the **flammable range** or **explosive range.**

explosive range. 1. The concentration of gas or vapor in air between the lower and upper explosive limits. 2. It is the range of concentrations in air in which ignition of the gas or vapor will occur. 3. Also called the **flammable range** or **explosive limits**.

exports. In a solid waste program, municipal solid waste and recyclables transported outside the state or locality where they originated.

exposure. 1. Any person or property exposed to a fire, hazmat incident, or other emergency. 2. Any contact with a hazardous chemical in the course of employment through any route of entry. 3. The concentration of a material in the air to which a worker can come into contact, which is usually measured near the nose of the worker. 4. The amount of radiation or pollutant present in a given environment that represents a potential health threat to living organisms. 5. Concerning radioactivity, it is the quantity used to indicate the amount of ionization in air produced by X-ray or gamma-ray radiation.

exposure assessment. The identification of the pathways by which toxicants may reach individuals, and the estimation of how much of a chemical an individual is likely to be exposed to, and the estimation of the number likely to be exposed.

exposure concentration. The concentration of a chemical or other pollutant representing a health threat in a particular environment.

exposure level. The amount (concentration) of a chemical at the absorptive surfaces of an organism.

exposure limit. The amount of material to which a worker may be exposed with no injury. Usually stated as threshold limit value–time-weighted average (TLV-TWA), permissible exposure limit (PEL), short-term exposure limit (STEL), and ceiling limit (C).

exposure pathway. The path from sources of pollutants via, soil, water, or food to man and other species or settings.

exposure-response relationship. The relationship between exposure level and the incidence of adverse effects.

exposure route. The way a chemical or pollutant enters an organism after contact; i.e., by ingestion, inhalation, or dermal absorption.

extender. *See* **filler**.

extinguishing media. The firefighting agents that should be used to extinguish fires.

extractant. A solvent that is used to separate a material from a mixture or solution.

extraction procedure (toxicity). The determination of toxicity by a procedure that simulates leaching.

extraction well. A discharge well used to remove groundwater or air.

extrapolation, low dose. An estimate of the response at a point below the range of the experimental data, generally through the use of a mathematical model.

extremely hazardous substance. 1. EPA substances listed in appendices A and B of 40 CFR Part 355, et seq., and constantly revised. 2. The chemicals required for facility notification under Section 302 and for emergency notification under Section 304. 3. The substances were determined based upon their acute toxicity and have corresponding threshold planning quantities (TPQ) and reportable quantities (RQ).

extrudate. The end product of the extrusion process. May be a sheet, film, rod, or a formed product called a *profile.*

extruder. A machine that forms continuous sheet, film, rods, or profiles by the action of a rotating screw (or in a much older machine, a ram or reciprocating plunger) inside a heated barrel, and carrying forward and forcing the fused plastic mass through a die that imparts the shape to the plastic as it cools.

extrusion. The process whereby a shape is imparted to a plastic material by forcing the molten mass through a die.

extrusion blow molding. The plastics process in which a *parison,* or hollow tube, is extruded and placed in a mold, and then is forced to assume the shape of the mold by a blast of air inside the parison.

eye hazard. A chemicals that affects the eye or visual capacity.

F

fabric filter. A cloth device that catches dust particles from industrial emissions.

facilities plans. Plans and studies related to the construction of treatment works necessary to comply with the Clean Water Act or RCRA.

facility. All buildings, equipment, structures, and other stationary items that are located on a single site, or on contiguous or adjacent sites, and which are owned or operated by the same person (or by any person who controls, is controlled by, or under common control with, such person).

facility emergency coordinator. The representative of a facility covered by environmental law who participates in the emergency reporting process with the local emergency planning committee (LEPC).

factitious. Made artificially or synthetically, rather than naturally.

facultative bacteria. Bacteria that can live under aerobic or anaerobic conditions.

Fahrenheit scale. 1. The temperature scale devised in 1717 by D. G. Fahrenheit and denoted by °F. 2. The normal freezing point of water is 32°F, and the normal boiling point of water is 212°F. *See also* **Celsius scale**, **Kelvin scale**, and **Rankine scale**.

fallout. Radioactive particles that fall from the sky after a nuclear explosion or accident.

family effect. All the elements in certain main groups on the periodic table of the elements have the same chemical characteristics.

faraday. A unit of electricity equal to the total charge of a mole of electrons; 1 faraday (F) is approximately equivalent to 96,500 coulombs.

fast attack. A firefighting strategy whereby the first arriving engine company attacks the fire using water carried in its booster tank, relying on the second arriving company to secure a water supply.

fatty acid. 1. Any organic monobasic compound with the general formula $C_nH_{2n+1}COOH$. 2. Fatty acids occur naturally as waxes, fats, and essential oils, and are usually found in animal and plant materials.

fauna. Animals or animal life of a particular region or a particular time.

feasibility study. 1. Analysis of the practicability of a proposal. 2. A small-scale investigation of a problem to ascertain whether a proposed research approach is likely to provide useful data.

fecal coliform bacteria. Bacteria found in the intestinal tracts of mammals.

federal implementation plan. A federally implemented plan to achieve attainment of air quality standards, used when a state is unable to develop an adequate plan.

federally permitted release. Releases in compliance with a permit issued under the Federal Water Pollution Control Act, Clean Air Act, Safe Drinking Water Act, and Solid Waste Disposal Act.

Federal Motor Vehicle Control Program. 1. The collection of federal actions aimed at controlling pollution from motor vehicles. 2. A federally designated area that is required to meet and maintain federal ambient air quality standards.

Federal Radiological Monitoring and Assessment Center (FRMAC). Part of Nuclear Incident Response Team (NIRT); focuses on radiological consequence management.

Federal Response Plan. A plan that includes multiple federal agencies under FEMA's oversight to respond to presidentially declared disasters; now called the **National Response Plan** (NRP).

feedlot. A confined area for the controlled feeding of animals.

femto-. The prefix that means "multiply by 10^{-15}"; f.

fen. A type of wetland that accumulates peat deposits.

fermium. A solid metallic element, symbol Fm, with atomic number 100, and atomic weight 257.

ferrous metal. A magnetic metal derived from iron or steel.

ferrum. Latin for "iron," hence the symbol, Fe.

FEV$_1$. *See* **forced expiratory volume**.

field operations guide. The document that will determine the proper setup of the incident command system.

FIFRA pesticide ingredient. An ingredient of a pesticide that must be registered with EPA under the Federal Insecticide, Fungicide, and Rodenticide Act. Products making pesticide claims must register under FIFRA and may be subject to labeling and use requirements.

fill. Man-made deposits of natural soils or rock products and waste materials.

filler. 1. A material added to a resin or plastic to alter its properties, but usually to reduce its cost. 2. May also be called an *extender*.

filling. Depositing dirt, mud or other materials into aquatic areas to create more dry land, usually for agricultural or commercial development purposes.

filling orbital. The orbital of an element that is only partially filled with electrons when an atom is at a neutral state electrically.

fill valve. An inlet valve assembly used for loading product into a cargo tank.

film. Sheet with a maximum thickness of 0.01 inch (10 mils).

film blowing. The extrusion of a hollow tube followed by continuous inflation of the tube by internal air pressure (no mold involved) to form a film.

film casting. The pouring of a fluid plastic compound or resin on an endless carrier, followed by removal of the solidified film from the carrier.

filter strip. Strip or area of vegetation used for removing sediment, organic matter, and other pollutants from runoff and wastewater.

filtration. A treatment process, under the control of qualified operators, for removing solid (particulate) matter from water by means of porous media such as sand or a man-made filter. May also refer to the process that removes particles that contain pathogens.

financial assurance for closure. Documentation or proof that an owner or operator of a facility such as a landfill or other waste repository is capable of paying the projected costs of closing the facility and monitoring it afterwards as provided in Resource Conservation and Recovery Act (RCRA) regulations.

finding of no significant impact (FONSI). A document prepared by a federal agency showing why a proposed action would not have a significant impact on the environment and thus would not require preparation of an environmental impact statement.

fine chemicals. Chemicals that are required to be in a relatively pure state and are usually made in significantly smaller quantities, usually for reagent uses, pharmaceutical uses, and medical and biological uses.

finished water. Water is "finished" when it has passed through all the processes in a water treatment plant and is ready to be delivered to consumers.

fire. A rapid chemical reaction involving the combination of a material with oxygen or another oxidizer, usually giving off heat and light. *See* **combustion**.

fire behavior. Any physical changes that occur in a material or product when that material or product burns.

fire brigade. A group of employees of an industrial plant or other organization trained to use fire fighting equipment within the plant and to carry out fire prevention and extinguishment activities.

fire department. A paid or voluntary professional fire department with jurisdiction over a facility or geographical area controlled by a governmental unit.

fire detection device. An alarm or other device installed in a building to produce an early detection of heat, smoke, or flame.

fire effluent. The total amount of gases, particulates, and aerosols liberated during combustion or pyrolysis.

fire endurance. A measure of the elapsed time during which a material or assemblage continues to exhibit fire resistance (ASTM E 176).

fire exposure. The heat flux of a fire, with or without direct flame impingement, to which a material, product, building element, or assembly is exposed (ASTM E 176).

fire extinguishment. 1. The breaking or interruption of the chemical chain reaction of fire, which most often means removing the oxidizing agent (usually the oxygen in air). Fire may also be extinguished by removing the fuel and/or lowering the temperature.

firefighting fog. *See* **water spray**.

firefighting gear. Turnout gear including footwear, trousers, a coat, gloves, a helmet, and respiratory protection (NFPA 472).

fire gases. The airborne products emitted by a material undergoing combustion or pyrolysis, which, at the relevant temperature, exist in the gas phase (ASTM E 176).

fire guard. *See* **fire watch**.

fire hazard. The potential for harm associated with a particular fire.

fire load. The total amount of combustible (or flammable) material present in a precisely defined area where a fire might occur.

fire mark. A distinctive metal marker once produced by insurance companies to identify their policyholders' buildings.

fire performance characteristic. A response of a material, product, or assembly to a prescribed source of heat or flame under controlled fire conditions. Such characteristics include ease of ignition, flame spread, smoke generation, fire endurance, and toxicity of smoke (ASTM E 176).

fire performance test. A procedure that measures a response of a material product or assembly to heat or flame under controlled fire conditions (ASTM E 176).

fire phase. One of three degrees of flame progression:

1. Fire in incipient stage and beginning to grow.
2. Free burning, with flame propagation at its greatest.
3. Oxygen deficient in the burn area, producing smoldering.

fire point. 1. The lowest temperature at which a liquid produces sufficient vapor to flash near its surface and then continue to burn. 2. It is usually a few degrees above the flash point. 3. *Contrast with* **flash point**.

fire prevention. The branch of the science of fire protection that deals with preventing the outbreak of fire by eliminating fire hazards through inspection, education, and investigation programs.

fire resistance. The property of a material or assemblage to withstand fire or give protection from it (ASTM E 176).

fire retardant chemical. A chemical, which when added to a combustible material, delays ignition and combustion of the resulting material when exposed to fire (ASTM E 176).

fire-retarded treatment. The use of a fire-retardant chemical or a fire-resistant coating (ASTM E 176).

fire risk. The probability that a fire will occur, and the potential for harm to life and damage to property resulting from its occurrence (ASTM E 176). To calculate the fire risk, there should be at least three measurements: the potential for harm; the probability that the fire will occur; and the probability of exposure of people, animals, property, systems, and the environment.

fire risk assessment standard. A standardized method of assessing fire risk of a material, product, or assembly in a specific environment or application. Formerly called *fire hazard standard* (ASTM E 176).

fire stop. A through-penetration fire stop is a specific construction consisting of the materials that fill the openings around penetrating items such as cables, cable trays, conduits, ducts, pipes, and their means of support through the wall or floor opening to prevent the spread of fire (ASTM E 814).

fire test. A procedure, not necessarily a standard test method, in which the response of materials to heat or flame, or both, is measured under controlled conditions or otherwise controlled (ASTM E 800).

fire tetrahedron. *See* **tetrahedron of fire**.

fire triangle. A theory of fire that states that if fuel, energy, and an oxidizer are brought together in proper amounts, a fire *will* occur.

firetube boiler. 1. A boiler in which combustion gases pass through the tubes, and water circulates around the tubes. 2. *Contrast with* **watertube boiler**.

fire watch. 1. The vigil maintained by individuals to watch for fires and life safety for specific periods or events. 2. Sometimes called a *fire guard*.

first draw. The water that comes out when a tap is first opened, likely to have the highest level of lead contamination from plumbing materials.

first ionization potential. The minimum amount of energy needed to remove the outermost (highest energy) electron from a neutral atom in the gaseous state. Also called *first ionization energy*.

first responder. The individual who arrives first at the scene of a hazardous materials incident with the responsibility to act.

fission. The splitting of an atomic nucleus by bombardment with neutrons.

fix a sample. A sample is "fixed" in the field by adding chemicals that prevent water quality indicators of interest in the sample from changing before laboratory measurements are made.

fixation. The process by which waterborne wood preservatives [such as chromated copper arsenate (CCA)] chemically react with wood, causing water-soluble metal oxides to be chemically reduced to less toxic metal complexes bonding with the wood cellulose.

fixed-location monitoring. The sampling of an environmental or ambient medium for pollutant concentration at one location continuously or repeatedly.

flame. A hot, usually luminous zone of gas, or particulate matter in gaseous suspension, or both, undergoing combustion (ASTM E 176).

flame front. The leading edge of a flame propagating through a gaseous mixture or across the surface of a liquid or a solid (ASTM E 176).

flame ionization detector (FID). *See* organic vapor analyzer.

flame length. The distance between the flame tip and the midpoint of the flame depth at the base of the flame.

flame propagation rate. The velocity at which combustion travels through a gas or over the surface of a liquid or solid.

flame resistance. The ability to withstand flame impingement or give protection from it (ASTM E 176).

flame retardance. The ability of a material to suppress, reduce, or delay the propagation of flame through a material or product.

flame-retardant. 1. A substance, that when added to another substance, material, or product, will suppress, reduce, or delay the propagation of flame through that substance, material, or product. 2. A reactive flame retardant is built chemically into the polymer molecule, while an additive flame retardant is added to the plastic after polymerization.

flame speed. Propagation of a flame front per unit time through a gaseous fuel and oxidizer mixture relative to a fixed reference point (ASTM E 176).

flame spread. 1. The propagation of the flame away from the source of ignition across the surface of a liquid or solid (ASTM E 176). 2. The tendency of a material to spread flame as it burns.

flame spread index. A number or classification indicating a comparative measure derived from observations made during the progress of the boundary of a zone of flame under defined test conditions (ASTM E 176).

flaming combustion. *See* **space burning**.

flammability. 1. A measure of a material's propensity to burn, or conversely, its resistance to ignition. 2. The ability of a substance to burn under specified test conditions.

flammability, degree of. There are four general categories used to characterize degree of flammability:

- Flammable; NFPA flammability hazard class 1.
- Very flammable; NFPA flammability hazard class 2.
- Highly flammable; NFPA flammability hazard class 3.
- Extremely flammable; NFPA flammability hazard class 4.

flammable. 1. Any material that ignites easily and will burn rapidly. 2. Subject to easy ignition and rapid flaming combustion (ASTM E 176).

flammable gas. A gas that at ambient temperature and pressure forms a flammable mixture with air at concentrations of 13% by volume or less. [In other words, a gas that has a lower explosive limit (LEL) of 13% or less.] 2. A gas that at ambient temperature and pressure has a flammable range (FR) that is at least 12% by volume, regardless of the LEL (FR = UEL – LEL). *See also* **flammable range**.

flammable liquid. A liquid with a flash point below 100°F (37.8°C). There are three divisions of class I flammable liquids:

- Class IA: flash points below 73°F and having a boiling point below 100°F.
- Class IB: flash points below 73°F and having a boiling point at or above 100°F.
- Class IC: flash points at or above 73°F and having a boiling point at or below 100°F.

flammable range (FR). 1. The concentration of gas or vapor in air between the lower and upper flammable limits. 2. It is the range of concentrations in air in which ignition of the gas or vapor will occur.

flammable solid. 1. A solid (other than an explosive) that ignites readily and continues to burn. 2. A flammable solid is liable to cause fires under ordinary conditions or during transportation through friction or retained heat from manufacturing or processing. Flammable solids burn so vigorously and persistently as to create a serious transportation hazard.

flare. A control device that burns hazardous materials to prevent their release into the environment; may operate continuously or intermittently, usually on top of a stack.

flashback. 1. A condition in which vapors of a flammable or combustible liquid may travel from a spill or leak to a source of ignition, ignite, and then travel back to the source of the fuel. 2. The tendency of flammable liquid fires to reignite from a source of ignition after they have been extinguished.

flash fire protective ensemble. A compliant vapor-protective ensemble that is also certified as being compliant with the additional requirements for limited protection against chemical flash fire for escape only [National Fire Protection Association (NFPA) Standard #1991].

flashover. The phenomenon that may occur during a fire whereby the surface of everything in a compartment appears to break into flame at the same time. This is caused by a condition in which heat radiated back to the floor by superheated gases near the ceiling causes the entire room to burst into flame, almost instantaneously.

flash point. The minimum temperature of the material at which it produces vapors sufficient to form an ignitable mixture with the air at the surface of the liquid or near the container. The lower the flash point, the more flammable the material.

floating roof. A special type of steel tank roof that floats upon the surface of the liquid in the tank, thereby eliminating tank breathing and reducing evaporation losses.

floc. A clump of solids formed in sewage by biological or chemical action.

flocculation. Process by which clumps of solids in water or sewage aggregate through biological or chemical action so they can be separated from water or sewage.

floodplain. The flat or nearly flat land along a river or stream or in a tidal area that is covered by water during a flood.

floor sweep. Capture of heavier-than-air gases that collect at floor level.

flora. Plant life of a specific region or particular period.

flowable. Pesticide and other formulations in which the active ingredients are finely ground insoluble solids suspended in a liquid. They are mixed with water for application.

flowmeter. A gauge indicating the velocity of wastewater moving through a treatment plant or of any liquid moving through various industrial processes.

flow rate. The rate, expressed in gallons or liters per hour, at which a fluid escapes from a hole or fissure in a tank.

flue gas. The air coming out of a chimney after combustion in the burner it is venting. Also called *stack gas.*

flue gas desulfurization. A technology that employs a sorbent, usually lime or limestone, to remove sulfur dioxide from the gases produced by burning fossil fuels.

fluid. A substance that flows freely. Gases and liquids are fluids.

fluid drachm. *See* **fluid dram**.

fluid dram. Unit of volume equal to 3.55 mL (60 minims). Also called *fluid drachm.*

fluidized. A mass of solid particles that is made to flow like a liquid by injection of water or gas.

fluidized bed incinerator. An incinerator that uses a bed of hot sand or other granular material to transfer heat directly to waste.

flume. A natural or man-made channel that diverts water.

fluorescence. The absorption of high-energy radiation by a substance and its subsequent emission of visible light.

fluoridation. The addition of a chemical to increase the concentration of fluoride ions in drinking water in order to reduce the incidence of tooth decay in humans.

fluorides. Gaseous, solid, or dissolved compounds containing the fluorine ion that result from industrial processes.

fluorinate. 1. The act of adding fluorine to a molecule. 2. A chemical reaction in which fluorine becomes attached to a molecule of some other material.

fluorinated ethylene propylene. A thermoplastic copolymer of tetrafluoroethylene and hexafluoropropylene.

fluorine. A highly toxic, corrosive, pale yellow, gaseous, nonmetallic element, symbol F, with atomic number 9, and atomic weight 18.998. It is a halogen, and therefore a very powerful oxidizing agent.

fluorocarbon polymers. The family of polymers made from monomers whose molecules contain at least carbon, hydrogen, and fluorine.

fluorocarbons (FCs). Any of a number of organic compounds analogous to hydrocarbons in which one or more hydrogen atoms are replaced by fluorine, and are now usually found mainly in coolants and some industrial processes. FCs containing chlorine are called *chlorofluorocarbons (CFCs). See also* **chlorofluorocarbons**.

flush. 1. To open a cold-water tap to clear out all the water that may have been sitting for a long time in the pipes. In new homes, to flush a system means to send large volumes of water gushing through the unused pipes to remove loose particles of solder and flux. 2. To force large amounts of water through a system to clean out piping or tubing, and storage or process tanks.

flux. 1. A flowing or flow. 2. A substance used to help metals fuse together. 3. To make fluid by melting or fusing. A fluxed material is not in the liquid state, but rather is in a "doughy" plastic state. 4. The rate of continuous change, flow, or movement of liquid, particles, or energy.

flux profile. The curve relating incident radiant heat energy on the specimen plane to distance of the point of initiation of flaming ignition (0 cm) (ASTM E 648).

fly ash. Noncombustible residual particles expelled by flue gas, usually obtained by burning powdered coal.

foam. 1. A colloidal suspension of a gas in a liquid or solid. 2. Firefighting foam consists of small bubbles that are produced by the mixing of air, water, and a foaming agent concentrate (often a surfactant or detergentlike material), which acts as a blanket, excluding air and blocking the escape of volatile vapor. Foam may be protein, synthetic, aqueous-film forming, high expansion, or alcohol type.

foam eductor. A device for mixing foam concentrate in proper proportions with a stream of water to produce foam solution.

fog. A suspension of liquid droplets in air.

fogging. Applying a pesticide by rapidly heating the liquid chemical so that it forms very fine droplets that resemble smoke or fog.

fog pattern. A water stream of finely divided particles used for fire control.

food chain. A sequence of organisms, each of which uses the next, lower member of the sequence as a food source.

food processing waste. Food residues produced during agricultural and industrial operations.

food waste. Uneaten food and food preparation wastes from residences and commercial establishments such as grocery stores, restaurants, and produce stands; institutional cafeterias and kitchens; and industrial sources like employee lunchrooms.

food web. The feeding relationships by which energy and nutrients are transferred from one species to another.

forced expiratory volume. The volume of air that can be forcibly exhaled during the first second of expiration following a maximal inspiration; FEV_1.

forced vital capacity (FVC). The maximal volume of air that can be exhaled as forcibly and rapidly as possible after a maximal inspiration.

formaldehyde. A colorless, pungent, and irritating gas, used chiefly as a disinfectant and preservative and in synthesizing other compounds like resins. Chemical formula is HCHO.

formalin. Water solution of formaldehyde.

formula. 1. Pertaining to a chemical formula, it is the chemical composition of the compound written out using the symbols of elements, showing the number of atoms or ions of each element present in the compound. 2. The shorthand used to signify what elements or ions are present in a compound, and how many of each.

formulation. The substances comprising all active and inert ingredients in a pesticide or other mixture.

formula weight. *See* **molecular weight.**

fossil fuel. 1. Fuel derived from ancient organic remains; e.g., peat, coal, crude oil, and natural gas. 2. Fuels such as coal, oil, and natural gas that were formed over millions of years from decayed plants and animals.

fracture. A break in a rock formation due to structural stresses.

francium. A solid, unstable, radioactive, metallic element, symbol Fr, with atomic number 87, and atomic weight 223. It is a member of the alkali metal family.

frangible disc. A safety relief device on a container holding a substance under pressure, which bursts when the pressure in the container reaches a predetermined level, emptying the container of its contents. *See also* **rupture disc.**

frank-effect level (FEL). A level of exposure or dose that produces irreversible, adverse effects at a statistically or biologically significant increase in frequency or severity between those exposed and those not exposed.

freeboard. 1. Vertical distance from the normal water surface to the top of a confining wall. 2. Vertical distance from the sand surface to the underside of a trough in a sand filter.

free burning. The second phase of burning in which materials burn in the presence of adequate oxygen.

free product. A petroleum hydrocarbon in the liquid-free or nonaqueous phase. *See also* **nonaqueous phase liquid.**

free radical. 1. A molecular fragment possessing at least one unpaired electron that is very active chemically and must react with another free radical rapidly to form a compound. 2. An atom or chemically combined group of atoms having at least one unpaired election, useful in polymerization processes due to its high reactivity. 3. An atom or group of atoms bound together chemically with at least one unpaired electron. A free radical is formed by the introduction of energy to a covalently bonded molecule, and that molecule is broken apart by the energy. It cannot exist free in nature for very long, and therefore must react quickly with other free radicals present.

freeze. To change from a liquid state to a solid state.

freezing point. The temperature at which a liquid changes to a solid.

freon 11. Trichlorofluoromethane; CCl_3F.

freon 12. Dichlorodifluoromethane; CCl_2F_2.

fresh water. Water that generally contains less than 1,000 milligrams per liter (mg/L) of dissolved solids.

friable. Capable of being crumbled, pulverized, or reduced to powder by hand pressure.

friable asbestos. Any material containing more than 1% asbestos, and that can be crumbled or reduced to powder by hand pressure.

frostbite. Injury caused to skin or other tissue by very low temperatures and/or cold materials.

fuel. Anything that will burn.

fuel cell. A device that produces electricity directly from a chemical reaction between oxygen and a gaseous fuel such as hydrogen or carbon monoxide.

fuel economy standard. The Corporate Average Fuel Economy (CAFE) Standard effective in 1978. It enhanced the national fuel conservation effort, imposing a miles-per-gallon floor for motor vehicles.

fuel efficiency. The proportion of energy released by fuel combustion that is converted into useful energy.

fuel load. The amount and distribution of combustibles in an occupancy (ASTM E 931).

fuel switching. 1. A precombustion process whereby a low sulfur coal is used in place of a higher sulfur coal in a power plant to reduce sulfur dioxide emissions. 2. Illegally using leaded gasoline in a motor vehicle designed to use only unleaded.

fugitive emissions. Emissions not caught by a capture system.

full face respirator. A respirator that covers the entire face from chin to hairline and from ear to ear.

full protective clothing. Clothing that prevents skin, eye, and respiratory contact with gases, vapors, fumes, liquids, mists, and dusts. Includes positive-pressure self-contained breathing apparatus (SCBA).

full-time employee. An employee with 2,000 hours per year of full-time equivalent employment.

full turnouts. Often called *bunker gear* or *structural firefighting clothing,* the protective clothing normally worn by firefighters during structural firefighting operations.

fulminate. A compound containing the $C_2N_2O_2^{-1}$ ion, named because such compounds are explosive. From Latin, *fulminare,* "to strike with lightning."

fume. 1. A very fine solid particle condensed from a liquid that is then dispersed in air, such as a metal fume. 2. Also may be the manifestation of a liquid that has evaporated and is condensing in air, such as an acid fume. 3. Tiny particles trapped in vapor in a gas stream.

fumigant. A pesticide vaporized to kill pests, usually used in buildings and greenhouses.

fuming. 1. The evolution of visible fumes by some highly reactive substance (usually a liquid) on contact with air. 2. The generation of vapors, usually of the gases dissolved in the acid or water. 3. Fuming may also occur as the result of a chemical reaction.

fuming acid. A very concentrated solution of the acid that liberates fumes.

functional equivalent. Term used to describe EPA's decision-making process and its relationship to the environmental review conducted under the National Environmental Policy Act (NEPA).

functional group. 1. An atom or group of atoms, bound together chemically, that has an unpaired electron, which when it attaches itself to the hydrocarbon backbone, imparts special properties to the new compound thus formed. 2. A molecular fragment, that when attached to another molecular fragment or a hydrocarbon backbone, will impart specific properties to the new compound. 3. May also be called a *radical.* 4. *See also* **radical** and **free radical**.

functional residual capacity (FRC). The lung volume at the end of tidal expiration [total lung capacity (TLC) – inspiratory capacity (IC)].

fungi. 1. Plantlike organisms that lack chlorophyll and are usually nonmobile, filamentous, and multicellular. They must obtain their food by microscopic, rootlike filaments that penetrate wood tissue and absorb its energy-rich chemicals. 2. Includes molds, mildews, yeasts, mushrooms, and puffballs. 3. Some grow in soil, while others attach themselves to decaying trees and other plants, from whence they obtain nutrients. Some are pathogens; others stabilize sewage and digest composted waste. 4. The singular form is *fungus.*

fungicide. Substances that are used to control, deter, or destroy fungi.

fungistat. A chemical that keeps fungi from growing.

furrow irrigation. Irrigation method in which water travels through the field by means of small channels between each group of rows.

fuse. 1. A device used to detonate an explosive charge. 2. A small piece of metal that will melt when an electrical circuit becomes overloaded, thus breaking the circuit. 3. Also, to make fluid by melting or fluxing. A fused material is not in the liquid state, but rather is in a "doughy" plastic state.

fusee. A colored flare designed as a railway warning device and used widely in other emergency situations.

fusible link. A piece of material (usually low melting point metals) designed to fail under elevated temperatures, in a fire, or under stress to activate a safety device such as a fire door.

fusible plug. A safety relief device on a container holding a substance under pressure that melts when the temperature of the container reaches a predetermined level, emptying the container of its contents.

fusion. The act of melting.

future liability. Refers to potentially responsible parties' obligations to pay for additional response activities beyond those specified in the record of decision or consent decree.

G

gadolinium. A silvery white, solid, metallic element, symbol Gd, with atomic number 64, and atomic weight 157.25. A rare earth metal.

G-agents. A name for the first three nerve agents: sarin, tabun, and soman.

gallium. A blue-gray, solid (silvery when liquid at room temperature), metallic element, symbol Ga, with atomic number 31, and atomic weight 69.72.

gallon. 1. Unit of liquid measure. 2. One U.S. gallon (3.785 L) has the volume of 231 $in.^3$ (3,785 m^3). 3. One imperial gallon (4.546 L) equals 1.201 U.S. gallons (4.546 L).

galvanic cell. *See* **voltaic cell**.

galvanization. The deposition of a thin layer of zinc on a ferrous material to prevent corrosion of the underlying surface.

gamma radiation. *See* **gamma rays**.

gamma rays. 1. Electromagnetic radiation of high energy. 2. Gamma rays are the most penetrating type of radiation and represent the major external hazard. 3. Extremely short wavelength and intensely high-energy electromagnetic radiation. 4. Gamma rays originate from an atom's nucleus and normally accompany alpha and beta particles as part of the emissions of the radioactive decay of an atom and always accompany nuclear fission. 5. Because gamma rays are energy and not matter, they are very penetrating and can cause damage to animal and plant tissues. 6. Also called *gamma radiation* or denoted as *γ-radiation*.

garbage. Animal and vegetable waste resulting from the handling, storage, sale, preparation, cooking, and serving of foods.

gas. A state of matter defined as a fluid with a vapor pressure of 40 psia or more at 100°F.

gas chromatograph/mass spectrometer (GC/MS). Instrument that identifies the molecular composition and concentrations of various chemicals in water and soil samples.

gasification. Conversion of solid material such as coal into a gas for use as a fuel.

gas laws. The laws that govern the behavior of gases when the variables are pressure, temperature, and volume. Specifically, they are Boyle's, Charles', and Gay-Lussac's laws.

gasohol. Mixture of gasoline and ethanol derived from fermented agricultural products containing at least 9% ethanol.

gasoline. A highly flammable liquid made up of pentane, hexane, heptane, octane, and nonane (and additives), with a flash point as low as –40°F.

gasoline volatility. 1. The property of gasoline whereby it evaporates into a vapor. Gasoline vapor is a mixture of volatile organic compounds.

Geiger counter. An instrument used to detect and measure radiation. Also called a *Geiger-Müller counter*, a *GM counter*, or a *GM meter*.

Geiger-Müller counter. *See* **Geiger counter**.

gel. A two-phase colloidal system consisting of a solid and a liquid in more solid form (jellylike) than an aerosol.

gelatin dynamite. Normal dynamite (nitroglycerine plus an inert filler) to which nitrocellulose has been added to lessen sensitivity.

general formula. The general molecular formula for an analogous series of compounds that will give the actual molecular formula for any member of the series as long as the number of carbon atoms in the compound is known. This number is substituted for the "n" in the formula. A formula that algebraically expresses the formula for every compound in an analogous family. For alkanes, the general formula is C_nH_{2n+2}.

generally recognized as safe (GRAS). Designation by the FDA that a chemical or substance (including certain pesticides) added to food is considered safe by experts, and so is exempted from the usual Federal Food, Drug, and Cosmetic Act (FFDCA) food additive tolerance requirements.

general permit. A permit applicable to a class or category of dischargers.

general reporting facility. A facility having one or more hazardous chemicals above the 10,000-pound threshold for planning quantities. Such facilities must file material safety data sheet (MSDS) information and emergency inventory information with the state emergency response commission (SERC), local emergency planning committee (LEPC), and local fire departments.

generator. 1. A facility or mobile source that emits pollutants into the air or releases hazardous waste into water or soil. 2. Any person, by site, whose act or process produces regulated medical waste or whose act first causes such waste to become subject to regulation. Where more than one person (e.g., doctors with separate medical practices) are located in the same building, each business entity is a separate generator. 3. A device that uses mechanical energy to create electrical energy.

genetic engineering. A process of inserting new genetic information into existing cells in order to modify a specific organism for the purpose of changing one of its characteristics.

genotoxic. 1. Damaging to DNA. 2. Pertaining to agents known to damage DNA.

geochemistry. The study of materials and chemical reactions in rocks, minerals, magma, seawater, and soil.

geographic information system (GIS). A computer system designed for storing, manipulating, analyzing, and displaying data in a geographic context.

geological log. A detailed description of all underground features (depth, thickness, and type of formation, etc.) discovered during the drilling of a well.

geophysical log. A record of the structure and composition of the Earth encountered when drilling a well or similar type of test hole or boring.

geothermal heat pump. Underground coils used to transfer heat from the groundwater to the inside of a building.

germanium. A brittle, silvery gray, solid, metallic element, symbol Ge, with atomic number 32, and atomic weight 72.64. It is in the same family as carbon and is a good semiconductor.

germicide. Any compound that kills disease-causing microorganisms.

Giardia lamblia. Protozoan in the feces of humans and animals that can cause severe gastrointestinal ailments.

glacial. 1. Glasslike, crystallized. 2. Adjective usually applied to acids that have a freezing point near or slightly below room temperature when pure. 3. The usage persists in terms such as *glacial acetic acid* and *glacial phosphoric acid.*

glass. 1. Generally referred to as a "super-cooled" liquid, glass is classified as a ceramic material, or noncrystalline solid with no definite melting point. 2. The principal ingredient is silicon dioxide (sand).

glass containers. For recycling purposes, containers like bottles and jars for drinks, food, cosmetics, and other products.

glass fiber. Fibers that have been drawn from molten glass.

global climate change. *See* **climate change**.

Globally Harmonized System (GHS). A UN system of classification and labeling of chemicals for MSDS.

global warming. An increase in the near-surface temperature of the Earth.

global warming potential. The ratio of the warming caused by a substance to the warming caused by a similar mass of carbon dioxide.

glove bag. A polyethylene or polyvinyl chloride baglike enclosure affixed around an asbestos-containing source, permitting the material to be removed while minimizing release of airborne fibers to the surrounding atmosphere.

glowing combustion. 1. The direct combination of an oxidizer with a solid fuel on the surface of the fuel. There will be no flame present, but heat and light may be emitted. 2. Also called **surface burning**.

glycerol. A series of substituted hydrocarbons with three hydroxyl radicals substituted for hydrogen atoms.

glycol. A hydrocarbon derivative with two hydroxyl groups substituted for two hydrogen atoms.

GM counter. *See* **Geiger counter**.

GM meter. *See* **Geiger counter**.

gold. A soft, heavy, yellow, solid, metallic element, symbol Au, with atomic number 79, and atomic weight 196.967.

gooseneck. 1. A portion of a water service connection between the distribution system water main and a meter. 2. Sometimes called a *pigtail.*

grab sample. A single sample collected at a particular time and place that represents the composition of the water, air, or soil only at that time and place.

grain. A unit of mass. The English grain was equal to 1/7,000 the mass of a pound avoirdupois, or 0.0648 grams.

grain alcohol. Ethyl alcohol or ethanol.

grain loading. The rate at which particles are emitted from a pollution source. Measurement is made by the number of grains per cubic foot of gas emitted.

gram. One thousandth of a kilogram. There are approximately 28.3495 grams (g) in an ounce.

gram-molecular weight (GMW). The atomic weight of an element or the molecular weight of a compound expressed in grams instead of atomic mass units.

granular activated carbon treatment (GAC). A filtering system often used in small water systems and individual homes to remove organics. Can be used by municipal water treatment plants.

graphite. A crystalline allotrope of carbon.

grasscycling. Source reduction activities in which grass clippings are left on the lawn after mowing.

grassed waterway. Natural or constructed watercourse or outlet that is shaped or graded and established in suitable vegetation for the disposal of runoff water without erosion.

gravity. The natural force exerted on a body toward the Earth's surface or between two bodies, depending on the masses of the bodies involved and the distance between them.

gray. The SI unit of absorbed dose; 1 gray = 100 rads.

gray water. Domestic wastewater composed of wash water from kitchen, bathroom, and laundry sinks, tubs, and washers. Also called **sanitary water**.

greenhouse effect. The warming of the Earth's atmosphere attributed to a buildup of carbon dioxide or other gases.

greenhouse gas. A gas that absorbs strongly in the infrared region of the spectrum. Infrared radiation is then reflected and emitted by the Earth's surface as heat and causes a fairly large warming effect when trapped by these gases in the atmosphere. In order of abundance and importance as greenhouse gases are: water vapor, carbon dioxide, ozone, nitrous oxide, methane, and chlorofluorocarbons (CFCs).

green vitriol. An archaic name for iron(II) sulfate ($FeSO_4 \cdot 7H_2O$).

grinder pump. A mechanical device that shreds solids and raises sewage to a higher elevation through pressure sewers.

gross alpha/beta particle activity. The total radioactivity due to alpha or beta particle emissions as inferred from measurements on a dry sample.

gross power-generation potential. The installed power generation capacity that landfill gas can support.

ground cover. Plants grown to keep soil from eroding.

grounding. A method whereby activities that may generate static electricity will be prevented from discharging a spark and thereby not produce an ignition point.

ground-penetrating radar. A geophysical method that uses high-frequency electromagnetic waves to obtain subsurface information.

ground source heat pump. Underground coils used to transfer heat from the ground to the inside of a building. *Contrast with* **water source heat pump**.

groundwater. The supply of fresh water found beneath the Earth's surface, usually in aquifers, which supply wells and springs.

groundwater discharge. Groundwater entering near coastal waters that has been contaminated by landfill leachate, deep well injection of hazardous wastes, or septic tanks, etc.

Ground Water Disinfection Rule. A 1996 amendment of the Safe Drinking Water Act requiring EPA to promulgate national primary drinking water regulations requiring disinfection for all public water systems, including surface waters and groundwater systems.

groundwater under the direct influence (UDI) of surface water. Any water beneath the surface of the ground with:

1. Significant occurrence of insects or other microorganisms, algae, or large-diameter pathogens.
2. Significant and relatively rapid shifts in water characteristics such as turbidity, temperature, conductivity, or pH, which closely correlate to climatological or surface water conditions.

group. 1. The vertical columns (major classes or divisions) into which elements are arranged in the periodic table of elements that all have similar chemical properties. 2. A substructure that imparts characteristic chemical behaviors to a molecule.

guidelines (human health risk assessment). Official, peer-reviewed documentation stating current U.S. EPA methodology in assessing risk of harm from environmental pollutants to populations.

gully erosion. Severe erosion in which trenches are cut to a depth greater than 30 cm (1 ft).

guncotton. Cellulose nitrate.

gypsum. Natural calcium sulfate.

H

habitat. The place where a population lives and its surroundings, both living and nonliving.

habitat indicator. A physical attribute of the environment measured to characterize conditions necessary to support an organism, population, or community in the absence of pollutants.

hafnium. A silvery, solid, metallic element, symbol Hf, with atomic number 72, and atomic weight 178.49.

half-life. 1. The time required for a pollutant to lose one-half of its original concentration. 2. The time required for one-half of the atoms of a radioactive element to undergo self-transmutation or decay. 3. The time required for the elimination of one-half a total dose from the body. 4. The time it takes for a radioactive particle to decompose to one-half its mass.

halide. A binary compound containing a halogen. A halogenated compound.

Halligan tool. 1. An all-purpose steel prying bar used as a forcible entry tool. 2. A forcible entry tool with a claw on one end and a spike or point at a right angle to a narrow wedge on the other.

halocarbon. Covalent compounds containing a halogen, carbon, and sometimes hydrogen.

halocarbon plastics. Plastics made from monomers containing only carbon and a halogen or halogens.

halogen. 1. An element of group VIIA on the periodic table: fluorine, chlorine, bromine, iodine, and astatine. 2. A type of incandescent lamp with higher energy efficiency than standard ones. 3. Fluorine and chlorine are the halogens present in some polymer molecules. Astatine is also a halogen, but it is so rare it will never be encountered in plastics.

halogen acid. Hydrofluoric acid, hydrochloric acid, hydrobromic acid, or hydriodic acid, all with the general formula HX.

halogen acid gas. Hydrogen fluoride, hydrogen chloride, hydrogen bromide, or hydrogen iodide, all with the general formula HX.

halogenated. The incorporation of a halogen (fluorine, chlorine, bromine, or iodine) into a chemical compound.

halogenated hydrocarbon. A hydrocarbon compound that has had one or more hydrogen atoms replaced by a halogen (fluorine, chlorine, bromine, or iodine).

halogenation. The chemical reaction whereby a halogen is substituted for another atom, usually a hydrogen atom.

Halon. The trade-marked name of bromine-containing compounds with long atmospheric lifetimes; their breakdown in the stratosphere causes depletion of ozone. Halons are used in firefighting.

Halon-2402. Dibromotetrafluoroethane ($C_2F_4Br_2$). Commonly used as a fire extinguishing agent, it is a known ozone-depleting chemical.

hammer mill. A high-speed machine that uses hammers and cutters to crush, grind, chip, or shred solid waste.

hardener. A substance that brings about the curing of a plastic (thermosetting).

hard water. Alkaline water containing dissolved salts that interfere with some industrial processes and prevent soap and detergents from being effective.

hashish. The extract of marijuana, which is more concentrated than the original drug from which it was extracted.

hassium. A solid metallic element, symbol Hs, with atomic number 108, and atomic weight 265.

hauler. Garbage collection company that offers complete refuse removal service. Many will also collect recyclables.

hazard. 1. Potential for radiation, a chemical, or other pollutant to cause human illness or injury. 2. In the pesticide program, the inherent toxicity of a compound. Hazard identification of a given substances is an informed judgment based on verifiable toxicity data from animal models or human studies. 3. A potential source of risk, danger, or harm.

hazard and operability study (HAZOP). A systematic technique for identifying hazards or operability programs throughout an entire facility.

hazard assessment. 1. The evaluation of the effects of a stressor or determining a margin of safety for an organism by comparing the concentration that causes toxic effects with an estimate of exposure to the organism. 2. The process of determining whether exposure to an agent can cause an increase in the incidence of a particular adverse health effect and whether the adverse health effect is likely to occur in humans.

Hazard Assessment Computer System (HACS). Computerized data system available through the National Response Center (NRC). It is a part of the Chemical Hazards Response Information System (CHRIS).

hazard category. These categories include:

1. "Immediate (acute) health hazard," including "highly toxic," "toxic," "irritant," "sensitizer," "corrosive" (as defined under Section 1910.1200 of 29 CFR), and other hazardous chemicals that cause an adverse effect to a target organ; this effect usually occurs rapidly as a result of short-term exposure and is of short duration.
2. "Delayed (chronic) health hazard," including "carcinogens" (as defined under Section 1910.1200 of 29 CFR) and other hazardous chemicals that cause an adverse effect to a target organ; this effect generally occurs as a result of long-term exposure and is of long duration.
3. "Fire hazard," including "flammable," "combustible liquid," "pyrophoric," and "oxidizer" (as defined under Section 1910.1200 of 29 CFR).
4. "Sudden release of pressure," including "explosive" and "compressed gas" (as defined under Section 1910.1200 of 29 CFR).
5. "Reactive," including "unstable reactive," "organic peroxide," and "water reactive" (as defined under Section 1910.1200 of 29 CFR).

hazard class. One of nine classes of hazardous materials as categorized and defined by the Department of Transportation in 49 CFR. The nine classes of hazardous materials are as follows:

- Class 1 explosives
- Class 2 compressed gas
- Class 3 flammable liquids
- Class 4 flammable solids
- Class 5 oxidizers/organic peroxides
- Class 6 toxic (poisonous)/infectious substances
- Class 7 radioactive material
- Class 8 corrosives
- Class 9 miscellaneous dangerous goods

Hazard Communication Standard (HCS). 1. The OSHA regulation that requires chemical manufacturers, suppliers, and importers to assess the hazards of the chemicals that they make, supply, or import, and to inform employers, customers, and workers of these hazards through MSDS information. 2. The OSHA standard cited in 29 CFR 1910.1200.

hazard evaluation. A component of risk evaluation that involves gathering and evaluating data on the types of health injuries or diseases that may be produced by a chemical and on the conditions of exposure under which such health effects are produced.

hazard identification. Determining if a chemical or a microbe can cause adverse health effects in humans and what those effects might be.

Hazard Information Transmission (HIT). A program that provides digital transmission of a CHEMTREC emergency chemical report to first responders at the scene of a hazardous materials incident.

hazardous air pollutants. Air pollutants that are not covered by ambient air quality standards but which, as defined in the Clean Air Act, may present a threat of adverse human health effects or adverse environmental effects.

Hazardous and Solid Waste Amendments of 1984 (HSWA). Public Law 98-616, which significantly expanded both the scope and the coverage of the Resource Conservation and Recovery Act of 1976 (RCRA).

hazardous chemical. 1. An EPA designation for any hazardous material requiring an MSDS under OSHA's Hazard Communication Standard. Hazardous chemicals are distinct from hazardous waste. *See* **hazardous waste**.

hazardous material (HM). 1. A substance or material that has been determined by the secretary of the Department of Transportation (DOT) to be capable of posing an unreasonable risk to health, safety, and property when transported in commerce, and which has been so designated (DOT). 2. Any material, that when it escapes its container, can cause damage to life, health, the environment, or property. 3. Any material that can cause damage to life, health, the environment, or property.

hazardous materials company. Any piece of equipment having the capabilities, personal protective equipment (PPE), equipment, and complement of personnel as specified in the regulations concerning hazardous materials company types and minimum capabilities.

hazardous materials incident. Uncontrolled, unlicensed release of hazardous materials during storage or use from a fixed facility or during transport outside a fixed facility that may impact public health, safety, and/or the environment.

Hazardous Materials Information Exchange (HMIX). A national data repository and "bulletin board" for states to use regarding planning, training courses, regional activities, and recent legislation or regulatory updates; (312) 972-3275.

Hazardous Materials Information System (HMIS). A central system for the collection, maintenance, and dissemination of data contained in the manufacturer's material safety data sheets and other sources of information designed by NPCA (National Paint and Coatings Association).

hazardous materials response team. An organized group of individuals that is trained and equipped to perform work to control actual or potential leaks, spills, discharges, or releases of hazardous materials, requiring possible close approach to the material.

Hazardous Materials Transportation Act (HMTA). Act that governs the commercial shipment of such materials by the Department of Defense; established broad authority under which the Department of Transportation regulates the transportation/safety of all hazardous materials in commerce.

hazardous ranking system (HRS). The principal screening tool used by EPA to evaluate risks to public health and the environment associated with abandoned or uncontrolled hazardous waste sites.

hazardous substance. 1. Any material that poses a threat to human health and/or the environment. Typical hazardous substances are toxic, corrosive, ignitable, explosive, or chemically reactive. 2. Any substance designated by EPA to be reported if a designated quantity of the substance is spilled in the waters of the United States or is otherwise released into the environment.

hazardous warning. Words, pictures, symbols, or any other depiction or combination thereof, that will transmit an indication of the hazard related to the product under consideration.

hazardous waste. 1. Byproducts of society that can pose a substantial or potential hazard to human health or the environment when improperly managed. 2. Product or chemical designated as such by the Resource Conservation and Recovery Act (RCRA) regulations of the EPA. 3. A material becomes a hazardous waste when it can no longer be used for its originally intended purpose, and it possesses at least one of four characteristics (ignitability, corrosivity, reactivity, or toxicity) or appears on special EPA lists. 4. It must be on the list of specific hazardous waste streams or chemicals, or else it must exhibit one or more of certain specific characteristics, including flammability, corrosivity, reactivity, and toxicity.

hazardous waste landfill. An excavated or engineered site where hazardous waste is deposited and covered.

hazardous waste manifest. The shipping document, originated and signed by the uniform (EPA usage) waste generator or an authorized representative, that contains the information required and that must accompany shipments of hazardous waste (40 CFR 262, subpart B).

hazardous waste minimization. The act of reducing the amount of toxicity or waste produced by a facility via source reduction or environmentally sound recycling.

Hazardous Waste Operations and Emergency Response Standard (HAZWOPER). The OSHA standard cited in 29 CFR 1910.120(a)(1)(i–v) and 1926.65(a)(1)(i–v).

hazard quotient. The ratio of estimated site-specific exposure to a single chemical from a site over a specified period to the estimated daily exposure level, at which no adverse health effects are likely to occur.

hazard rating. A rating system of one to four that indicates the severity of hazard with respect to health, flammability, and reactivity.

hazard ratio. A term used to compare an animal's daily dietary intake of a pesticide to its lethal dose (LD_{50}) value. A ratio greater than 1.0 indicates that the animal is likely to consume a dose amount that would kill 50% of animals of the same species. *See* **lethal dose**.

hazards. 1. Dangerous or unwanted outcomes to life, the environment, or property. 2. The inherent characteristics of a material that may cause incapacitation, injury, or mortality by contact, inhalation, or ingestion.

hazards analysis. Procedures used to:

1. Identify potential sources of release of hazardous materials from fixed facilities or transportation accidents.
2. Determine the vulnerability of a geographical area to a release of hazardous materials.
3. Compare hazards to determine which present greater or lesser risks to a community.

hazards identification. Providing information on which facilities have extremely hazardous substances, what those chemicals are, how much there is at each facility, how the chemicals are stored, and whether they are used at high temperatures.

hazard warning. Any words, pictures, symbols, or combination thereof appearing on a label or other appropriate form of warning that conveys the hazards of the chemical(s) in the container(s).

hazard zones. *See* **inhalation hazard zones.**

hazmat. Shortened form of "hazardous material(s)."

hazmat foam. A special vapor-suppressing mix that can be applied to liquids or solids to prevent off-gassing.

hazmat incident. Actual or potential unplanned release of a hazardous material.

hazmat task force. A group of resources with common communications and a leader.

hazmat trained and equipped. The level of training and equipment defined by the Occupational Safety and Health Administration (OSHA) and the National Fire Protection Association (NFPA).

headspace. The vapor mixture trapped above a solid or liquid in a sealed vessel.

health advisory level. A nonregulatory health-based reference level of chemical traces in drinking water at which there are no adverse health risks when ingested over various periods of time.

health assessment. An evaluation of available data on existing or potential risks to human health posed by a Superfund site.

health hazard. A substance for which there is statistically significant evidence based on at least one study conducted in accordance with established scientific principles that acute or chronic health effects may occur in exposed employees.

heat. 1. A form of energy. 2. The total amount of vibration in a group of molecules.

heat exhaustion. Results from compromise of the body's ability to cool down properly from prolonged exposure to intense heat; causes excessive sweating and sodium deficiency.

heat flux. 1. A measure of heat impinging onto a surface per unit time, usually from a radiant heating device. 2. The rate of flow of heat energy onto a measured area.

heat island effect. A "dome" of elevated temperatures over an urban area caused by structural and pavement heat fluxes, as well as pollutant emissions.

heat of combustion. The total amount of energy released during the complete combustion of the material.

heat of condensation. The amount of heat that must be removed from 1 g of a vapor at its condensation point to condense the vapor with no change in temperature.

heat of crystallization. The amount of heat generated or absorbed when a crystal is formed from a saturated solution of the substance.

heat of dilution. The amount of heat that evolves when 1 mole of solute is diluted from one concentration to another.

heat of formation. The amount of heat generated or absorbed when 1 mole of a compound is formed in its standard state from constituents in their standard states.

heat of fusion. 1. The energy required to convert a solid into a liquid with no temperature change. 2. This is also called the *latent heat of fusion* or *melting*.

heat of hydration. The amount of heat generated or absorbed when a hydrate of a compound is formed, or when ions in a solution are hydrated.

heat of reaction. The amount of heat generated or absorbed when a chemical reaction occurs.

heat of solution. The amount of heat generated or absorbed when a substance is dissolved in a solvent.

heat of sublimation. The amount of heat generated or absorbed when a material is converted directly from the solid state to the vapor state, bypassing the liquid state.

heat of transition. The amount of heat generated or absorbed when a known mass of a substance is converted from one crystalline form to another.

heat of vaporization. The energy required to convert a substance from the liquid to the gaseous state with no temperature change. This is also called the **latent heat of vaporization**.

heat pump. An electric device with both heating and cooling capabilities. *See also* **ground source heat pump** and **water source heat pump**.

heat sink. Any system or device that will absorb heat from a thermal system.

heat stress. The adverse effects in humans exposed to heated atmospheres or radiant heat in a fire.

heat stroke. A life-threatening condition that can occur during prolonged exposure to intense heat. The body is unable to sweat, resulting in extremely high body temperature and collapse.

heat transfer. Transmission of heat energy from one location to another by convection, conduction, or radiation.

heavy metals. 1. Metallic elements with high atomic weights (e.g., mercury, chromium, cadmium, arsenic, and lead) that can damage living things at low concentrations and tend to accumulate in the food chain. 2. The group of metallic elements that are precipitated from solution by hydrogen sulfide. 3. Generally, those metals with atomic numbers greater than 24.

heavy water. Deuterium oxide (D_2O). Heavy water is about 11% denser than ordinary water.

helium. 1. A nonflammable, gaseous, nonmetallic element, symbol He, with atomic number 2, and atomic weight 4.0026. A member of group VIII on the periodic table of the elements, the inert (or noble) gases. 2. It is the second lightest gas and is used in lighter-than-air aircraft.

hematopoietic. Referring to the process of blood formation in the body.

hematotoxin. A substance toxic to the blood or organs where blood is made.

hemihydrate. A hydrate that contains two parts of the compound to one part water.

hemoglobin (Hb). A protein in red blood cells that carries oxygen from the lungs to the tissues where it exchanges it for carbon dioxide.

hepatotoxin. A substance toxic to the liver.

heptachlor. An insecticide that was banned on some food products in 1975 and in all of them 1978.

heptyl. The radical ($-C_7H_{15}$) formed when a hydrogen is removed from heptane (C_7H_{16}).

herbicide. A chemical pesticide designed to control or destroy plants, weeds, or grasses.

herbivore. An animal that feeds on plants.

heterocyclic. A closed-ring structure of either five or six elements, at least one of which is not carbon.

heterogeneous. A mixture or material that is not the same composition throughout.

heterotrophic organisms. Species that are dependent on organic matter for food.

hexyl. The radical ($-C_6H_{13}$) formed when one hydrogen is removed from hexane (C_6H_{14}).

high-angle rescue. *See* **rope rescue**.

high-density polyethylene. A polymer used to make plastic bottles and other products.

high-end exposure (dose) estimate. An estimate of exposure or dose level received by anyone in a defined population that is greater than the 90th percentile of all individuals in that population, but less than the exposure at the highest percentile in that population.

high-expansion foam. A detergent-based foam (low water content) that expands at ratios of about 1,000 to 1.

highest dose tested. The highest dose of a chemical or substance tested in a study.

high explosive. 1. An explosive that may or may not be combustible. 2. Most high explosives, with the exception of primary and secondary explosives, are relatively insensitive to heat and shock. 3. It ordinarily detonates, usually by means of a primary explosive. 4. Also called the *main charge.*

high-intensity discharge. A generic term for mercury vapor, metal halide, and high-pressure sodium lamps and fixtures.

high-level nuclear waste facility. Plant designed to handle disposal of used nuclear fuel, high-level radioactive waste, and plutonium waste.

high-level radioactive waste (HLRW). Waste generated in core fuel of a nuclear reactor, found at nuclear reactors or by nuclear fuel reprocessing. It is a serious threat to anyone who comes near the waste without shielding.

high-line jumpers. Pipes or hoses connected to fire hydrants and laid on top of the ground to provide emergency water service for an isolated portion of a distribution system.

highly toxic. A chemical falling within any of the following three categories:

1. A chemical that has a median lethal dose (LD_{50}) of 50 mg or less per kg of body weight when administered orally to albino rats weighing between 200 g and 300 g each.
2. A chemical that has a median lethal dose of 200 mg or less per kg of body weight when administered by continuous contact for 24 hours (or less if death occurs within 24 hours) with the bare skin of albino rabbits weighing between 2 kg and 3 kg each.
3. A chemical that has a median lethal concentration in air of 200 ppm by volume or less of gas or vapor, or 2 mg/L or less of mist, fume, or dust, when administered by continuous inhalation for 1 hour (or less if death occurs within 1 hour) to albino rats weighing between 200 g and 300 g each.

high-pressure container. Any container designed to withstand pressures from 100 psi to 3,000 psi.

high-risk community. A community located within the vicinity of numerous sites of facilities or other potential sources of environmental exposure or health hazards that may result in high levels of exposure to contaminants or pollutants.

high sulfur coal. *See* **noncompliance coal.**

high-to-low-dose extrapolation. The process of prediction of low exposure risk to humans and animals from the measured high-exposure/high-risk data involving laboratory animals.

holding pond. A pond or reservoir, usually made of earth, built to store polluted runoff.

holding time. The maximum amount of time a sample may be stored before analysis.

hollow stem auger drilling. Conventional drilling method that uses augurs to penetrate the soil.

holmium. A silvery white, solid, metallic element, symbol Ho, with atomic number 67, and atomic weight 164.93. It is a member of the rare earth group.

homeowner water system. Any water system that supplies piped water to a single residence.

homogeneous. A substance or material that is the same composition throughout.

homogeneous area. In accordance with Asbestos Hazard and Emergency Response Act (AHERA) definitions, an area of surfacing materials, thermal surface insulation, or miscellaneous material that is uniform in color and texture.

homopolymer. The polymer produced by polymerization of a single monomer.

hood capture efficiency. Ratio of the emissions captured by a hood and directed into a control or disposal device, expressed as a percent of all emissions.

horsepower. The English system unit used to measure mechanical power, equal to 746 watts.

host. 1. In genetics, the organism, typically a bacterium, into which a gene from another organism is transplanted. 2. In medicine, an animal infected or parasitized by another organism.

hot zone. The clearly marked and controlled area immediately surrounding a dangerous goods or hazardous materials incident that extends far enough to prevent adverse effects from released hazardous materials to personnel outside the zone. This zone is also referred to as the *exclusion zone*, *red zone*, or *restricted zone* in other documents (EPA Standard Operating Safety Guidelines, OSHA 29 CFR 1910.120, and NFPA 472).

household bleach. A dilute solution of sodium hypochlorite or calcium hypochlorite that kills bacteria and destroys colored organic materials by oxidizing them.

household hazardous waste. Hazardous products used and disposed of by residential as opposed to industrial consumers.

household waste. Solid waste, composed of garbage and rubbish, that normally originates in a private home or apartment house. Household waste may contain a significant amount of toxic or hazardous waste. Also called *domestic waste*.

human equivalent concentration (HEC). The human concentration (for inhalation exposure) of an agent that is believed to induce the same magnitude of toxic effect as the experimental animal species concentration or dose. *See also* **human equivalent dose**.

human equivalent dose (HED). A dose that, when administered to humans by routes of exposure other than inhalation, produces an effect equal to that produced by a dose in animals. *See also* **human equivalent concentration**.

human exposure evaluation. Describing the nature and size of the population exposed to a substance and the magnitude and duration of their exposure.

human health risk. The likelihood that a given exposure or series of exposures may have damaged or will damage the health of individuals.

humectant. A material that absorbs or retains moisture, usually added to another material to keep it from drying out.

humidity. The moisture content of air.

hydrargyrum. Latin for "mercury," hence the symbol, Hg.

hydrate. 1. A chemical compound that contains one or more water molecules attached to it, which usually can be removed by heating without destroying the compound. It is attached as a molecule and can be driven off by heat. 2. Water attached this way is referred to as *water of hydration*, and molecules with this water attached are said to be *hydrated*.

hydrated. Water that is attached to the molecule of another substance.

hydrated lime. Calcium hydroxide $Ca(OH)_2$.

hydraulic conductivity. The rate at which water can move through a permeable medium (i.e., the coefficient of permeability).

hydraulic fluid. A liquid usually composed of paraffinic and cycloparaffinic liquids plus additives.

hydraulic gradient. In general, the direction of groundwater flow due to changes in the depth of the water table.

hydraulics. The study of the use and movement of fluids at rest or in motion.

hydrides. 1. A group or family of ionic chemical compounds containing a metal and hydrogen. 2. May also be covalent when hydrogen combines with a nonmetal. 3. The inorganic hydrides are flammable, water-reactive, and are very dangerous fire risks.

hydrocarbon (HC). 1. Chemical compounds that consist entirely of carbon and hydrogen. 2. A covalent chemical compound containing only carbon and hydrogen.

hydrocarbon backbone. The molecular fragment that remains after a hydrogen atom is removed from a hydrocarbon. 2. The hydrocarbon portion of a hydrocarbon derivative. *See* **hydrocarbon radical**.

hydrocarbon derivative. A covalent compound made up of a hydrocarbon backbone and a functional group.

hydrocarbon plastics. Plastics made from resins or monomers containing only hydrogen and carbon.

hydrocarbon radical. 1. A molecular fragment that began as a hydrocarbon molecule and had one or more hydrogen atoms removed, leaving a free radical. 2. Also called a **hydrocarbon backbone**. 3. In general formulas, "R" stands for a hydrocarbon radical.

hydrocracking. The cracking of long-chain hydrocarbons in petroleum in the presence of hydrogen.

hydrocyanic acid. Hydrogen cyanide (HCN).

hydrogen. 1. A colorless, tasteless, odorless, gaseous, nonmetallic element, symbol H, with atomic number 1, and atomic weight 1.0079. 2. It is the lightest of all the elements and is extremely flammable.

hydrogenate. 1. To add hydrogen to a molecule. 2. Usually refers to the addition of hydrogen atoms to an unsaturated hydrocarbon molecule to cause the compound to change from a liquid to a solid.

hydrogenated. The addition of hydrogen to an organic molecule.

hydrogenation. The chemical reaction in which hydrogen atom(s) are added to an organic molecule.

hydrogen bond. 1. An electrostatic attraction of the positive (hydrogen) end of a molecule to the negative end (unpaired electron) of another molecule, usually oxygen. 2. The hydrogen bond is the force responsible for water existing as a liquid under standard temperature and pressure. 3. The hydrogen bond is 10 times stronger than van der Waals force.

hydrogen cyanide. A chemical blood agent (HCN); agent AC.

hydrogen halide. 1. A binary compound of hydrogen and a halogen. 2. The acid gases hydrogen fluoride, hydrogen chloride, hydrogen bromide, and hydrogen iodide, all represented by the general formula HX.

hydrogen sulfide. Gas emitted during organic decomposition. Also a by-product of oil refining and burning. Smells like rotten eggs and, in heavy concentration, can kill or cause illness; H_2S. A chemical blood agent.

hydrogeological cycle. The natural process recycling water from the atmosphere down to (and through) the surface of the Earth and back to the atmosphere again.

hydrogeology. The geology of groundwater, with particular emphasis on the chemistry and movement of water.

hydrologic cycle. Movement or exchange of water between the atmosphere and the Earth.

hydrology. The science dealing with the properties, distribution, and circulation of water.

hydrolysis. The breakdown of a chemical by interaction with water.

hydrolyze. A substance reacting with water to form two or more new substances. The reaction is called **hydrolysis**.

hydrometer. An instrument used to measure the density of liquids.

hydronic. A ventilation system using heated or cooled water pumped through a building.

hydronium ion. Formed by capture of a hydrogen ion by a water molecule. A strong covalent bond is formed between the hydrogen ion and water oxygen. All hydrogen ions in aqueous solution are bound inside hydronium ions (H_3O^{+1}).

hydrophilic. Having a strong affinity for water.

hydrophobic. Having a strong aversion for water.

hydropneumatic. A water system, usually small, in which a water pump is automatically controlled by the pressure in a compressed air tank.

hydrosphere. The portion of the atmosphere that contains water in the liquid, solid, or gaseous phase.

hydroxide ion. The anion (OH^{-1}) associated with bases.

hydroxyl. 1. A radical (-OH) that, when combined with a hydrocarbon backbone, produces a class of chemicals called alcohols. 2. The functional group of the alcohols; the structural formula is -O-H, usually written -OH.

hygroscopic. The ability to absorb moisture from the environment.

hypergolic. The property of reacting with another substance immediately upon coming in contact with that substance; both materials must be hypergolic.

hypersensitivity diseases. 1. Diseases characterized by allergic responses to pollutants. 2. Diseases most clearly associated with indoor air quality are asthma, rhinitis, and pneumonic hypersensitivity.

hyperventilation. Rapid breathing that overly oxygenates the blood.

hypo. Sodium thiosulfate solution.

hypobromite. 1. Any compound containing the hypobromite ion (BrO^{-1}). 2. Derived from hypobromous acid (HOBr). 3. Usually a strong oxidizing agent.

hypochlorite. 1. Any compound containing the hypochlorite ion (ClO^{-1}). 2. Derived from hypochlorous acid (HOCl). 3. Usually a strong oxidizing agent.

hypolimnion. Bottom waters of a thermally stratified lake. The hypolimnion of a eutrophic lake is usually low or lacking in oxygen.

hypoxia. A deficiency of oxygen reaching body tissues.

hypoxic waters. Waters with dissolved oxygen concentrations of less than 2 ppm, the level generally accepted as the minimum required for most marine life to survive and reproduce.

I

IC_{50}. *See* **incapacitating concentration.**

ice. A crystalline allotrope of water (H_2O).

-ide. 1. A suffix used in naming compounds that contain two elements. 2. When a metal forms a compound with a nonmetal, the metal retains its name, and the second part of the name is the nonmetal with its name changed to end in "ide."

identification code. The unique code assigned to each generator, transporter, and treatment, storage, or disposal facility by regulating agencies to facilitate identification and tracking of chemicals or hazardous waste. Also called *EPA ID number*.

ignitability. The ease with which a substance will ignite.

ignitable. Capable of burning or causing a fire.

ignitable mixture. A mixture of fuel and air within the flammable range.

ignition. 1. The initiation of combustion (ASTM E 176). 2. The beginning of flame propagation or burning. 3. The start of a fire.

ignition continuity. The continuation of burning caused by the radiated heat of the flame.

ignition source. Any energy source that will raise the material to its ignition temperature. Examples are light, heat, friction, or spark.

ignition temperature. The minimum temperature to which a material must be raised before combustion will occur. At this temperature, no ignition source need be present. Also referred to as *autoignition temperature. See also* **autoignition**.

Imhoff cone. A clear, cone-shaped container used to measure the volume of settleable solids in a specific volume of water.

imide. A covalent acid containing nitrogen with two double bonds.

imine. A covalent compound containing a carbon-to-nitrogen double bond. It is highly reactive.

immediately dangerous to life or health (IDLH). 1. The maximum level to which a healthy individual can be exposed to a chemical for 30 minutes and escape without suffering irreversible health effects or impairing symptoms. Used as a "level of concern" (*See* **level of concern**). 2. The amount of material, usually expressed as parts per million (ppm) of air or other material, or milligrams per cubic meter (mg/m^3) of air that will pose an immediate life- or health-threatening situation to the exposed person.

imminent hazard. One that would likely result in unreasonable adverse effects on humans or the environment or risk unreasonable hazard to an endangered species during the time required for a pesticide registration cancellation proceeding.

imminent threat. A high probability that exposure is occurring.

immiscibility. 1. The inability of two or more substances or liquids to readily dissolve into one another, such as oil and water.

immiscible. 1. Not able to readily dissolve into one another. 2. Sometimes means that a material does not mix readily with water.

impact modifier. Materials added to brittle polymers or compounds to improve their resistance to breaking under impact.

impact resistance. The relative ease with which plastic parts break under high-speed stress applications. Also called *impact strength*.

impact strength. *See* **impact resistance.**

impermeable. 1. Not easily penetrated. 2. The property of a material or soil that does not allow, or allows only with great difficulty, the movement or passage of water.

impervious. Preventing the penetration of, or passage through, one material by another.

import. To cause a chemical to be imported into the customs territory of the United States.

imports. Municipal solid waste and recyclables that have been transported to a state or locality for processing or final disposition, but that did not originate in that state or locality.

impoundment. A body of water or sludge confined by a dam, dike, floodgate, or other barrier.

incapacitating agent. A substance that produces temporary effects that renders a person incapable of performing normal functions.

incapacitating concentration. It is the concentration of gas or smoke that will produce incapacitation in 50% of the test animals within a specified exposure time; IC_{50}.

incendiary gel. Thermite mixed in an oil and made into a gel by the addition of a soap that will spontaneously ignite on exposure to air.

incidence. The number of new cases of a disease that develop within a specified population over a specified period of time.

incidence rate. The ratio of new cases within a population to the total population at risk given a specified period of time.

incident. The occurrence of an emergency event that requires response by emergency personnel to minimize damage to the population, environment, property, or systems.

incident commander (IC). 1. The person responsible for the management and coordination of all incident operations. 2. The person in charge at the scene of an incident, who uses an ICS to manage operational personnel.

incident command post (ICP). A facility located at a safe distance from an emergency site, where the incident commander, key staff, and technical representatives can make decisions and deploy emergency manpower and equipment.

incident command system (ICS). 1. The organizational arrangement in which one person, normally the fire chief of the impacted district, or in some cases, the first responding chief officer, is in charge of an integrated, comprehensive emergency response organization and the emergency incident site. 2. It is a management system of specific procedures for controlling personnel, facilities, equipment, and communications from different agencies to work together towards a common goal in an effective and efficient manner. 3. It is the chain of command and leadership at the scene of an emergency.

incident management system (IMS). The flexible on-scene system that identifies key roles and tasks that must be filled to safely manage an emergency incident. It stipulates that one person (the incident commander) is responsible for overall operations during the incident.

incineration. A treatment technology involving destruction of waste by controlled burning at high temperatures.

incineration at sea. Disposal of waste by burning at sea on specially-designed incinerator ships.

incinerator. A furnace for burning waste under controlled conditions.

incipient fire stage. The first phase of the burning process where the substance being oxidized is producing some heat, but the heat has not spread to other substances nearby.

incompatibility. The chemical makeup of a material such that it cannot be mixed with another material without starting a chemical reaction.

incompatible waste. A waste unsuitable for mixing with another waste or material because it may react to form a hazard.

indemnification. In the pesticide program, legal requirement that EPA pay certain end-users, dealers, and distributors for the cost of stock on hand at the time a pesticide registration is suspended.

indicator. 1. In biology, any biological entities, processes, or communities with characteristics that show the presence of specific environmental conditions. 2. In chemistry, a substance that shows a visible change, usually of color, at a desired point in a chemical reaction. 3. A device that indicates the result of a measurement; e.g., a pressure gauge or a moveable scale.

indirect application. A method of extinguishing fire by putting water fog into a closed superheated atmosphere to obtain the maximum heat absorption and steam generation for smothering and cooling the fire area.

indirect discharge. Introduction of pollutants from a nondomestic source into a publicly owned waste-treatment system. Indirect dischargers can be commercial or industrial facilities with wastes that enter local sewers.

indirect source. Any facility or building, property, road, or parking area that attracts motor vehicle traffic and indirectly causes pollution.

indium. A solid metallic element, symbol In, with atomic number 49, and atomic weight 114.82.

individual risk. The probability that an individual will experience an adverse effect.

indoor air. The breathable air inside a habitable structure or conveyance.

indoor air pollution. Chemical, physical, or biological contaminants in indoor air.

indoor climate. Temperature, humidity, lighting, air flow, and noise levels in a habitable structure or conveyance.

industrial chemical. A chemical manufactured for use in industrial operations.

industrial pollution prevention. Combination of industrial source reduction and toxic chemical use substitution.

industrial process waste. Residues produced during manufacturing operations.

industrial sludge. Semiliquid residue or slurry remaining from treatment of industrial water and wastewater.

industrial source reduction. Practices that reduce the amount of any hazardous substance, pollutant, or contaminant entering any waste stream or otherwise released into the environment, including equipment or technology modifications, substitution of raw materials, and improvements in housekeeping, maintenance, training, or inventory control.

industrial waste. Unwanted materials from an industrial operation, which may be liquid, sludge, solid, or hazardous waste.

inert. A term used to indicate that a substance does not take part in chemical reactions easily.

inert gases. The elements of group VIIIA: helium, neon, argon, krypton, xenon, and radon. 2. Also known as the *noble gases.*

inertia. The tendency of a body to maintain its state of rest or uniform motion.

inertial separator. A device that uses centrifugal force to separate waste particles.

inert ingredient. Pesticide components, such as solvents, carriers, dispersants, and surfactants, that are not active against target pests.

infectious agent. Any organism, such as a pathogenic virus, parasite, or bacterium, that is capable of invading body tissues, multiplying, and causing disease.

infectious waste. Hazardous waste capable of causing infections in humans. Also called *red bag waste.*

infiltration. 1. The penetration of water through the ground surface into subsurface soil, or the penetration of water from the soil into sewer or other pipes through defective joints, connections, or manhole walls. 2. The technique of applying large volumes of wastewater to land in order to penetrate the surface and percolate through the underlying soil. *See also* **percolation.**

infiltration gallery. A subsurface groundwater collection system, typically shallow in depth, constructed with open-jointed or perforated pipes that discharge collected water into a watertight chamber from which the water is pumped to treatment facilities and into the distribution system.

infiltration rate. The quantity of water that can enter the soil in a specified time interval.

inflow. Entry of extraneous rainwater into a sewer system from sources other than infiltration, such as basement drains, manholes, storm drains, and street washing.

influent. Water, wastewater, or other liquid flowing into a reservoir, basin, or treatment plant.

information collection request (ICR). A description of information to be gathered in connection with rules, proposed rules, surveys, and guidance documents that contain information-gathering requirements.

information file. In the Superfund program, a file that contains accurate, up-to-date documents on a Superfund site.

infrared. The region of the electromagnetic spectrum with wavelengths longer than visible light but shorter than microwave radiation [0.7 microns (μm) to 300 μm].

infrared spectroscopy. A technique for determining the structure (and sometimes concentration) of molecules by observing how infrared radiation is absorbed by a sample. Also called *IR spectroscopy*.

ingestion. Taking a substance into the body through the mouth.

inhalable particles. All dust capable of entering the human respiratory tract.

inhalation. The breathing in of a substance in the form of a gas, vapor, fume, mist, or dust.

inhalation hazard zone. One of the four hazard zones as designated by lethal concentration (LC_{50}) are:

- *Hazard zone A.* LC_{50} of less than or equal to 200 ppm.
- *Hazard zone B.* LC_{50} greater than 200 ppm and less than or equal to 1,000 ppm.
- *Hazard zone C.* LC_{50} greater than 1,000 ppm and less than or equal to 3,000 ppm.
- *Hazard zone D.* LC_{50} greater than 3,000 ppm and less than or equal to 5,000 ppm.

inhibited. A material containing a small amount of another substance included to prevent the first material from reacting with itself or other things in its environment.

inhibitor. 1. Any substance used to slow down or prevent any chemical reaction. 2. A chemical added to a monomer to prevent polymerization during transportation or storage. 3. Materials used to prevent or slow up the polymerization reaction. 4. May also be called a **stabilizer**. 5. In the polymerization reactor, an initiator (or starter) is used to overcome the inhibitor and start the reaction.

initial attack. The actions taken by the first resources to arrive at a fire to protect lives and property, and prevent further extension of the fire.

initial compliance period (water). The first full three-year compliance period that begins at least 18 months after promulgation.

initiation. The first stage of carcinogenesis.

initiator. A chemical added to a monomer that will overcome the stabilization action of the inhibitor to allow the polymerization reaction to begin. May also be called a *starter*.

injection blow molding. The process by which a parison (or hollow) plastic part is formed by injection molding or extrusion and is then formed by a blast of air forcing the parison into the shape of the mold.

injection molding. The process by which plastic parts are formed by forcing fused or molten resin or compound into a mold by use of a ram and/or reciprocating screw.

injection well. A well into which fluids are injected for purposes such as waste disposal, improved recovery of crude oil, or solution mining.

injection zone. A geological formation receiving fluids through a well.

in-line filtration. Pretreatment method in which chemicals are mixed by the flowing water.

inner transition metals. The elements of the lanthanides and actinides series, which are subseries of the transition metals.

innovative technologies. New or inventive methods to effectively treat hazardous waste and reduce risks to human health and the environment.

innovative treatment technologies. Technologies whose routine use is inhibited by lack of data on performance and cost. *Contrast with* **established treatment technologies**.

inoculum. 1. Bacteria or fungi injected into compost to start biological action. 2. A medium containing organisms, usually bacteria or a virus, that is introduced into cultures or living organisms. 3. Plural form is *inocula*.

inorganic. 1. Pertaining to or composed of chemical compounds that do not contain carbon as the principal element (except carbonates, carbides, carbon oxides, carbon disulfide, cyanides, and cyanates). 2. Matter other than plant or animal.

inorganic acid. Usually called mineral acids. They are ionic in composition, and all contain the hydrogen (H^+) ion. Some are strong acids.

inorganic arsenical. A waterborne wood preservative, such as chromated copper arsenate (CCA), ammoniacal copper arsenate (ACA), and ammoniacal copper zinc arsenate (ACZA).

inorganic chemicals. Chemical substances of mineral origin, not of basically carbon structure.

inorganic compound. 1. Inorganic refers to all those compounds that are not compounds of carbon, with the exception of carbon disulfide, carbides, cyanides, cyanates, the carbon oxides, and the carbon-containing oxysalts. 2. Inorganic chemistry is usually referred to as the chemistry of minerals and compounds made from them. 3. The vast majority of inorganic compounds will not burn.

inorganic peroxides. Inorganic compounds containing the peroxy anion, O_2^{-2}. 2. They are oxidizing agents that give up their oxygen with such ease that they are very dangerous.

inorganic pigments. 1. Natural occurring or synthesized colorants that are ionic in nature. 2. They may be oxides, sulfides, or other salts. 3. They may also be man-made.

inorganic polymer. A polymer without carbon in its backbone.

input heat. In a fire, the amount of heat required to produce the evolution of vapors from a solid or liquid.

insecticide. A pesticide compound specifically used to kill or prevent the growth of harmful insects.

in situ. In its original place. Something unmoved or unexcavated, remaining at the site or in the subsurface.

in-situ flushing. Introduction of large volumes of water, at times supplemented with cleaning compounds, into soil, waste, or groundwater to flush hazardous contaminants from a site.

in-situ oxidation. Technology that oxidizes contaminants dissolved in groundwater, converting them into insoluble compounds.

in-situ stripping. Treatment system that removes or "strips" volatile organic compounds from contaminated groundwater or surface water by forcing an airstream through the water and causing the compounds to evaporate.

in-situ vitrification. Technology that treats contaminated soil in place at extremely high temperatures (3,000°F or higher).

insoluble. A substance that does not dissolve in a solvent to any significant degree (usually less than 1%).

inspection. *See* **original AHERA inspection.**

inspection and maintenance (I/M). 1. Activities to ensure that vehicles' emission controls work properly. 2. Also applies to wastewater treatment plants and other antipollution facilities and processes.

institutional waste. Waste generated at institutions such as schools, libraries, hospitals, and prisons, etc.

instream use. Water use taking place within a stream channel.

insulator. 1. Any material that prevents the flow of electrons. 2. A poor conductor of electricity and heat.

Integrated Emergency Management Information System (IEMIS). A group of related computer programs that provides for text processing, electronic communications, database development and management, modeling of weather information, evacuation dynamics, and graphics display.

integrated emergency management system (IEMS). A long-term, all-hazard concept for improving the development and implementation of emergency management capabilities at the state and local levels.

integrated exposure assessment. Cumulative summation (over time) of the magnitude of exposure to a toxic chemical in all media.

integrated pest management (IPM). A mixture of chemical and other (non-pesticide) methods to control pests.

Integrated Risk Information System (IRIS). An electronic database containing EPA's latest descriptive and quantitative regulatory information on chemical constituents.

integrated waste management. Using a variety of practices to handle municipal solid waste, including source reduction, recycling efforts, incineration, and landfill usage.

interceptor sewers. Large sewer lines that, in a combined system, control the flow of sewage to the treatment plant.

interface. The common boundary between two substances such as a water and a solid, water and a gas, or between two liquids, such as water and oil.

interfacial tension. The strength of the film separating two immiscible fluids (e.g., oil and water) measured in dynes (or millidynes) per centimeter.

interim (permit) status. Period during which treatment, storage, and disposal facilities coming under RCRA in 1980 are temporarily permitted to operate while awaiting a permanent permit. Permits issued under these circumstances are usually called *part A permits* or *part B permits*.

intermediate. 1. A chemical compound that is used in the production of another chemical compound. 2. A chemical that is produced in a chemical reaction and is then further reacted.

internal belly valve. The excess flow valve in a tank truck, designed to close automatically if the external belly valve is sheared off.

internal dose. In exposure assessment, the amount of a substance penetrating the absorption barriers (e.g., skin, lung tissue, and gastrointestinal tract) of an organism through either physical or biological processes. *See also* **absorbed dose.**

internal floater. A liquid bulk storage tank with a roof that moves in relation to the level of liquid within.

International Air Transport Association (IATA). Organization of airline members that have adopted the rules set forth by the International Civil Aviation Organization (ICAO) and other additional requirements that are more restrictive, reflecting industry standard practices or operational considerations.

International Air Transport Association Dangerous Goods Regulations. Rules set forth by the International Air Transport Association (which publishes an annual *Dangerous Goods Regulations* manual) for the transport of dangerous goods by international and domestic air.

International Civil Aviation Organization (ICAO). Organization that sets the standards for international transport of dangerous goods by air.

International Maritime Dangerous Goods (IMDG) Code. Regulatory document that implements the requirements of the IMO.

International Maritime Organization (IMO). Organization that sets the standards for international transport of dangerous goods by vessel.

International Union of Pure and Applied Chemistry (IUPAC). An organization that sets international standards for chemical nomenclature, atomic weights, and the names of newly discovered elements.

interspecies dose conversion. The process of extrapolating from animal doses to human equivalent doses.

interstate carrier water supply. A source of water for drinking and sanitary use on planes, buses, trains, and ships operating in more than one state.

Interstate Commerce Clause. A clause of the U.S. Constitution that reserves to the federal government the right to regulate the conduct of business across state lines.

interstate district. An emergency response planning district with responsibility for facilities in two or more states.

interstate waters. Waters that flow across or form part of state or international boundaries, such as the Great Lakes, the Mississippi River, or coastal waters.

interstitial monitoring. The continuous surveillance of the space between the walls of an underground storage tank.

intracerebral. Inside the brain.

intrastate product. Pesticide products once registered by states for sale and use only in the state.

intubation. Insertion of an endotracheal tube to help an unconscious patient breathe.

intumescent. The property of swelling and producing a cellular surface when exposed to high temperatures.

inventory. Inventory of chemicals produced pursuant to Section 8 (b) of the Toxic Substances Control Act.

inventory form. The tier I or tier II emergency and hazardous chemical inventory form used for hazardous chemical reporting.

inverse square law. The relationship that states that electromagnetic radiation intensity is inversely proportional to the square of the distance from a point source.

inversion. A layer of warm air that prevents the rise of cooling air and traps pollutants beneath it. Can cause an air pollution episode.

in vitro. Testing or action outside an organism (e.g., inside a test tube or culture dish).

iodate ion. 1. Any compound containing the iodate ion (IO_3^{-1}). Derived from iodic acid (HIO_3), it is usually a strong oxidizing agent.

iodine. A toxic, highly corrosive, dark gray to purplish black, solid, nonmetallic element, symbol I, with atomic number 53, and atomic weight 126.9045. It is a member of the halogen family and is a strong oxidizer.

ion. 1. An electrically charged atom or group of atoms. 2. An atom or group of atoms, bound together chemically, that have gained or lost one or more electrons, and that are electrically charged according to how many electrons were gained or lost.

ion exchange treatment. A water-softening method that uses calcium compounds to precipitate out unwanted metals.

ionic. 1. A type of bonding where the parts of the compound are electrically charged and are called *ions*. 2. Ionic bonding differs from covalent bonding in that the parts of an ionic compound (the ions) are held together by the electrostatic attraction of the opposite charges on the ions.

ionic bond. The electrostatic attraction of oppositely charged ions to each other. Also called *electrostatic bond* or *electrovalent bond*.

ionic compound. A chemical combination of oppositely charged ions, held together by the electrostatic attraction of opposite charges.

ionization. 1. The process by which ions are formed. 2. Production of charged particles in a medium. 3. An orbital electron is stripped from a neutral atom or molecule, producing an ion pair (a negatively charged electron and a positively charged atom molecular fragment).

ionization chamber. A device that measures the intensity of ionizing radiation.

ionization energy. The minimum energy needed to remove an electron from an atom.

ionizing radiation. 1. Radiation that can strip electrons from atoms; e.g., alpha, beta, and gamma radiation. 2. Electromagnetic (X-ray and gamma) or particulate (alpha and beta) radiation capable of producing ions or charged particles.

ionomer. A thermoplastic composed mainly of polyethylene; contains both covalent and ionic bonds.

iridium. A brittle, silver-white, solid, metallic element, symbol Ir, with atomic number 77, and atomic weight 192.2.

IRIS. *See* **Integrated Risk Information System**.

iron. A solid metallic element, symbol Fe, with atomic number 26, and atomic weight 55.845. An easily oxidized metal used to make steel.

irradiated food. Food subject to brief radioactivity, usually gamma rays, to kill insects, bacteria, and mold, and to permit storage without refrigeration.

irradiation. 1. Exposure to radiation of wavelengths shorter than those of visible light (gamma, X-ray, or ultraviolet) for medical purposes, to sterilize milk or other foodstuffs, or to induce polymerization of monomers or vulcanization of rubber. 2. Exposure to ionizing radiation.

irreversible effect. Effect characterized by the inability of the body to partially or fully repair injury caused by a toxic agent.

irrigation. Applying water or wastewater to land areas to supply the water and nutrient needs of plants.

irrigation efficiency. The amount of water stored in the crop root zone compared to the amount of irrigation water applied.

irrigation return flow. Surface and subsurface water that leaves the field following application of irrigation water.

irritant. 1. A substance that is not classified as a poison but may cause injury by irritation of the eyes, skin, or mucous membranes. 2. A substance that can cause irritation of the skin, eyes, or respiratory system. Effects may be acute from a single high-level exposure, or chronic from repeated low-level exposures to such compounds as chlorine, nitrogen dioxide, and nitric acid. 3. A chemical that is not corrosive but causes a reversible inflammatory effect on living tissue by chemical action at the site of contact. 4. A chemical is a skin irritant if, when tested on the intact skin of albino rabbits by the methods of 16 CFR 1500.41 for four hours' exposure or by other appropriate techniques, it results in an empirical score of five or more. 5. A chemical is an eye irritant if so determined under the procedure listed in 16 CFR 1500.42 or other appropriate techniques.

irritating materials. Liquids or solid substances that, upon contact with fire or when exposed to air, give off dangerous or intensely irritating fumes, but not any poisonous material of class A poison classification.

IR spectroscopy. *See* **infrared spectroscopy**.

iso-. The prefix (meaning "the same") given to a compound having the same number and kind of atoms as another compound, as in *isomer*.

isoconcentration. More than one sample point exhibiting the same isolate concentration.

isocyanate. A compound containing the isocyanate radical (-NCO).

isocyanide. A compound containing the cyanide radical (-NC) or cyanide ion (CN^{-1}).

isolation. 1. The process of separating a person or thing from others. 2. A method of decontamination in which contaminated equipment and materials are bagged or covered and set aside, usually for subsequent shipment to an approved landfill for disposal.

isomer. One of two or more chemical compounds with the same molecular formula but a different structural formula, possessing different chemical and physical properties.

isopleth. The line or area represented by an isoconcentration.

isopropanol. Legal label name for isopropyl alcohol (2-propanol).

isopropyl alcohol. *See* **rubbing alcohol**.

isopropyl ester (of methylphosphonofluoridic acid). Chemical name for **sarin.**

isopropyl methylphosphanofluoridate. Chemical name for **sarin**.

isotactic. A polymeric molecular structure having a sequence of regularly spaced asymmetric atoms arranged similarly along the polymer chain. *Contrast with* **atactic**.

isotope. 1. A form of the same element, having identical chemical properties, but a different number of neutrons in the nucleus of its atoms. 2. A variation of an element that has the same atomic number of protons but a different weight because of the number of neutrons. Various isotopes of the same element may have different radioactive behaviors, some being highly unstable.

isotropy. The condition in which the hydraulic or other properties of an aquifer are the same in all directions.

-ite. A suffix used to indicate the presence of oxygen in the compound.

Izod. An impact testing device that uses a notched-bar sample of the material to be tested.

J

jar test. A laboratory procedure that simulates a water treatment plant's coagulation/flocculation units with differing chemical doses, mix speeds, and settling times to estimate the minimum or ideal coagulant dose required to achieve certain water quality goals.

jet-A. Aviation fuel commonly referred to as a "type of high-grade kerosene," used primarily in civilian air operations. Fuel used in jet engines and turbine style power plants. Flashpoint is 100°F–150°F (NFPA).

jeweler's rouge. Ferric oxide.

joint and several liability. Under CERCLA, this legal concept relates to the liability for Superfund site cleanup and other costs on the part of more than one potentially responsible party.

joist. A supporting member used in building construction to support a floor, roof, or ceiling.

joule. A unit of energy or work; 1 joule (J) = 1 kg-m^2/s^2.

JP-4. Aviation fuel blending hydrocarbon fuels such as gasoline and kerosene to gain specific characteristics acute to both fuels. Due to the additional hazards associated with this fuel, it is used primarily in military operations. Flashpoint is –10°F to +30°F (NFPA).

jurisdiction. The area over which legal authority extends.

K

kalium. Latin for "potassium," hence the symbol, K.

karst. A geologic formation of irregular limestone deposits within sinks, underground streams, and caverns.

Kelly tool. A firefighter's metal forcible-entry tool similar to the claw tool, but with an adze blade.

Kelvin scale. An absolute temperature scale in which absolute zero is assigned the value zero. One kelvin (denoted simply K, or sometimes in older sources, °K) is the same size as a Celsius degree, so the normal freezing point of water is 273.15 K, and the normal boiling point is 373.15 K. Compare with **Celsius scale**, **Fahrenheit scale**, and **Rankine** scale.

kerosene. A mixture of liquid alkanes that produces a combustible liquid with a flash point between 100°F and 150°F.

ketone. An organic hydrocarbon derivative with the general formula R-CO-R', where the R- is a hydrocarbon radical or backbone, the -R' is either the same hydrocarbon radical, or a different one, and the -C=O is the carbonyl radical.

Kevlar. Special lightweight chemical and fire-resistant clothing material.

kilo-. The prefix that means "one thousand" or 10^3; k.

kilogram. One thousand grams. One kilogram (kg) equals approximately 2.2 pounds.

kilowatt. A unit of electrical power equal to 1,000 watts.

kilowatt-hour. A unit of electrical energy equal to the amount of that consumed by electrical appliances that use 1 kilowatt (kW) for a period of 1 hour (hr); kWh.

kinetic energy. Energy possessed by a moving object or water body.

kinetic molecular theory. 1. A theory that states that all molecules are in constant motion at any temperature above absolute zero. 2. As energy is absorbed by the molecules, their speed of motion or vibration will increase, and as energy is withdrawn, molecular motion will decrease.

kinetic rate coefficient. A number that describes the rate at which a water constituent such as a biochemical oxygen demand or dissolved oxygen rises or falls, or at which an air pollutant reacts.

kinetics. The study of how fast chemical reactions occur and the influence of physical and chemical conditions on these rates.

knockdown. 1. The firefighting activity designed to reduce flame and heat and prevent the danger of further extension of fire. 2. To bring a fire under control.

knot. Unit of speed in navigation; the rate of 1 nautical mile (6,080 feet, 1.15 miles, or 1,852 meters) per hour.

krypton. A nonflammable, gaseous, nonmetallic element, symbol Kr, with atomic number 36, and atomic weight 83.8. It is a member of group VIII on the periodic table of the elements (the inert, or "noble," gases).

L

L. Liter.

label. A written notice of the name and other information about the substance in the container.

laboratory animal studies. Investigations using animals as surrogates for humans.

lachrymation. The excessive tearing of the eyes.

lachrymator. Any material that will cause tearing of the eyes.

lagoon. 1. A shallow pond where sunlight, bacterial action, and oxygen work to purify wastewater. 2. May be used for storage of wastewater or spent nuclear fuel rods. 3. A shallow body of water, often separated from the sea by coral reefs or sandbars.

laminate. A bonding together of two or more layers of materials, usually either all plastic or plastic and nonplastic materials.

lampblack. Carbon.

land application. Discharge of wastewater onto the ground for treatment or reuse.

land ban. Phasing out of land disposal of most untreated hazardous wastes, as mandated by the 1984 RCRA amendments.

land disposal restrictions. Rules that require hazardous wastes to be treated before disposal on land to destroy or immobilize hazardous constituents that might migrate into soil and groundwater.

land farming (of waste). A disposal process in which hazardous waste deposited on or in the soil is degraded naturally by microbes.

landfill, class I. A disposal facility or part of a facility where hazardous waste is placed in or on land and which is not a land treatment facility, surface impoundment, or injection well.

landfills. 1. Sanitary landfills are disposal sites for nonhazardous solid wastes spread in layers, compacted to the smallest practical volume, and covered by material applied at the end of each operating day. 2. Secure chemical landfills are disposal sites for hazardous waste, selected and designed to minimize the chance of release of hazardous substances into the environment.

landscape. 1. The traits, patterns, and structure of a specific geographic area, including its biological composition, its physical environment, and its anthropogenic or social patterns. 2. An area where interacting ecosystems are grouped and repeated in similar form.

landscape characterization. Documentation of the traits and patterns of the essential elements of the landscape.

landscape ecology. The study of the distribution patterns of communities and ecosystems, the ecological processes that affect those patterns, and changes in patterns and processes over time.

landscape indicator. A measurement of the landscape, calculated from mapped or remotely sensed data, used to describe spatial patterns of land use and land cover across a geographic area.

land treatment facility. A facility or part of a facility at which hazardous waste is applied onto or incorporated into the soil surface. Such facilities are disposal facilities if the waste remains after closure.

Langelier Index (LI). An index reflecting the equilibrium pH of a water with respect to calcium and alkalinity; used in stabilizing water to control both corrosion and scale deposition.

lanthanides. 1. Of the rare earth metals, the 14 elements of the upper row on the inner transition metals on the periodic table that follow the element lanthanum (#57 to #71). 2. For all of these elements, the filling orbital is 4f. 3. This series is a subseries of the transition metals.

lanthanum. A solid metallic element, symbol La, with atomic number 57, and atomic weight 138.91. It is a rare earth metal.

large quantity generator. Person or facility generating more than 2,200 pounds of hazardous waste per month.

large water system. A water system that services more than 50,000 customers.

laser-induced fluorescence. A method for measuring the relative amount of soil and/or groundwater with an in-situ sensor.

latency. Time from the first exposure of a chemical until the appearance of a toxic effect or the development of a disease.

latency period. The time between first exposure to an agent and manifestation or detection of a health effect of interest.

latent heat. The amount of energy liberated or absorbed when a substance changes state.

latent heat of fusion. *See* **heat of fusion**.

latent heat of vaporization. The amount of heat a substance must absorb when it changes from a liquid to a vapor or gas. *See* **heat of vaporization**.

lateral sewers. Pipes that run under city streets and receive the sewage from homes and businesses, as opposed to domestic feeders and main trunk lines.

latex. A water dispersion of a polymeric material.

laughing gas. Nitrous oxide (N_2O).

laundering weir. Sedimentation basin overflow weir.

lawrencium. A solid, radioactive, metallic element, symbol Lr, with atomic number 103, and atomic weight 256.

lay-up molding. A process whereby fluid resin is applied to a layer of reinforcing material, cured, and then formed with or without the use of pressure.

LC_{50}. *See* **lethal concentration**.

LD_{50}. *See* **lethal dose**.

LD_{Lo}. *See* **lethal dose low**.

leachate. Water that collects contaminants as it trickles through wastes, pesticides, or fertilizers. Leaching may occur in farming areas, feedlots, and landfills, and may result in hazardous substances entering surface water, groundwater, or soil.

leachate collection system. A system that gathers leachate and pumps it to the surface for treatment.

leaching. The process by which soluble constituents are dissolved and filtered through the soil by a percolating fluid. *See also* **leachate**.

lead. A solid metallic element, symbol Pb, with atomic number 82, and atomic weight 207.2. A heavy metal that is hazardous to health if breathed or swallowed. Its use in gasoline, paints, and plumbing compounds has been sharply restricted or eliminated by federal laws and regulations. *See also* **heavy metals**.

lead service line. A service line made of lead that connects the water to the building inlet and any lead fitting connected to it.

LED_{10}. *See* **lower limit on effective dose**.

Legionella. A genus of bacteria, some species of which have caused a type of pneumonia called Legionnaires' disease.

lethal concentration. 1. A standard measure of toxicity. 2. The concentration of gas or smoke that will produce lethality in 50% of the test animals within a specified exposure and postexposure time (LC_{50}).

3. The amount of gases, vapors, fumes, dusts, and other particulates that will cause death to half the test animals exposed to the material within a specified time.

lethal dose. 1. The dose of a toxicant or microbe that will kill 50% of the test organisms within a designated period. The lower the lethal dose (LD_{50}), the more toxic the compound. 2. The weight of product, relative to body weight of the animal, that will produce lethality in 50% of the test animals within a specified exposure and post-exposure time. 3. The amount of material, usually expressed as milligrams per kilogram of body weight (mg/kg), that will cause death to half the test animals to which the material was administered (usually fed) during the test period, usually 14 days.

lethal dose low. The lowest dose in an animal study at which lethality occurs; LD_{Lo}.

leukocyte. A white blood cell.

level of concern (LOC). The concentration of an extremely hazardous substance (EHS) in air above which there may be serious irreversible health effects or death as a result of a single exposure for a relatively short time.

level of incidents. There are three general levels of incidents:

- *Level one incident.* Hazardous materials incidents that can be correctly contained, extinguished, and/or abated utilizing equipment, supplies, and resources immediately available to first responders having jurisdiction, and whose qualifications are limited to and do not exceed the scope of training as explained in 29 CFR 1910, with reference to "first responder, operational level."

- *Level two incident.* Hazardous materials incidents that can only be identified, tested, sampled, contained, extinguished, and/or abated utilizing the resources of a hazardous materials response team (HMRT), which requires the use of specialized chemical protective clothing, and whose qualifications are explained in 29 CFR 1910, with reference to "hazardous materials, technician level."

- *Level three incident.* A hazardous materials incident that is beyond the controlling capabilities of an HMRT (technician or specialist level) whose qualifications are explained in 29 CFR 1910; and/or requires the use of two or more HMRTs, and/or must be additionally assisted by qualified specialty teams or individuals.

level of protection. Personal protective equipment is divided into four categories based on the degree of protection afforded:

- *Level A.* The greatest level of skin, respiratory, and eye protection. A totally encapsulating chemical protective suit, meaning a full body garment that is constructed of protective clothing materials, covers the wearer's torso, head, arms, and legs, has boots and gloves that may be an integral part of the suit, or separate and tightly attached, and completely encloses the wearer in combination with the wearer's respiratory equipment. All components of a totally encapsulating chemical protective (TECP) suit, such as relief valves, seams, and enclosure assemblies, should provide equivalent chemical resistance protection.

- *Level B.* The highest level of respiratory protection necessary, but a lesser level of skin protection is needed. Often referred to as a *splash suit.*

- *Level C.* The concentration(s) and type(s) of airborne substances(s) are known, and the criteria for using air purifying respirators are met. Level C protection is more common in industry than emergency response.

- *Level D.* A work uniform affording minimal protection, used for nuisance contamination only. Should be used only when the atmosphere contains no known hazard.

Lewis dot formula. *See* **dot method**.

lewisite. A vesicant or blister agent ($C_2H_2AsCl_3$). Agent L.

life cycle of a product. All stages of a product's development, from extraction of fuel for power to production, marketing, use, and disposal.

life-safety. The joint consideration of both the life and the well-being of the population.

lifetime average daily dose. A figure for estimating excess lifetime cancer risk.

lifetime exposure. Total amount of exposure to a substance that a human would receive in a lifetime (usually assumed to be 70 years).

lift. In a sanitary landfill, a compacted layer of solid waste and the top layer of cover material.

lifting station. *See* **pumping station**.

light-emitting diode (LED). A long-lasting illumination technology, used for exit signs, that requires very little power.

light nonaqueous phase liquid (LNAPL). A nonaqueous phase liquid with a specific gravity less than 1.0. Because the specific gravity of water is 1.0, most LNAPLs float on top of the water table. Most common petroleum hydrocarbon fuels and lubricating oils are LNAPLs.

lime. Calcium oxide (CaO).

limestone scrubbing. Use of a limestone and water solution to remove gaseous stack-pipe sulfur before it reaches the atmosphere.

limewater. A saturated aqueous solution of calcium hydroxide; $Ca(OH)_2$.

limited access zone. *See* **warm zone.**

limited degradation. An environmental policy permitting some degradation of natural systems but terminating at a level well beneath an established health standard.

limited evidence. A term used in evaluating study data for the classification of a carcinogen by the 1986 U.S. EPA guidelines for carcinogen risk assessment.

limiting factor. A condition that if absent, or present in excessive concentrations, is incompatible with the needs or tolerance of a species or population. It may have a negative influence on their ability to thrive.

limiting oxygen index (LOI). The minimum concentration of oxygen in the atmosphere necessary for sustained combustion. A material with an LOI of more than 21 should not burn in air at room temperature.

limit of detection (LOD). The minimum concentration of a substance being analyzed that has a 99% probability of being identified.

limnology. The study of the physical, chemical, hydrological, and biological aspects of freshwater bodies.

lindane. A pesticide that causes adverse health effects in domestic water supplies and is toxic to freshwater fish and aquatic life.

linear. The molecular structure characterized by a straight, branchless chain. *Contrast with* **branched**.

linear dose response. A pattern of frequency or severity of biological response that varies proportionately with the amount of dose of an agent.

linearized multistage procedure. A modification of the multistage model, used for estimating carcinogenic risk, that incorporates a linear upper bound on extra risk for exposures below the experimental range.

linear polymer. A polymer that has the appearance of a chain, with little or no side branching.

liner. 1. A relatively impermeable barrier designed to keep leachate inside a landfill. Liner materials include plastic and dense clay. 2. An insert or sleeve for sewer pipes to prevent leakage or infiltration.

lipid solubility. The maximum concentration of a chemical that will dissolve in fatty substances. Lipid-soluble substances are insoluble in water. They will very selectively disperse through the environment via uptake in living tissue.

liquefaction. Changing a solid into a liquid.

liquefied gas. A gas that has been converted to a liquid by pressure and/or cooling.

liquid. A fluid with a vapor pressure no higher than 40 pounds per square inch absolute (psia).

liquid crystal. A substance that has liquidlike long-range disorder, but some crystallike aspects of short-range order.

liquid injection incinerator. Commonly used system that relies on high pressure to prepare liquid wastes for incineration by breaking them up into tiny droplets to allow easier combustion.

liquid petroleum gas (LPG). A group of easily liquefied hydrocarbon gases; the most common are propane and butane. Less common are: 1-butene, 2-butene, isobutane, isobutylene, and propylene.

liquid splash-protective ensemble. Multiple elements designed to provide a degree of protection for emergency response personnel from adverse exposure to the inherent risks of liquid-chemical exposure occurring during hazardous materials (hazmat) emergencies and similar operations. The liquid splash-protective ensemble is either an encapsulating or nonencapsulating ensemble [National Fire Protection Association (NFPA) Standard # 1992].

listed waste. Wastes listed as hazardous under RCRA but that have not been subjected to the toxic characteristics listing process because the dangers they present are considered self-evident.

liter. The volume of 1,000 g (1 kg) of water at 4°C. One liter (L) equals 1.05 quarts, or 0.26 gallons.

litharge. Yellow lead(II) oxide (PbO).

lithium. A soft, silvery white, solid, metallic element, symbol Li, with atomic number 3, and atomic weight 6.941. It is the lightest of the alkali metals and extremely water-reactive.

lithology. The branch of mineralogy that deals with grain size, texture, and other physical properties of granular soil, sediment, or rock.

lithopone. An inorganic white pigment used in plastics made from barium sulfate, zinc oxide, and zinc sulfide.

lithosphere. The outer, rigid shell of the Earth, containing the Earth's crust, continents, and plates.

litmus paper. Paper impregnated with litmus, usually cut in narrow strips. Dipping red litmus paper into a basic solution turns it blue, and dipping blue litmus paper into an acidic solution turns it red.

litter. 1. The highly visible portion of solid waste carelessly discarded outside the regular garbage and trash collection and disposal system. 2. Leaves and twigs fallen from forest trees.

littoral zone. 1. That portion of a body of fresh water extending from the shoreline lakeward to the limit of occupancy of rooted plants. 2. A strip of land along the shoreline between the high and low water levels.

loading level. The amount of additive added to a plastics compound.

loading valve. Any valve used to bring product into a tank; may be located anywhere on the tank.

local education agency (LEA). In the asbestos program, an educational agency at the local level that exists primarily to operate schools or to contract for educational services, including primary and secondary public and private schools.

local emergency planning committee (LEPC). A committee appointed by the state emergency response commission (SERC), as required by SARA Title III, to formulate a comprehensive emergency plan for its jurisdiction.

lockout. A procedure to prevent use of any equipment that should not be used, generally tagged and locked closed or off.

long ton. A unit of weight in the UK that equals 1,016 kg or 2,240 pounds.

low-angle rescue. *See* **rope rescue**.

low density polyethylene (LDPE). Plastic material used for both rigid containers and plastic film applications.

low emissivity (low-E) windows. New window technology that lowers the amount of energy loss through windows by inhibiting the transmission of radiant heat while still allowing sufficient light to pass through.

lower detection limit. The smallest signal above background noise an instrument can reliably detect.

lower explosive limit (LEL). 1. The concentration of a compound in air below which the mixture will not ignite. 2. The minimum concentration of gas or vapor in air below which it is not possible to ignite the vapors. 3. Also called the **lower flammable limit (LFL)**.

lower flammable limit (LFL). 1. The minimum percentage of gas or vapor in air below which ignition will not occur (the mixture is too lean). 2. Also called the **lower explosive limit (LEL)**.

lower limit on effective dose. The 95% lower confidence limit of the dose of a chemical needed to produce an adverse effect in 10% of those subjects exposed to the chemical, relative to control; LED_{10}.

lowest acceptable daily dose (LADD). The largest quantity of a chemical that will not cause a toxic effect, as determined by animal studies.

lowest achievable emission rate (LAER). Under the Clean Air Act, the rate of emissions that reflects whichever is more stringent of the following:

1. The most stringent emission limitation in the implementation plan of any state for such source unless the owner or operator demonstrates such limitations are not achievable.
2. The most stringent emissions limitation achieved in practice. A proposed new or modified source may not emit pollutants in excess of existing new source standards.

lowest effect level (LEL). *See* **lowest observed effect level.**

lowest observed adverse effect level (LOAEL). The lowest level of a stressor that causes statistically and biologically significant differences in test samples as compared to other samples subjected to no stressor.

lowest observed effect level (LOEL). In a study, the lowest dose or exposure level at which a statistically or biologically significant effect is observed in the exposed population compared with an appropriate unexposed control group.

low explosive. 1. Explosives that usually deflagrate and do not usually detonate unless confined. 2. Also called **propellants**.

low-level radioactive waste (LLRW). Wastes less hazardous than most of those associated with a nuclear reactor; generated by hospitals, research laboratories, and certain industries.

low-NO_x burners. One of several combustion technologies used to reduce emissions of nitrogen oxides (NO_x).

low-pressure container. A container designed to withstand pressures from 5 to 100 psi.

LPG. *See* **liquid petroleum gas**.

lubricant. Any material that reduces friction between two surfaces.

lumber. Logs that have been sawed into boards, planks, or structural members, such as beams.

lumen. A unit used to measure how much light is being produced.

lutetium. A silvery white, solid, metallic element, symbol Lu, with atomic number 71, and atomic weight 174.97. It is a lanthanide rare earth metal.

lye. A strong solution of sodium hydroxide (NaOH) or potassium hydroxide solution (KOH) in water.

M

m. Meter.

macromolecule. The giant molecule formed by polymerization.

macropores. Secondary soil features such as root holes or desiccation cracks that can create significant conduits for movement of nonaqueous phase liquids (NAPL) and dissolved contaminants, or vapor-phase contaminants.

magazine. A special storage area, room, or container that is used to store explosives.

magnesia. Magnesium oxide.

magnesium. A light, silvery white, solid, metallic element, symbol Mg, with atomic number 12, and atomic weight 24.305. It burns with a brilliant white light.

magnetic separation. Use of magnets to separate ferrous materials from a mixed municipal waste stream.

main charge. *See* **high explosive**.

main group elements. 1. The elements of the tall groups on the periodic table, excluding the transition elements and the rare earth elements. 2. Those elements of the groups with an "A" after the Roman numeral. 3. The vertical columns headed by hydrogen, beryllium, boron, carbon, nitrogen, oxygen, fluorine, and helium. 4. Also known as the *representative elements.*

main-line valve. A device that controls air flow to the regulator on supplied-air respirators.

majors. Publicly owned treatment works with flows of 1 million gallons or more per day. *Contrast with* **minors**.

malignant tumor. An abnormal growth of tissue that can invade adjacent or distant tissues.

malleable. The property of being able to be hammered into sheets. Metals are typical malleable materials.

management plan. Under the Asbestos Hazard Emergency Response Act (AHERA), a document that each local education agency (LEA) is required to prepare, describing all activities planned and undertaken by a school to comply with AHERA regulations, including building inspections to identify asbestos-containing materials, response actions, and operations and maintenance programs to minimize the risk of exposure.

managerial controls. Methods of nonpoint source pollution control based on decisions about managing agricultural wastes or application times or rates for agrochemicals.

mandatory recycling. Programs that by law require consumers to separate trash so that some or all recyclable materials are recovered for recycling rather than going to landfills.

manganese. A brittle, grayish white, solid, metallic element, symbol Mn, with atomic number 25, and atomic weight 54.938. It is used to alloy steel.

manifest. 1. A document containing a full list of a ship's cargo, extracted from the bills of lading. 2. A one-page form used by haulers transporting waste that lists EPA identification numbers, type, and quantity of waste, the generator from which it originated, the transporter that shipped it, and the storage or disposal facility to which it is being shipped. It includes copies for all participants in the shipping process.

manifest system. Tracking of hazardous waste from generation through disposal with accompanying documents known as *manifests*. Also called **cradle-to-grave system**.

man-made beta particle and photon emitters. All anthropogenic radionuclides emitting beta particles and/or photons listed in *Maximum Permissible Body Burdens and Maximum Permissible Concentrations of Radionuclides in Air and Water for Occupational Exposure*.

mannitol. A natural sugar that acts as a diuretic, used in cases of drug overdoses and cerebral swelling.

manual separation. Hand sorting of recyclable or compostable materials in waste.

manufacture. 1. To produce, prepare, import, or compound a chemical, raw material, or product. 2. Also applies to substances that are produced coincidentally during the manufacture, processing, use, or disposal of another substance or mixture, including by-products and coproducts that are separated from that other substance or mixture, and impurities that remain in that substance or mixture.

manufacturer's formulation. A list of substances or component parts as described by the maker of a coating, pesticide, or other product containing chemicals or other substances.

manufacturing use product. Any product intended (labeled) for formulation or repackaging into other pesticide products.

manway. A large opening in the top of a railroad tank car that allows access to the interior of the tank.

marble. Calcium carbonate.

margin of exposure (MOE). 1. The ratio of the no-observed-adverse-effect level to the estimated exposure dose. 2. The LED_{10} or other point of departure divided by the actual or projected environmental exposure of interest.

margin of safety (MOS). Maximum amount of exposure producing no measurable effect in animals (or studied humans) divided by the actual amount of human exposure in a population.

marine sanitation device. Any equipment or process installed on board a vessel to receive, retain, treat, or discharge sewage.

marsh. A type of wetland that does not accumulate appreciable peat deposits and is dominated by herbaceous vegetation; may be either fresh or saltwater, tidal or nontidal.

marsh gas. Methane (CH_4).

mass. 1. The quantity of matter contained in a particle, body, or substance. 2. Mass is constant throughout the universe, while weight is dependent on gravitational force.

mass balance. An accumulation of the annual quantities of chemicals transported to or from a facility; produced, consumed, used, accumulated, or released at a facility; or transported from a facility as a waste or as a commercial product or by-product component of a commercial product or by-product.

mass burning rate. Mass loss per unit time by materials burning under specified conditions (ASTM E 176).

mass explosion. An explosion that affects almost all of the explosive material present virtually instantaneously.

mass median aerodynamic diameter (MMAD). Median of the distribution of airborne particle mass with respect to the aerodynamic diameter.

mass number. The sum of the numbers of protons and neutrons in an atom.

mass percentage. The concentration of a component in a mixture or an element in a compound; (w/w)%.

mass spectrometer. An instrument that measures the masses and relative abundances of a sample that has been vaporized and ionized.

mass spectrometry. A method for experimentally determining isotopic masses and isotopic abundances. The mass of the ions can be determined, and the relative number of ions (the isotopic abundance) can be determined. Also called *mass spectroscope of elements*.

masterbatch. 1. A plastics compound containing a very high concentration of an active ingredient. 2. Also an old term for rubber compounds containing a very high concentration of an active ingredient. 3. Also called **concentrate**.

material category. In the asbestos program, broad classification of materials into thermal surfacing insulation, surfacing material, and miscellaneous material.

material safety data sheet (MSDS). 1. A compilation of information required under the OSHA Communication Standard on the identity of hazardous chemicals, health, and physical hazards, exposure limits, and precautions. 2. Section 311 of SARA requires facilities to submit MSDSs under certain circumstances. 3. A nonuniform document that must contain, at a minimum, certain information about a substance. 4. It must be provided by all manufacturers, distributors, and importers of hazardous materials (as defined by the OSHA Hazard Communication Standard) to all nonretail users of the substance. 5. By law, the MSDS must contain certain information describing the hazardous properties of the substance.

materials recovery facility (MRF). A facility that processes residentially collected mixed recyclables into new products available for market.

material type. Classification of suspect material by its specific use or application.

matter. Anything that has mass and occupies space.

maximally exposed individual. The person with the highest exposure in a given population. Also called *most exposed individual.*

maximum acceptable toxic concentration. For a given ecological effects test, the range (or geometric mean) between the no-observable-adverse-effect level (NOAEL) and the lowest observable adverse effect level (LOAEL).

maximum available control technology (MACT). The emission standard for sources of air pollution requiring the maximum reduction of hazardous emissions, taking cost and feasibility into account, as defined in the Clean Air Act Amendments of 1990.

maximum contaminant level (MCL). The maximum permissible level of a contaminant in water delivered to any user of a public system.

maximum contaminant level goal (MCLG). Under the Safe Drinking Water Act, a nonenforceable concentration of a drinking water contaminant, set at the level at which no known or anticipated adverse effects on human health occur and that allows an adequate safety margin.

maximum exposure range. Estimate of exposure or dose level received by an individual in a defined population that is greater than the 98th percentile dose for all individuals in that population, but less than the exposure level received by the person receiving the highest exposure level.

maximum likelihood estimate (MLE). *See* **maximum likelihood method**.

maximum likelihood (ML) method. Statistical method for estimating model parameters. Generally provides a mean or central tendency estimate, as opposed to a confidence limit on the estimate.

maximum residue level. Comparable to a U.S. tolerance level, the maximum residue level is the enforceable limit on food pesticide levels in some countries.

maximum safe storage temperature (MSST). The highest storage temperature for specific chemicals such as organic peroxides. Temperatures above this level may result in slow decomposition or explosion.

maximum tolerated dose. The maximum dose that an animal species can tolerate for a major portion of its lifetime without significant impairment or toxic effect other than carcinogenicity.

mean lethal dose. The dose of chemical that will kill 50% of exposed, unprotected, and untreated personnel.

measurement endpoint. *See* **measure of effect.**

measure of effect. A measurable characteristic of an ecological entity that can be related to an assessment endpoint.

measure of exposure. A measurable characteristic of a stressor used to help quantify the exposure of an ecological entity or individual organism.

mechanical aeration. Use of mechanical energy to inject air into water to cause a waste stream to absorb oxygen.

mechanical foam. A substance introduced into the water line by various means at a specified concentration, after which air is then introduced to yield a firefighting foam.

mechanical separation. Using mechanical means to separate waste into various components.

mechanical turbulence. Random irregularities of fluid motion in air caused by buildings or other nonthermal processes.

media. Specific environments, such as air, water, and soil, that are the subject of regulatory concern and activities.

median tolerance unit. A designation of a toxic material's concentration at which 50% of the test subjects, usually aquatic, survive; TL_m. Sometimes called *medium tolerance unit.*

medical surveillance. A periodic comprehensive review of a worker's health status.

medical waste. Any solid waste generated in the diagnosis, treatment, or immunization of human beings or animals, in research pertaining thereto, or in the production or testing of biologicals, excluding hazardous waste identified or listed under 40 CFR Part 261 or any household waste as defined in 40 CFR Subsection 261.4 (b)(1).

medium-size water system. A water system that serves 3,300 to 50,000 customers.

mega-. The prefix meaning "multiply by 10^6"; M.

megawatt. A unit of electrical power equal to 1,000,000 watts; MW.

meitnerium. A synthetic, radioactive, metallic element, symbol Mt, with atomic number 109, and atomic weight 266.

melt index. 1. The measurement of the amount of a material that can be forced through a particular opening (0.0825 in.) by a specific weight (2,160 g) in a specified time (10 min) at a specified temperature (190°C or 374°F) (ASTM D 1238). 2. It is a measurement of the viscosity of a thermoplastic polymer.

melting. A solid turning into a liquid. *See also* **heat of fusion.**

melting point. The temperature at which a solid turns to a liquid.

mendelevium. A synthetic, radioactive, metallic element, symbol Md, with atomic number 101, and atomic weight 258.

meniscus. The curved top of a column of liquid in a small tube.

-mer. The repeating molecular unit in any polymer.

mercaptan. 1. A class of chemicals resembling alcohols, but having the oxygen in the hydroxyl radical replaced by sulfur. 2. The general formula is R-SH, where the R- is a hydrocarbon radical. 3. Most members of this chemical class are flammable, toxic, and have strong odors. 4. Also called **thiols**.

mercury. 1. A bright, silvery, liquid, metallic element, symbol Hg, with atomic number 80, and atomic weight 200.59. 2. It is a heavy metal that can accumulate in the environment and is highly toxic if breathed or swallowed. 3. Also called *quicksilver*.

mesosphere. The region immediately between the stratosphere and the thermosphere from about 31 miles high to about 50 miles high.

mesotrophic. Reservoirs and lakes that contain moderate quantities of nutrients and are moderately productive in terms of aquatic animal and plant life.

meta-. A term that refers to a particular arrangement of functional groups attached to a particular molecule.

metabolism. The chemical reactions that go on in the body to provide the energy and nutrients to maintain life.

metabolites. Any substances produced by biological processes, such as those from pesticides.

metalimnion. The middle layer of a thermally stratified lake or reservoir. Also called a **thermocline**.

metalizing. The application of a thin coating of metal to a nonmetallic surface.

metallic. 1. As in metallic compounds, these are salts that contain a metal ion and a simple or complex nonmetal ion. 2. All salts are inorganic metallic compounds.

metallic bonding. The electrostatic bonding within metals due to the electrical attraction of positively charged metal ions for mobile electrons that belong to the crystalline structure as a whole.

metallic compounds. Compounds that contain at least one metallic element.

metallic hydroxides. Ionic compounds that contain a metallic (or the ammonium) ion and the hydroxide ion.

metallization. The process by which metal particles are deposited permanently on the surface of another material.

metalloids. 1. Elements with properties intermediate between metals and nonmetals. 2. Boron, silicon, germanium, arsenic, antimony, tellurium, and polonium. 3. They are now are called **semiconductors**. 4. Some lists include carbon, selenium, and phosphorus.

metallurgy. The science of extracting metals from their ores, or of purifying metals.

metals. 1. The elements to the left of and below the line on the periodic table of the elements. 2. Metallic elements lose electrons easily to form cations. 3. About 80% of the known chemical elements are metals.

metastasis. The dissemination or secondary growth of a malignant tumor at a site distant from the primary tumor.

meteorology. The science of the atmosphere, its direct effects upon the Earth's surface, and the weather.

meter. Unit of length in the metric system; 1 meter (m) is equal to approximately 39.37 in.

methane. 1. A colorless, nontoxic, flammable gas (CH_4) created by the anaerobic decomposition of organic compounds. 2. A major component of natural gas used in the home.

methanol. 1. Methyl alcohol (CH_3OH). 2. An alcohol that can be used as an alternative fuel or as a gasoline additive. It is less volatile than gasoline, and when blended with gasoline, it lowers the carbon monoxide emissions but increases hydrocarbon emissions. Toxic to humans and animals if ingested.

methemoglobin. An abnormal form of hemoglobin that will not carry oxygen in the blood.

Method 18. An EPA test method that uses gas chromatographic techniques to measure the concentration of volatile organic compounds in a gas stream.

Method 24. An EPA reference method to determine density, water content, and total volatile content (water and VOC) of coatings.

Method 25. An EPA reference method to determine the VOC concentration in a gas stream.

method detection limit (MDL). *See* **limit of detection.**

methoxychlor. Pesticide that causes adverse health effects in domestic water supplies and is toxic to freshwater and marine aquatic life.

methyl. The hydrocarbon radical ($-CH_3$), formed by removing one hydrogen from methane (CH_4).

methyldichloroarsine. A vesicant or blister agent; agent MD.

methylene. The hydrocarbon radical ($-CH_2$) formed by removing two hydrogens from methane (CH_4).

methyl methacrylate (MMA). The monomer of polymethyl methacrylate (PMMA). Its formula is $CH_2=CCH_3COOCH_3$.

methyl orange alkalinity. A measure of the total alkalinity in a water sample in which the color of methyl orange reflects the change in level.

methylphosphonofluoridic acid. A chemical name for sarin; *see also* **sarin.**

metric ton. A unit of weight equal to 1,000 kilograms or 2,204.6 pounds.

micro-. The prefix meaning "one millionth of" (10^{-6}); μ.

microbial growth. The amplification or multiplication of microorganisms such as bacteria, algae, diatoms, plankton, and fungi.

microbial pesticide. A microorganism that is used to kill a pest but is of minimum toxicity to humans.

microclimate. 1. Localized climate conditions within an urban area or neighborhood. 2. The climate around a tree or shrub or a stand of trees.

microenvironmental method. A method for sequentially assessing exposure for a series of microenvironments that can be approximated by constant concentrations of a stressor.

microenvironments. Well-defined surroundings such as the home, office, or kitchen that can be treated as uniform in terms of stressor concentration.

microgram. One millionth of a gram (10^{-6}); μg.

micrometer. One millionth of a meter (10^{-6}); μm. Also called a *micron.*

micron. *See* **micrometer.**

microwave. Electromagnetic radiation with wavelength between 3 mm and 30 cm.

migration. *See* **bleeding.**

mil. One thousandth (10^{-3} or 0.001) of an inch.

milk of magnesia. An aqueous suspension of magnesium hydroxide, $Mg(OH)_2$.

milli-. Prefix used in the SI system meaning "one thousandth of" (10^{-3}); m.

milliampere. One thousandth of an ampere.

millibar. One thousandth of a bar.

milligram. One thousandth of a gram; mg.

milliliter. One thousandth of a liter (10^{-3}). One milliliter (mL) is equal to 1 cubic centimeter (cc).

millimeter. One thousandth of a meter, or 0.03937 in. One inch equals 25.4 millimeters (mm).

millimicron. One thousandth of a micron, or 1 nanometer (10^{-9} meter); mμ.

million gallons per day (MGD). A measure of water flow.

mineral acid. 1. An acid that ionizes in water, usually called an inorganic acid, as opposed to organic acids, which do not ionize in water. 2. Mineral acids are generally more corrosive than organic acids at the same concentration. Examples of mineral acids are sulfuric, nitric, hydrochloric, hydrofluoric, hydrobromic, hydriodic, perchloric, and phosphoric acids, among many others.

mineral oil. Any oil distilled from a mineral, usually from petroleum.

minimization. A comprehensive program to minimize or eliminate wastes, usually applied to wastes at their point of origin.

mining of an aquifer. Withdrawal, over a period of time, of groundwater that exceeds the rate of recharge of the aquifer.

mining waste. Residues resulting from the extraction of raw materials from the Earth.

minors. Publicly owned treatment works with flows less than 1 million gallons per day. *Contrast with* **majors**.

minor source. New emissions sources or modifications to existing emissions sources that do not exceed NAAQS emission levels.

miscellaneous asbestos-containing material (ACM). Interior asbestos-containing building material or structural components, members, or fixtures, such as floor and ceiling tiles. Does not include surfacing materials or thermal system insulation.

miscellaneous materials. Interior building materials on structural components, such as floor or ceiling tiles.

miscibility. 1. The ability of a liquid to dissolve in another liquid. 2. Under some circumstances, it may mean that a material mixes readily with water. 3. It may also refer to solids that may not be able to be evenly mixed together.

miscible. Two or more materials that can be mixed and will remain mixed under normal conditions.

missed detection. The situation that occurs when a test indicates that a tank is "tight," when in fact, it is leaking.

mist. Liquid particles measuring 40 to 500 micrometers (μm) that are formed by condensation of vapor. By comparison, fog particles are smaller than 40 μm.

mitigation. 1. Measures taken to reduce adverse impacts on the environment. 2. The act of trying to control a situation so that the outcome will be positive, or at least less negative than the current situation.

mixed funding. Settlements in which potentially responsible parties and EPA share the cost of a response action.

mixed glass. Recovered container glass not sorted into categories, such as color or grade.

mixed liquor. A mixture of activated sludge and water containing organic matter undergoing activated sludge treatment in an aeration tank.

mixed metals. Recovered metals not sorted into categories such as aluminum, tin, or steel cans or ferrous or nonferrous metals.

mixed municipal waste. Solid waste that has not been sorted into specific categories, such as plastic, glass, or yard trimmings.

mixed paper. Recovered paper not sorted into categories such as old magazines, old newspapers, or old corrugated boxes, etc.

mixed plastic. Recovered plastic that is unsorted by category.

mixture. 1. A substance made up of two or more compounds, physically mixed together. 2. A mixture may also contain elements and compounds mixed together, or elements mixed together. 3. A heterogeneous association of substances where the various individual substances retain their identities and can usually be separated by mechanical means. Includes solutions or compounds but does not include alloys or amalgams.

Mobile Air Transportable Telecommunications System (MATTS). System deployed to disaster sites to reestablish emergency communications.

Mobile Emergency Response System (MERS). System deployed to disaster sites to provide on-site management of disaster response activities.

mobile incinerator systems. Hazardous waste incinerators that can be transported from one site to another.

mobile source. Any nonstationary source of air pollution such as cars, trucks, motorcycles, buses, airplanes, and locomotives.

modacrylic. Any synthetic fiber containing more than 35% but less than 85% acrylonitrile (CH_2=CHCN).

mode. Any of the following transportation methods: rail, highway, air, or water.

model. A mathematical function with parameters that can be adjusted so the function closely describes a set of empirical data.

model plant. A hypothetical plant design used for developing economic, environmental, and energy impact analyses as support for regulations or regulatory guidelines.

modified bin method. Way of calculating the required heating or cooling for a building based on determining how much energy the system would use if outdoor temperatures were within a certain temperature interval and then multiplying the energy use by the time the temperature interval typically occurs.

modified source. An increase in a major stationary pollutant source. The enlargement of a major stationary pollutant source is often referred to as *modification*, implying that more emissions will occur.

modifying factor (MF). A factor used in the derivation of a reference dose or reference concentration.

moiety. A characteristic portion of a molecule.

moisture content. 1.The amount of water lost from soil upon drying to a constant weight, expressed as the weight per unit of dry soil or as the volume of water per unit bulk volume of the soil. For a fully saturated medium, moisture content indicates the porosity. 2. Water equivalent of snow on the ground; an indicator of snowmelt flood potential. 3. The weight of water contained in wood, expressed as a percentage of the oven-dried weight of the wood.

molality. The number of moles of solute dissolved in 1 kilogram (kg) of solvent; m. *Contrast with* **molarity**.

molarity. 1. The number of moles of a solute dissolved in a liter of solvent; M. 2. Molality is represented by a lower-case "m," whereas molarity is represented by an upper-case "M" (sometimes italicized). *Contrast with* **molality**.

molar mass. 1. The unit that enables scientists to calculate the weight of any chemical substance, whether it is an element or a compound. 2. Molar mass is the sum of all of the atomic masses in a formula.

mold. To shape a plastic by confining it in a closed cavity.

mole. 1. The basic unit of measurement in chemistry. 2. By definition, 1 mole (mol) represents the number of carbon atoms in exactly 12 g of carbon-12 (^{12}C). 3. One mole of molecules has a mass equal to the molecular weight of the compound in grams.

molecular formula. 1. The use of chemical symbols to show what atoms (or ions) and how many of them are present in a compound. 2. A method of representing a molecule by a written formula, listing which atoms and how many of them are in the molecule, without showing how they are bonded to each other. *See also* **chemical formula**.

molecular mass. The sum of the atomic masses of all the atoms in the molecule.

molecular orbital (MO). An orbital (or ring) resulting from overlap and mixing of atomic orbitals (or rings) on different atoms. An MO belongs to the molecule as a whole, rather than to individual atoms.

molecular orbital theory. 1. The theory of chemical bonding based upon the existence of molecular orbitals. 2. A combination of atomic orbitals on those atoms that make up the molecule.

molecular sieve. A material that contains many small cavities interconnected with pores of precisely uniform size.

molecular weight. 1. The total weight of a molecule, calculated by adding up the atomic weights of all the atoms in the molecule. 2. Also known as *formula weight*.

molecule. 1. The smallest particle of a covalent compound that can still be identified as that compound. 2. The smallest division of a compound that still retains or exhibits all the properties of the substance. 3. Also, two or more atoms, bound together chemically by covalent bonds; electrically neutral.

mole fraction. The number of moles of a substance in a mixture divided by the total number of moles of the mixture.

molten salt reactor. A thermal treatment unit that rapidly heats waste in a heat-conducting fluid bath of carbonate salt.

molybdenum. A silvery, solid, metallic element, symbol Mo, with atomic number 42, and atomic weight 95.94. Used to alloy steel.

monatomic. Elements that are present in the gaseous state as single atoms. These elements are the noble gases: helium, neon, argon, krypton, xenon, and radon.

monitor. A self-supporting firefighting nozzle that can function unattended. It delivers a large volume of fire suppressant material, usually water.

monitoring. 1. Periodic or continuous surveillance or testing to determine the level of compliance with statutory requirements and/or pollutant levels in various media or in humans, plants, and animals. 2. Determining the amount of ionizing radiation or radioactive contamination present. 3. Also referred to as *surveying*.

monitoring badge. An instrument that detects or "counts" radiation, such as alpha particles, beta particles, gamma rays, or X-rays.

monitoring well. 1. A well used to obtain water quality samples or measure groundwater levels. 2. A well drilled at a hazardous waste management facility or Superfund site to collect groundwater samples for the purpose of physical, chemical, or biological analysis to determine the amounts, types, and distribution of contaminants in the groundwater beneath the site.

mono-. The prefix that means "one."

monobasic. Concerning acids, those having only one displaceable hydrogen atom for each molecule of the acid.

monoclonal antibodies (mAbs, also MCAs). 1. Man-made clones of a molecule, produced in quantity for medical or research purposes. 2. Molecules of living organisms that selectively find and attach to other molecules to which their structure conforms exactly.

monomer. A "tiny" molecule that possesses the unusual chemical property of being able to react with itself to form a polymer.

monomeric. Having the properties of a monomer.

monomictic. Lakes and reservoirs that are relatively deep, do not freeze over during winter, and undergo a single stratification and mixing cycle during the year, usually in the fall.

monsoon. Heavy winds characterized by a pronounced seasonal change in direction.

Monte Carlo technique. A repeated random sampling from the distribution of values for each of the parameters in a calculation (e.g., lifetime average daily exposure), to derive a distribution of estimates of exposures in the population.

Montreal Protocol. Treaty, signed in 1987, that governs stratospheric ozone protection and research, and the production and use of ozone-depleting substances. It provides for the end of production of ozone-depleting substances such as CFCs.

moratorium. During the negotiation process, a period of 60 to 90 days during which EPA and potentially responsible parties may reach settlement, but no site response activities can be conducted.

morbidity. Rate of disease incidence.

mortality. Death rate.

most exposed individual. *See* **maximally exposed individual**.

most probable number. An estimate of microbial density per unit volume of water sample, based on probability theory.

motor carrier (MC). The Department of Transportation specifies various highway transportation containers for selected commodities.

mouthpiece escape respirator. A disposable respirator equipped with inhalation and exhalation valves and a one-piece plastic body with a belt clip or neck strap, designed for emergency escape protection against a variety of toxic gases.

muck soils. Earth made from decaying plant materials.

mud balls. Round material that forms in filters and gradually increases in size when not removed by backwashing.

mulch. A layer of material such as wood chips, straw, or leaves placed around plants to hold moisture, prevent weed growth, and enrich or sterilize the soil.

multimedia approach. Joint approach to several environmental media, such as air, water, and land.

multimeter. A device that can measure voltage, current, and resistance; may also be called a **volt-ohm meter (VOM)**.

multiple bond. A double or triple covalent bond.

multiple chemical sensitivity. A diagnostic label for people who suffer multisystem illnesses as a result of contact with, or proximity to, a variety of airborne agents and other substances.

multiple use. Use of land for more than one purpose. Also applies to use of bodies of water for recreational purposes, fishing, and water supply.

multistage remote sensing. A strategy for landscape characterization that involves gathering and analyzing information at several geographic scales, ranging from generalized levels of detail at the national level through high levels of detail at the local scale.

multiunit tank car. A tank car consisting of a number of separate tanks or containers used for transporting liquids in bulk.

municipal discharge. Discharge of effluent from wastewater treatment plants that receive wastewater from households, commercial establishments, and industries in the coastal drainage basin, including combined or separate sewer wastewater and storm overflows.

municipal sewage. Wastes (mostly liquid) originating from a community; may be composed of domestic wastewaters and/or industrial discharges.

municipal sludge. Semiliquid residue remaining from the treatment of municipal water and wastewater.

municipal solid waste. Common garbage or trash generated by industries, businesses, institutions, and homes.

municipal waste combustor. *See* **waste-to-energy facility.**

muriatic acid. Hydrochloric acid; HCl.

muriatic gas. Hydrogen chloride gas; HCl.

mustard. 1. Dichlorodiethyl sulfide (bis-2-chloroethylsulfide); $(ClCH_2CH_2)_2S$. 2. A vesicant or blister agent; agent H or HD.

mustard gas. 1. Dichlorodiethyl sulfide (bis-2-chloroethylsulfide); $(ClCH_2CH_2)_2S$. Used as a chemical weapon in World War I. 2. A vesicant war gas. In addition to its toxicity and ability to be absorbed through the skin, it can cause blindness.

mustard lewisite. A chemical vesicant or blister agent; agent HL.

mustard oil. A family of compounds having the general formula R-N=C=S.

mustard T. A chemical vesicant or blister agent.

mutagen. An agent that causes a permanent genetic change in a cell other than that which occurs during normal growth.

mutagenic. Having the property of causing a mutation in a cell or another organism.

mutagenicity. Mutagenicity is the capacity of a chemical or physical agent to cause permanent changes in a cell.

mutual aid agreement. Written agreement between agencies and/or jurisdictions in which they agree to assist one another upon request, by furnishing personnel and equipment in emergencies.

N

NA identification number. A four-digit number assigned to some chemicals found in transport in North America.

nano-. Prefix meaning "10^{-9}."

nanometer. One billionth of a meter (10^{-9} m).

napalm. A thickening agent made from preparing an aluminum soap mixed with oleic, naphthenic, and coconut fatty acids. When mixed with gasoline, it forms a flammable jelly that adheres to almost anything.

naphtha. A general term for a flammable liquid that remains after petroleum is cracked to produce short-chain hydrocarbons.

narcosis. Deep unconsciousness caused by a drug or chemical.

narcotic. 1. A drug that can dull the senses, relieve pain, cause a person to sleep, or induce a comatose state. 2. It may be natural or synthetic, and is usually addictive.

National Ambient Air Quality Standards (NAAQS). Standards established by EPA that apply for outdoor air throughout the country.

National Chemical Response and Information Center (NCRIC). A CMA program that provides emergency response information nationally through CHEMTREC, CHEMNET, and the Chemical Referral Center (CRC).

National Contingency Plan (NCP). Shortened name of the National Oil and Hazardous Substances Contingency Plan. *See also* **National Oil and Hazardous Substances Contingency Plan.**

National Emissions Standards for Hazardous Air Pollutants (NESHAPS). Emissions standards set by EPA for an air pollutant not covered by NAAQS that may cause an increase in fatalities or in serious, irreversible, or incapacitating illness.

national environmental performance partnership agreements. System that allows states to assume greater responsibility for environmental programs based on their relative ability to execute them. A feature of the National Environmental Performance Partnership System of the EPA.

National Environmental Policy Act (NEPA). The basic national law for protection of the environment, enacted in 1969.

National Fire Danger Rating System (NFDRS). A uniform fire danger rating system that focuses on the environmental factors that control the moisture content of fuels.

National Fire Protection Association (NFPA). An organization dedicated to fire safety that produces many standards, including the four-color diamond (NFPA 704) used on labels to indicate hazard.

National Hazardous Materials Information Exchange (NHMIE). *See* **Hazardous Materials Information Exchange (HMIX).**

National Incident Management System (NIMS). A nationwide approach for federal, state, and local governments to work together to prepare for, respond to, and recover from domestic incidents, regardless of cause, size, or complexity.

National Institute for Environmental Health Sciences (NIEHS). A federal agency responsible for issues related to the environment.

National Institute for Occupational Safety and Health (NIOSH). A federal agency that, among other activities, tests and certifies respiratory protective devices and air sampling detector tubes, and recommends occupational exposure limits for various substances.

National Municipal Plan. A policy created by EPA and the states in 1984 to bring all publicly owned treatment works (POTWs) into compliance with Clean Water Act requirements.

National Oil and Hazardous Substances Contingency Plan (NOHSCP). The federal regulation that guides determination of the sites to be corrected under both the Superfund program and the program to prevent or control spills into surface waters or elsewhere. Also called the *National Contingency Plan (NCP).*

National Pollutant Discharge Elimination System (NPDES). A provision of the Clean Water Act that prohibits discharge of pollutants into waters of the United States unless a special permit is issued by EPA, a state, or, where delegated, a tribal government on an Indian reservation.

National Priorities List (NPL). EPA's list of the most serious uncontrolled or abandoned hazardous waste sites identified for possible long-term remedial action under Superfund.

National Response Center (NRC). The federal operations center that receives notifications of all releases of oil and hazardous substances into the environment. It is open 24 hours a day and is operated by the U.S. Coast Guard, which evaluates all reports and notifies the appropriate agency.

National Response Plan (NRP). A comprehensive plan established to enhance the ability of the United States to manage all domestic incidents, forming the basis of coordination among federal, state, local, and tribal governments as well as the private sector during incidents. Formerly called the *Federal Response Plan.*

National Response System (NRS). The national chemical emergency response system developed through the National Contingency Plan (NCP).

National Response Team (NRT). Representatives of 14 federal agencies that, as a team, coordinate federal responses to nationally significant incidents of pollution and provide advice and technical assistance to the responding agencies before and during a response action.

National Strike Force (NSF). A version of the original USCG strike teams.

natrium. Latin for "sodium," hence the symbol, Na.

natron. Sodium carbonate.

natural. When referring to a plastics compound, a natural compound is one that has no color or other special property additive included, but may contain a plasticizer, stabilizer, filler, or other additive.

natural gas. A colorless, odorless, tasteless, nontoxic, flammable gas that has an odorant added to it to make it detectable by smell well below its lower flammable limit. It is mostly methane (depending on its source, it may be as high as 90% methane), with ethane making up the vast majority of the balance of the mixture.

natural polymers. Those polymers produced in nature, as opposed to man-made polymers. Natural polymers include cellulose (the major ingredient in wood and plants), cotton (almost pure cellulose), wool, silk, leather, and human skin.

natural radiation. *See* **background radiation**.

nautical mile. Distance of one minute of longitude at the equator, approximately 6,076.115 ft, 1.15 mi, or 1,852 m.

navigable waters. Traditionally, waters sufficiently deep and wide for navigation by all, or specified, vessels.

necrosis. Death of plant or animal cells or tissues.

nematocide. A chemical agent that is destructive to nematodes.

nematode. A very tiny worm, usually microscopic, that is a parasite of plants and animals.

neo-. 1. A prefix given to an isomer of a compound. 2. It exists in compounds that were named long ago, and is used only when the compound it best known by its common name. 3. It also means "new."

neodymium. A silvery white, solid, metallic element, symbol Nd, with atomic number 60, and atomic weight 144.24. It is a member of the rare earth elements.

neon. A nonflammable, gaseous, nonmetallic element, symbol Ne, with atomic number 10, and atomic weight 20.18. It is a member of group VIII on the periodic table of the elements (the inert, or "noble," gases). It glows red when an electric current is passed through it.

neoplasm. An abnormal growth of tissue that may be benign or malignant.

Neoprene. The trade name for polychloroprene $(C_4H_5Cl)_n$.

nephelometric. Method of measuring turbidity in a water sample by passing light through the sample and measuring the amount of the light that is deflected.

nephrotoxins. Chemicals that produce kidney damage.

neptunium. A silvery, solid, radioactive, metallic element, symbol Np, with atomic number 93, and atomic weight 237. It is a member of the actinide series.

nerve agents. 1. Substances that interfere with the central nervous system. Exposure is primarily through contact with the liquid (via skin and eyes) and secondarily through inhalation of the vapor. 2. Tabun (GA), Sarin (GB), Cyclosarin (GF), Soman (GD), DMAEDMAPP (GP), DMAPDMAPP (EA5414), V-Gas (Vx), VM, and VX are nerve agents. 3. Symptoms include pinpoint pupils, extreme headache, severe tightness in the chest, dyspnea, runny nose, coughing, salivation, unresponsiveness, and seizures.

netting. A concept in which all emissions sources in the same area that are owned or controlled by a single company are treated as one large source, thereby allowing flexibility in controlling individual sources in order to meet a single emissions standard.

neurotoxins. Chemicals that produce their primary toxic effects on the nervous system and brain.

neutral. 1. Having no net electrical charge. Atoms and molecules are electrically neutral, but ions have either a positive or negative charge. 2. A solution containing equal concentrations of H^+ and OH^-.

neutralization. 1. Decreasing the acidity or alkalinity of a substance by adding alkaline or acidic materials, respectively. 2. A chemical reaction in which an acid and a base are reacted, bringing the resulting solution to a pH of 7.0 (neutral). 3. Any reaction caused by the reacting of two or more chemicals that results in a neutral solution.

neutralization reactants. 1. The chemical compounds produced in the chemical reaction in which an acid and a base are reacted, bringing the resulting solution to a pH of 7.0 (neutral). 2. Any chemical compounds produced in the reaction where two or more chemicals are reacted to make a solution neutral.

neutrino. 1. An elementary particle produced by certain nuclear decay processes. 2. Neutrinos have no charge and have extremely small masses compared to other subatomic particles.

neutron. A nuclear particle that has an atomic weight of 1 and is electrically neutral.

new source. Any stationary source built or modified after publication of final or proposed regulations that prescribe a given standard of performance.

New Source Performance Standards (NSPS). Uniform national EPA air emission and water effluent standards that limit the amount of pollution allowed from new sources or from modified existing sources.

New Source Review (NSR). A Clean Air Act requirement that state implementation plans must include a permit review that applies to the construction and operation of new and modified stationary sources in nonattainment areas to ensure attainment of National Ambient Air Quality Standards.

newton. A unit of force; a newton (N) is expressed in $kg\text{-}m/s^2$.

NFPA 704. National Fire Protection Association's standard for hazard warning for stationary containers.

nicad battery. *See* **nickel-cadmium cell.**

nickel. A silvery white, solid, metallic element, symbol Ni, with atomic number 28, and atomic weight 58.69. It is used in alloys and is resistant to corrosion.

nickel-cadmium cell. A dry cell in which the anode is Cd, the cathode is NiO_2, and the electrolyte is basic. Also called a *nicad battery.*

nickel carbonyl. A chemical choking agent; $Ni(CO)_4$.

nielsbohrium. 1. A synthetic, radioactive, solid, metallic element, symbol Ns, with atomic number 107, and atomic weight 262. 2. In a compromise, the accepted name is now *bohrium*, symbol Bh. *See also* **bohrium**.

niobium. A light gray, solid, metallic element, symbol Nb, with atomic number 41, and atomic weight 92.906. It is used in steel alloys.

NIOSH designation. *See* **Registry of Toxic Effects of Chemical Substances.**

niter. Potassium nitrate (KNO_3). Alternative spelling is "nitre."

nitrate. 1. A compound containing the nitrate ion (NO_3^{-1}) 2. A salt or ester of nitric acid. 3. Almost always an oxidizing agent. 4. Also, to add the nitrate radical to a compound by a chemical reaction.

nitration. A reaction in which a nitro group ($-NO_3$) replaces a hydrogen attached to a carbon atom in a hydrocarbon compound.

nitric acid. 1. Powerful corrosive and strong oxidizing agent. 2. A transparent, colorless to yellow liquid that may be releasing nitrogen dioxide. 3. Will attack almost all metals and will quickly destroy animal and plant tissue. 4. HNO_3.

nitric oxide. 1. A gas formed by combustion under high temperature and high pressure in an internal combustion engine. 2. It is converted by sunlight and photochemical processes in ambient air to nitrogen oxide. 3. Nitric oxide (NO) is a precursor of ground-level ozone pollution, or smog. 4. It is one of the nitrogen oxides. 5. Also called *nitrogen oxide* and *nitrogen monoxide. See also* **nitrogen oxide**.

nitride. A compound made up of a metal and nitrogen.

nitrification. The process whereby ammonia in wastewater is oxidized to nitrite and then to nitrate by bacterial or chemical reactions.

nitrile. 1. An organic compound containing the carbon triple-bond nitrogen group, the cyanide radical (-CN). 2. Most nitriles are toxic and may be flammable.

nitrile rubber. Polybutadiene copolymerized with acrylonitrile.

nitrilotriacetic acid (NTA). A compound now replacing phosphates in detergents.

nitrite. 1. A compound containing the nitrite ion (NO_2^{-1}). A salt or ester of nitrous acid. 2. Almost always an oxidizing agent.

nitrocellulose. Cellulose nitrate.

nitrogen. A colorless, odorless, tasteless, gaseous, nonmetallic element, symbol N, with atomic number 7, and atomic weight 14. It exists in the Earth's atmosphere at about 79% as molecular nitrogen (N_2).

nitrogen cycle. The complex series of reactions by which nitrogen is slowly but continually recycled in the atmosphere, lithosphere, and hydrosphere.

nitrogen dioxide. 1. The result of nitric oxide combining with oxygen in the atmosphere. 2. A major component of photochemical smog. 3. One of the nitrogen oxides (NO_2).

nitrogen monoxide. *See* **nitric oxide** and **nitrogen oxide**.

nitrogen mustard. 1. A family of compounds that are strong lachrymators and have a fishlike odor. 2. Their structures are somewhat similar to mustard gas.

nitrogen mustard-1. A vesicant or blister agent; agent HN-1.

nitrogen mustard-2. A vesicant or blister agent; agent HN-2.

nitrogen mustard-3. A vesicant or blister agent; agent HN-3.

nitrogenous waste. Animal or vegetable residue that contain significant amounts of nitrogen.

nitrogen oxide. A chemical choking agent and one of the nitrogen oxides (NO). Also called *nitrogen monoxide* and *nitric oxide. See also* **nitric oxide**.

nitrogen oxides. 1. A group of gases that contain only nitrogen and oxygen; NO_x. 2. They include dinitrogen tetraoxide (N_2O_4), dinitrogen pentoxide (N_2O_5), nitrous oxide (N_2O), nitric oxide (NO), nitrogen dioxide (NO_2), nitrogen sesquioxide (N_2O_3), and trinitrogen tetraoxide (N_3O_4). 3. Some of the gases are reddish-brown in color. 4. They are formed by photochemical reactions of nitric oxide in ambient air. 5. They are the major component of photochemical smog. 6. They are also formed as products of combustion from transportation and stationary sources and are a major contributor to the formation of ozone in the troposphere and to acid deposition.

nitrophenols. Synthetic organopesticides containing carbon, hydrogen, nitrogen, and oxygen.

nobelium. A solid, metallic, man-made, radioactive element, symbol No, with atomic number 102, and atomic weight 254.

noble gases. 1. The elements of group VIII: helium, neon, argon, krypton, xenon, and radon. They are also known as the *inert gases*, since they do not react with other atoms of elements.

noble metal. Chemically inactive metal such as gold; does not corrode easily.

no further remedial action planned. Determination made by EPA following a preliminary assessment that a site does not pose a significant risk and so requires no further activity under CERCLA.

noise. Product-level or product-volume changes occurring during a test that are not related to a leak but may be mistaken for one.

Nomex. 1. A trade name for an aramid (highly aromatic polyamide) fiber or fabric. 2. A fire-resistant material typically used in the manufacture of firefighting clothing.

non-. Prefix meaning "nine."

nonaqueous phase liquid (NAPL). Contaminants that remain undiluted as the original bulk liquid in the subsurface. *See also* **free product**.

nonattainment area. Area that does not meet one or more of the National Ambient Air Quality Standards for the criteria pollutants designated in the Clean Air Act.

nonbinding allocations of responsibility (NBAR). A process for EPA to propose a way for potentially responsible parties to allocate costs among themselves.

noncombustible. The property of not being capable of combustion under specified test conditions.

noncommunity water system. A public water system that is not a community water system.

noncompliance coal. 1. Any coal that emits greater than 3.0 pounds of sulfur dioxide per million Btu when burned. 2. It is also known as *high sulfur coal.*

noncontact cooling water. Water used for cooling that does not come into direct contact with any raw material, product, by-product, or waste.

nonconventional pollutant. Any pollutant not statutorily listed or that is poorly understood by the scientific community.

nondegradation. An environmental policy that disallows any lowering of naturally occurring quality regardless of preestablished health standards.

nondischarging treatment plant. A treatment plant that does not discharge treated wastewater into any stream or river.

nonelectrolyte. 1. A substance that does not ionize in solution. 2. A substance whose aqueous solutions do not conduct electricity.

nonferrous metals. Nonmagnetic metals such as aluminum, lead, and copper.

nonflammable. The property of not being capable of burning with a flame under specific test conditions.

nonfriable asbestos-containing material. Any material containing more than 1% asbestos that, when dry, cannot be crumbled, pulverized, or reduced to powder by hand pressure.

nonhazardous industrial waste. Industrial process waste in wastewater not considered municipal solid waste or hazardous waste under RCRA.

nonionizing electromagnetic radiation. 1. Radiation that does not change the structure of atoms but does heat tissue and may cause harmful biological effects. 2. Microwaves, radio waves, and low-frequency electromagnetic fields from high-voltage transmission lines. Also called *radio frequency radiation.*

nonlinear dose response. A pattern of frequency or severity of biological response that does not vary proportionately with the amount of dose of an agent.

nonmetallic elements. 1. Elements that are not metals. Also called *nonmetals.* 2. Elements that will accept electrons to form negatively charged ions. 3. Elements that will share electrons to form covalent compounds. 4. The nonmetallic elements are: hydrogen, boron, carbon, silicon, germanium, nitrogen, phosphorus, arsenic, antimony, oxygen, sulfur, selenium, tellurium, polonium, fluorine, chlorine, bromine, iodine, astatine, helium, neon, argon, krypton, xenon, and radon. All the other elements are metals.

nonmetals. The elements to the right of and above the line on the periodic table. *See* **nonmetallic elements**.

nonmethane hydrocarbon (NMHC). The sum of all hydrocarbon air pollutants except methane; significant precursors to ozone formation.

nonmethane organic gases (NMOG). The sum of all organic air pollutants, excluding methane, which account for aldehydes, ketones, alcohols, and other pollutants that are not hydrocarbons but are precursors of ozone.

nonpoint sources. Diffuse pollution sources, which include such common sources as agriculture, forestry, urban, mining, construction, dams, channels, land disposal, saltwater intrusion, and city streets.

nonpolar. Chemical species not having positive and negative ends.

nonpotable. Water that is unsafe or unpalatable to drink because it contains pollutants, contaminants, minerals, or infective agents.

nonroad emissions. Pollutants emitted by combustion engines on farm and construction equipment, gasoline-powered lawn and garden equipment, and power boats and outboard motors.

nontransient noncommunity water system. A public water system that regularly serves at least 25 of the same nonresident persons per day for more than six months per year.

nonyl. The radical ($-C_9H_{19}$) formed when one hydrogen is removed from nonane (C_9H_{20}).

no-observed-adverse-effect level (NOAEL). An exposure level at which there are no statistically or biologically significant increases in the frequency or severity of adverse effects between the exposed population and its appropriate control.

no-observed-effect level (NOEL). Exposure level at which there are no statistically or biologically significant differences in the frequency or severity of any effect in the exposed or control populations.

Nordhausen acid. Fuming sulfuric acid.

normal. 1. The designation given to a straight-chain compound that has isomers, and its designation in the molecular formula is an "n-" in front of the formula. 2. The straight-chain version of an isomer.

normality. A measure of solution concentration, defined as the number of equivalents of solute per liter of solution; N.

notice of deficiency. An EPA request to a facility owner or operator requesting additional information before a preliminary decision on a permit application can be made.

notice of intent to cancel. Notification sent to registrants when EPA decides to cancel registration of a product containing a pesticide.

notice of intent to deny. Notification by EPA of its preliminary intent to deny a permit application.

notice of intent to suspend. Notification sent to a pesticide registrant when EPA decides to suspend product sale and distribution because of failure to submit requested data in a timely and/or acceptable manner, or because of imminent hazard.

no-till. Planting crops into an existing cover crop, sod, or crop residues without prior seedbed preparation, and eliminating subsequent tillage operations.

not otherwise specified (n.o.s. or NOS). Used where the actual chemical name for a particular chemical is not listed in the regulations and a generic name must be used to describe it on shipping papers.

noxious. A material that may be harmful or injurious to health or physical well-being.

nuclear fission. The process in which a heavy nucleus splits into nuclei of intermediate masses and one or more protons are emitted.

nuclear fusion. A thermonuclear reaction in which nuclei of hydrogen fuse together to form helium.

nuclear particles. The proton and the neutron.

nuclear reaction. A way to produce heat that is different from combustion, occurring when the center of an atom, called a nucleus, either splits apart or joins together with the center of another atom. This involves a change in the composition of a nucleus and can evolve or absorb an extraordinarily large amount of energy.

nuclear reactors and support facilities. Uranium mills, commercial power reactors, fuel reprocessing plants, and uranium enrichment facilities.

Nuclear Regulatory Commission (NRC). The federal agency responsible for community and worker protection from radiation hazards.

nuclear winter. Prediction by some scientists that smoke and debris rising from massive fires of a nuclear war could block sunlight for weeks or months, cooling the Earth's surface and producing climate changes that could negatively affect world agricultural and weather patterns.

nucleons. Particles comprising the nucleus; protons and neutrons.

nucleus. 1. A subatomic particle that contains all the positive charge and essentially all the weight of the atom. 2. The subatomic particle that is the center of every atom. It contains protons (and therefore all the positive charge of the atom) and neutrons (with the exception of hydrogen). Both protons and neutrons each have an atomic weight of 1; therefore, the nucleus contains essentially all the weight of the atom.

nuclide. An atom characterized by the number of protons, neutrons, and energy in the nucleus. The term refers to a particular species.

nutrient. Any substance assimilated by living things that promotes growth. The term is generally applied to nitrogen and phosphorus in wastewater, but is also applied to other essential and trace elements.

nutrient pollution. Contamination of water resources by excessive inputs of nutrients. In surface waters, excess algal production is a major concern.

nylon. The generic name for polyamides, polymers that contain the amide group (-CONH). *See also* **polyamides**.

O

occupancy. The purpose for which a building or portion thereof is used or intended to be used (ASTM E 931).

Occupational Safety and Health Administration (OSHA). A federal agency charged with creating and enforcing laws regarding occupational safety and health.

ocean discharge waiver. A variance from Clean Water Act requirements for discharges into marine waters.

ocher. Inorganic pigments, mostly oxide minerals. Unmodified, ocher usually refers to an iron oxide. Also *ochre*.

octane number. The number representing antiknock properties of gasoline, obtained by the ratio of isooctane and n-heptane in the gasoline under test.

octet. A set of eight valence electrons.

octet rule. For an element to reach stability, it must gain, lose, or share electrons with other atom(s) until it has eight electrons in its outer ring. A special subset of the octet rule is the duet rule. *See also* **duet rule**.

octyl. 1. The radical ($-C_8H_{17}$) formed when one hydrogen is removed from octane (C_8H_{18}). 2. Also known as its 2-ethylhexyl isomer.

odds ratio (OR). A relative measure of the difference in exposure between the diseased individuals (cases) and not-diseased individuals (controls) in a case-control study. *See also* **case-control study**.

odorant. A substance that has a very powerful, distinctive, sometimes disagreeable odor, that when added to odorless materials, will alert exposed persons of their presence.

odor threshold. The minimum odor of a water or air sample that can just be detected after successive dilutions with odorless water. Also called *threshold odor* and *odor threshold value (OTV).*

odor threshold value. *See* **odor threshold**.

office paper. High-grade papers such as copier paper, computer printout, and stationary almost entirely made of uncoated chemical pulp, although some ground wood is used.

off-loading valve. An outlet valve for the discharge of product.

offsets. A concept whereby emissions from proposed new or modified stationary sources are balanced by reductions from existing sources to stabilize total emissions.

off-site facility. A hazardous waste treatment, storage, or disposal area that is located away from the generating site.

offstream use. Water withdrawn from surface or groundwater sources for use at another place.

Ohm's law. Voltage equals amps (current) divided by ohms (resistance); $V = I/R$.

oil. Generally viscous liquids that are not miscible with water. Oils may have their source as plant or animals, or as minerals, generally from petroleum.

oil and gas waste. Gas and oil drilling muds, oil production brines, and other waste associated with exploration for, and development and production of, crude oil or natural gas.

Oil and Hazardous Materials/Technical Assistance Data System (OHMTADS). A computerized database containing chemical, biological, and toxicological information about hazardous substances.

oil desulfurization. Widely used pre-combustion method for reducing sulfur dioxide emissions from oil-burning power plants. The oil is treated with hydrogen, which removes some of the sulfur by forming hydrogen sulfide gas.

oil fingerprinting. A method that identifies sources of oil and allows spills to be traced to their source.

oil of sulfur. An archaic term for sulfuric acid.

oil of vitriol. An archaic term for sulfuric acid.

oil of wintergreen. Methyl salicylate.

oil spill. An accidental or intentional discharge of oil that reaches bodies of water.

-ol. A suffix indicating one or more hydroxyl (-OH) groups are present in an organic compound.

olefin. A synonym for the alkene series.

olefin plastics. The polyolefins (polyetheylene, polypropylene, polybutylene, polyisobutylene, polybutadiene, and polymethylpentene).

oleum. Fuming sulfuric acid.

olfactory. A term that relates to the nose or sense of smell.

oligotrophic lakes. Deep, clear lakes with few nutrients, little organic matter, and a high dissolved-oxygen level.

O-mustard. A vesicant or blister agent; agent T.

onboard controls. Devices placed on vehicles to capture gasoline vapor during refueling and route it to the engines when the vehicle is starting so that it can be efficiently burned.

oncogenic. Resulting from a gene that can induce neoplastic transformations in the cell in which it occurs or into which it is introduced.

oncogenicity. The capacity to induce cancer.

one-hit model. A mathematical model based on the biological theory that a single "hit" of some minimum critical amount of a carcinogen at a cellular target (such as DNA) can start an irreversible series of events leading to a tumor.

on-scene commander (OSC). Predesignated federal representative found at the regional level, either from EPA or USCG. Provides federal direction and coordination of response and clean-up activities.

on-scene coordinator (OSC). The predesignated EPA, Coast Guard, or Department of Defense official who coordinates and directs Superfund removal actions or Clean Water Act oil- or hazardous-spill response actions.

on-site facility. A hazardous waste treatment, storage, or disposal area that is located on the generating site.

opacity. 1. The property of preventing light from passing through a medium. 2. The amount of light obscured by particulate pollution in the air.

opacity of smoke. The ratio of incident luminous flux (*I*) to transmitted luminous flux (*T*) through smoke under specified test conditions (ISO/IEC Guide 52.1989).

open burning. Uncontrolled fires in an open dump. *See* **open dump**.

open dump. An uncovered site used for disposal of waste without environmental controls.

operable unit. Term for each of a number of separate activities undertaken as part of a Superfund site cleanup.

operating conditions. Conditions specified in a RCRA permit that dictate how an incinerator must operate as it burns different waste types. A trial burn is used to identify operating conditions needed to meet specified performance standards.

operation and maintenance. 1. Activities conducted after a Superfund site action is completed to ensure that the action is effective. 2. Actions taken after construction to ensure that facilities constructed to treat wastewater will be properly operated and maintained to achieve normative efficiency levels and prescribed effluent limitations in an optimum manner. 3. Ongoing asbestos management plan in a school or other public building, including regular inspections, various methods of maintaining asbestos in place, and removal when necessary.

operations level. A level of training for those first responders who will respond to releases or potential releases of hazardous materials as part of the initial response to the incident for the purpose of protecting nearby persons, the environment, or property from the effects of the release. They shall be trained to respond in a defensive fashion to control the release from a safe distance and keep it from spreading (ANSI/NFPA 472).

operator certification. Certification of operators of community and nontransient noncommunity water systems, asbestos specialists, pesticide applicators, hazardous waste transporters, and other such specialists as required by the EPA or a state agency implementing an EPA-approved environmental regulatory program.

optical density of smoke. 1. A measure of the attenuation of a light beam passing through smoke, expressed as the common logarithm of the ratio of the incident flux, I_O, to the transmitted flux, *I*. Optical density of smoke (*D*) = $\log_{10}(I_o/I)$ (ASTM E 176). 2. Also the common logarithm of the opacity of smoke.

optimal corrosion control treatment. An erosion control treatment that minimizes the lead and copper concentrations at users' taps while also ensuring that the treatment does not cause the water system to violate any national primary drinking water regulations.

oral toxicity. Ability of a substance to cause injury when ingested.

Orange Book. Officially titled *Transport of Dangerous Goods*, this UN publication contains the modal regulations of the UN Committee of Experts on the transport of dangerous goods.

orbitals. The probability distributions of where electrons may be found in their atoms, as determined by the quantum number of each electron. Also called **rings**.

orbits. The "rings" around the nucleus that contain the orbiting electrons.

ordinance. Weaponry, guns, or armaments.

ore. A mineral from which one or more metals can be extracted.

organic. 1. Referring to or derived from living organisms. 2. In chemistry, any compound containing carbon, with certain exceptions. 3. Pertaining to organic chemistry, which is the chemistry of compounds that were part of living things. Generally recognized as the chemistry of carbon compounds, hydrocarbon compounds, and their derivatives.

organic acid. A covalent hydrocarbon derivative that contains the carboxyl (-COOH) group and does not ionize in water. Organic acids are weaker than inorganic or mineral acids of the same concentrations. Examples are acetic, acrylic, carbolic, formic, hydrocyanic, methacrylic, and butyric acids, among many others.

organic chemicals. Naturally occurring (animal or plant-produced) or synthetic substances containing mainly carbon, hydrogen, nitrogen, and oxygen. Also called **organic compounds**.

organic compounds. *Organic* pertains to chemical compounds that were once part of living things, but now may be made by man. These are generally the hydrocarbon compounds and their derivatives.

organic matter. Carbonaceous waste contained in plant or animal matter and originating from domestic or industrial sources.

organic peroxides. 1. A group of highly dangerous hazardous materials, used as initiators for thermoplastics and curing agents for thermosetting plastics. 2. They are highly reactive oxidizing agents that burn, and they can start their own decomposition process when contaminated, heated, or shocked. 3. A hydrocarbon derivative that contains the very unstable peroxide radical (-O-O-) between two hydrocarbon radicals.

organic pigments. 1. Colorants that are covalently bonded, not including dyes. 2. Organic pigments are generally not soluble in the plastic in which they are dispersed. 3. *Contrast with* **dyes**.

organic vapor analyzer. A type of monitoring equipment used to detect hydrocarbon and hydrocarbon derivatives. May also be referred to as an *FID* or *flame ionization detector*.

organism. Any form of animal or plant life.

Organization of Economic Cooperation and Development (OECD) guidelines. Testing guidelines prepared by the Organization of Economic and Cooperative Development of the United Nations.

organoleptic. Affecting or involving a sense organ such as that of taste, smell, or sight.

organometallic compound. A compound that contains a metal attached directly to a carbon atom.

organophilic. A substance that easily combines with organic compounds.

organophosphate. 1. An organic compound containing a phosphorus-oxygen double bond. 2. A pesticide that contains phosphorus. They are usually short-lived but can be toxic when first applied.

organotins. Chemical compounds used in antifoulant paints to protect the hulls of boats and ships, buoys, and pilings from marine organisms such as barnacles. Also used as stabilizers for some thermoplastics.

original AHERA inspection. Examination of school buildings arranged by local education agencies to identify asbestos-containing-materials, evaluate their condition, and take samples of materials suspected to contain asbestos; performed by EPA-accredited inspectors. Also referred to as *original inspection* and *inspection*.

original generation point. Where regulated medical or other material first becomes waste.

original inspection. *See* **original AHERA inspection**.

ORM-A. An obsolete U.S. Department of Transportation (DOT) designation for "other regulated materials." The "A" designation is for materials that have an anesthetic, irritating, noxious, toxic, or other similar property that can cause an extreme annoyance or discomfort to passengers or crew if a leak occurs during transportation.

ORM-B. An obsolete U.S. Department of Transportation (DOT) designation for "other regulated materials." The "B" designation is for materials that are capable of causing significant damage to an airplane from leakage during transportation. They are corrosive to aluminum only.

ORM-C. An obsolete U.S. Department of Transportation (DOT) designation for "other regulated materials." The "C" designation is for materials that have characteristics that make them unsuitable for shipment unless properly identified.

ORM-D. An obsolete U.S. Department of Transportation (DOT) designation for "other regulated materials." The "D" designation is for materials that are consumer commodities that present a limited hazard during transportation.

ORM-E. An obsolete U.S. Department of Transportation (DOT) designation for "other regulated materials." The "E" designation is for materials that are not included in any other hazard class, but are subject to DOT regulations. Includes hazardous wastes.

ortho-. A prefix that refers to a particular arrangement of elements within a chemical molecule.

ortho P. *See* **total dissolved phosphorous.**

osmium. A solid metallic element, symbol Os, with atomic number 76, and atomic weight 190.2.

osmosis. The passage of a liquid from a weak solution to a more concentrated solution, across a semipermeable membrane that allows passage of the solvent (water) but not the dissolved solids.

other ferrous metals. Recyclable metals from strapping, furniture, and metal found in tires and consumer electronics. Does not include metals found in construction materials or cars, locomotives, and ships.

other glass. Recyclable glass from furniture, appliances, and consumer electronics. Does not include glass from transportation products (cars, trucks, or shipping containers) and construction or demolition debris.

other nonferrous metals. Recyclable nonferrous metals such as lead, copper, and zinc from appliances, consumer electronics, and nonpackaging aluminum products. Does not include nonferrous metals from industrial applications and construction and demolition debris.

other paper. For recyclable paper from books, third-class mail, commercial printing, paper towels, plates, and cups; and other nonpackaging paper such as posters, photographic papers, cards and games, milk cartons, folding boxes, and paperboard. Does not include wrapping paper or shipping cartons.

other plastics. Recyclable plastic from appliances, eating utensils, plates, containers, toys, and various kinds of equipment.

other solid waste. Recyclable nonhazardous solid wastes, other than municipal solid waste, covered under Subtitle D of Resource Conservation and Recovery Act (RCRA). *See also* **solid waste**.

otherwise use. Any use of a toxic chemical that is not covered by the terms "manufacture" or "process" and includes use of a toxic chemical contained in a mixture or trade-name product.

other wood. Recyclable wood from furniture, consumer electronics cabinets, and other nonpackaging wood products. Does not include lumber and tree stumps recovered from construction and demolition activities, and industrial process waste such as shavings and sawdust.

outage. *See* **ullage**.

outdoor air supply. Air brought into a building from outside.

outermost zone. *See* **safe zone**.

outer shell. The ring or orbital furthest from the nucleus.

outfall. The place where effluent is discharged into receiving waters.

outgassing. The removal of a gas from a metal or other material by heating the material.

overburden. Rock and soil cleared away before mining.

overdraft. The pumping of water from a groundwater basin or aquifer in excess of the supply flowing into the basin; results in a depletion or "mining" of the groundwater in the basin.

overfire air. Air forced into the top of an incinerator or boiler to fan the flames.

overflow rate. One of the guidelines for design of the settling tanks and clarifiers in a treatment plant; used by plant operators to determine if tanks and clarifiers are overused or underused.

overhaul. Postfire operation of "cleaning up" after a fire. It is the process of putting a structure in the safest condition following a fire, and verifying that the fire has not extended into unknown areas; any hidden "hot spots" are extinguished.

overland flow. A land application technique that cleanses wastewater by allowing it to flow over a sloped surface. As the water flows over the surface, contaminants are absorbed, and the water is collected at the bottom of the slope for reuse.

overpack. 1. The act of putting a smaller container into a bigger one to prevent product leakage. 2. Also, the larger of two containers. The smaller fits into the larger, and the larger can be sealed.

oversized regulated medical waste. Medical waste that is too large for plastic bags or standard containers.

overturn. One complete cycle of top-to-bottom mixing of previously stratified water masses. This phenomenon may occur in spring or fall, or after storms, and results in uniformity of chemical and physical properties of water at all depths.

oxidant. 1. Any chemical species that readily accept electrons. 2. A collective term for some of the primary constituents of photochemical smog.

oxidation. 1. Originally defined as the combination of any substance with oxygen. The definition is now more complicated, having to do with the transfer of electrons. 2. The chemical addition of oxygen to break down pollutants or organic waste, as in the destruction of chemicals such as cyanides, phenols, and organic sulfur compounds in sewage by bacterial and chemical means. 3. A chemical reaction that used to mean the combination of a substance with oxygen or other oxidizer. 4. *Contrast with* **reduction**.

oxidation number. 1. The number of electrons to be added to or subtracted from an atom in a combined state to convert it to its elemental form. 2. The numerical charge on the ions of an element. Also called *oxidation state* or *valence*. *See also* **valence**.

oxidation pond. A man-made body of water in which waste is consumed by bacteria, used most frequently with other waste treatment processes; a sewage lagoon.

oxidation-reduction potential. 1. The electric potential required to transfer electrons from one compound or element (the oxidant) to another compound (the reductant). 2. Used as a qualitative measure of the state of oxidation in water treatment systems.

oxidation state. *See* **oxidation number**.

oxide. A binary chemical compound where metallic ions are chemically bound to oxygen.

oxidizer. 1. Substances that contain oxygen and give it up readily, or will otherwise support combustion. 2. The halogens are oxidizers that contain no oxygen. 3. Also, a substance that accepts electrons from another substance. It oxidizes another substance and is thereby reduced. Also called **oxidizing agents**. *Contrast with* **reducing agent.**

oxidizing agents. *See* **oxidizer.**

oxyanion. A complex ion containing oxygen and at least one other element; negatively charged.

oxygen. 1. A colorless, odorless, tasteless, gaseous, nonmetallic element, symbol O, with atomic number 8, and atomic weight 16. 2. Exists in the Earth's atmosphere at about 20.9% as molecular oxygen (O_2). 3. The principal oxidizing agent on Earth.

oxygenated fuel. Gasoline that has been blended with alcohols or ethers that contain oxygen in order to reduce carbon monoxide and other emissions.

oxygenated solvent. An organic solvent containing oxygen as part of the molecular structure. Alcohols and ketones are oxygenated compounds often used as paint solvents.

oxygen deficient. An atmosphere containing less than 19.5% oxygen.

oxygen enriched. An atmosphere containing more than 22% oxygen.

oxyhemoglobin. The red compound that forms when oxygen reacts with the hemoglobin of the blood.

oxysalt. An ionic compound made up of a metal (or complex cation) and an oxyanion.

ozonation. Application of ozone to water for disinfection or for taste and odor control.

ozonator. *See* **ozonation**.

ozone. An unstable, bluish, gaseous compound formed by three atoms of oxygen (O_3). It is a powerful oxidizer.

ozone depletion. Destruction of the stratospheric ozone layer that shields the Earth from ultraviolet radiation harmful to life.

ozone hole. A thinning break in the stratospheric ozone layer.

ozone layer. The protective layer in the atmosphere, about 15 miles above the ground, that absorbs some of the Sun's ultraviolet rays, thereby reducing the amount of potentially harmful radiation that reaches the Earth's surface.

P

packaging. The assembly of one or more containers and any other components necessary to ensure minimum compliance with a program's storage and shipment packaging requirements.

packed bed scrubber. An air pollution control device in which emissions pass through alkaline water to neutralize hydrogen chloride gas.

packed tower. A pollution control device that forces dirty air through a tower packed with crushed rock or wood chips while liquid is sprayed over the packing material.

packer. An inflatable gland, or balloon, used to create a temporary seal in a borehole, probe hole, well, or drive casing. It is made of rubber or nonreactive materials.

packing group. A grouping system according to the degree of danger presented by hazardous materials:

- *Packing group I.* Indicates great danger.
- *Packing group II.* Indicates medium danger.
- *Packing group III.* Indicates minor danger.
- *No packing group required.* Class 2, class 7, and ORM-D packing group is determined from the hazardous material tables (49 CFR, ICAO, IATA, IMDG). Some items, such as flammable liquids, may use packing group I, II or III. In this instance, the flammability (flashpoint and boiling point) of the material is used to determine the applicable packing group.

paired electrons. Electrons in orbit around the nucleus that are near to each other will tend to be attracted to each other in pairs.

palatable water. Water, at a desirable temperature, that is free from objectionable tastes, odors, colors, and turbidity.

palladium. A silvery white, solid, metallic element, symbol Pd, with atomic number 46, and atomic weight 106.4.

pandemic. A widespread epidemic throughout an area, nation, or the world.

paper. In the recycling business, refers to products and materials, including newspapers, magazines, office papers, corrugated containers, bags, and some paperboard packaging that can be recycled into new paper products.

paper processor/plastics processor. Intermediate facility where recovered paper or plastic products and materials are sorted, decontaminated, and prepared for final recycling.

para-. Refers to a particular arrangement of elements within a chemical molecule.

paraffinic. Of the nature of straight- and branched-chain saturated hydrocarbons of the general formula C_nH_{2n+2}. Also called **alkanes**.

paraffin series. An older name given to the alkanes. *See also* **alkanes**.

paramedic. A practitioner credentialed by a state to function at the advanced life support (ALS) level in the state emergency medical services (EMS) system.

parameter. A variable, measurable property, the value of which is a determinant of the characteristics of a system.

paraquat. A standard herbicide used to kill various types of crops, including marijuana.

Paris blue. Ferric ferrocyanide.

Paris green. Copper acetoarsenite.

parison. In blow molding, it is the hollow tube that is extruded or injection molded, placed inside a mold, heated, and is forced to assume the shape of the mold by an internal blast of air.

Paris white. Powdered calcium carbonate.

Parshall flume. Device used to measure the flow of water in an open channel.

part A permit. *See* **interim permit status**.

part B permit. *See* **interim permit status**.

partial pressure, law of. The pressure caused by each gas or vapor in a mixture of gases or vapors. Also known as *Dalton's law.*

participation rate. Portion of population participating in a recycling program.

particle count. Results of a microscopic examination of treated water with a special "particle counter" that classifies suspended particles by number and size.

particulate loading. The mass of particulates per unit volume of air or water.

particulates. 1. Fine liquid or solid particles such as dust, smoke, mist, fumes, or smog, found in air or emissions. 2. Very small solids suspended in water; they can vary in size, shape, density, and electrical charge and can be gathered together by coagulation and flocculation.

partition coefficient. 1. Measure of the sorption phenomenon, whereby a pesticide is divided between the soil and water phase. 2. Also referred to as *adsorption partition coefficient.*

parts per billion (ppb). Units commonly used to express contamination ratios, as in establishing the maximum permissible amount of a contaminant in water, land, or air.

parts per million (ppm). Units commonly used to express contamination ratios, as in establishing the maximum permissible amount of a contaminant in water, land, or air.

party wall. A wall common to two buildings.

pascal. The SI unit of pressure equal to a force of 1 newton (N)/m^2; 101,325 pascals (Pa) = 1 atmosphere; 105 pascals = 1 bar.

passive smoking. Inhalation of other smokers' tobacco smoke. Also called *secondhand smoke.*

passive treatment walls. Technology in which a chemical reaction takes place when contaminated groundwater comes in contact with a barrier such as limestone or a wall containing iron filings.

pathogen. A microorganism that can cause disease in humans, animals, and plants.

pathway. The physical course a chemical or pollutant takes from its source to the exposed organism.

Pauli exclusion principle. 1. No two electrons may have the same quantum numbers. 2. Only two electrons may occupy an orbital, but they must have opposite spins.

pay-as-you-throw. Systems under which residents pay for municipal waste management and disposal services by weight or volume collected, not a fixed fee. Also called *unit-based pricing.*

peak electricity demand. The maximum electricity used to meet the cooling load of a building or buildings in a given area.

peak levels. Levels of airborne pollutant contaminants much higher than average or occurring for short periods of time in response to sudden releases.

pear oil. Isoamyl acetate.

penetration. 1. The ability of a substance to pass through a barrier. 2. The flow of a chemical through zippers, stitched seams, pores, or imperfections in the material.

penta. 1. Abbreviation for pentachlorophenol, which is an oil-borne wood preservative widely used in the treatment of utility poles, vaulted ceiling beams, fresh water pilings, and bridge timbers. 2. Also a prefix meaning "five."

pentaerythritol tetranitrate (PETN). Mainly used in the manufacture of detonating fuses. May be called *Primacord,* a trademarked product that uses PETN in the production of detonating cord.

pentavalent arsenic. 1. A naturally occurring trace element present in soil, water, and air, as well as in the tissues of plants and animals (including humans). 2. The form of arsenic used in the wood preservative CCA.

pentyl. The radical ($-C_5H_{11}$) formed when one hydrogen is removed from pentane (C_5H_{12}).

peracid. An acid containing the peroxy (-O-O-) group. Examples are peracetic acid, perchromic acid, and persulfuric acid.

percent saturation. The amount of a substance that is dissolved in a solution compared to the amount that *could* be dissolved in it.

perched water. Zone of unpressurized water held above the water table by impermeable rock or sediment.

perchlorate. 1. Any compound containing the perchlorate ion (ClO_4^{-2}). 2. An ion derived from perchloric acid ($HClO_4$). 3. Always a very strong oxidizing agent.

perchloromethyl mercaptan. A chemical choking agent.

percolating water. Water that passes through rocks or soil under the force of gravity.

percolation. 1. The movement of water downward and radially through subsurface soil layers, usually continuing downward to groundwater. Can also involve upward movement of water. 2. Slow seepage of water through a filter. 3. The action by which a liquid will pass into and/or through a porous material.

percutaneous. Refers to being passed, done, or effected through the skin.

performance bond. Cash or securities deposited before a landfill operating permit is issued, which are held to ensure that all requirements for operating and subsequently closing the landfill are faithfully performed.

performance data. As relating to incinerators, the information collected during a trial burn on concentrations of designated organic compounds and pollutants found in incinerator emissions.

performance-oriented packaging (POP). A type of packaging based on the ability of packaging to perform to a specified level of integrity when subjected to performance tests.

performance standards. 1. Regulatory requirements limiting the concentrations of designated organic compounds, particulate matter, and hydrogen chloride in emissions from incinerators. 2. Operating standards established by EPA for various permitted pollution control systems, asbestos inspections, and various program operations and maintenance requirements.

periodicity. The regular repeating of chemical properties of the elements.

periodic law. 1. The electron configurations of the atoms of the elements vary periodically with their atomic number. 2. All properties of the elements that depend on their electron configuration tend also to change with the increasing atomic number in a periodic manner.

periodic table of the elements. A systematic arrangement of all the known elements by their atomic numbers, which demonstrates the periodicity, or regular repeating, of chemical properties of the elements.

periods (table of the elements). 1. The elements in a horizontal row of the periodic table constitute a period. 2. While groups are characterized by the number of electrons present in the outer shell, periods are characterized by the number of energy levels (shells) of electrons surrounding the nucleus. 3. Elements in period 1 have only one shell, elements in period 2 have two shells, and so on.

periphyton. Microscopic underwater plants and animals that are firmly attached to solid surfaces such as rocks, logs, and pilings.

permanganate. 1. A chemical compound containing the permanganate ion (MnO_4^{-1}), which has an intense purple color. 2. Permanganates are powerful oxidizing agents.

permeability. The rate at which liquids pass through soil or other materials in a specified direction.

permissible dose. The dose of a chemical that may be received by an individual without the expectation of a significantly harmful result.

permissible exposure limit (PEL). 1. The time-weighted average concentration for a normal 8-hour workday and a 40-hour work week, to which nearly all workers may be repeatedly exposed, day after day, without adverse effect (OSHA). 2. The ACGIH term is **threshold limit value–time-weighted average (TLV-TWA)**.

permit. An authorization, license, or equivalent control document issued by EPA or an approved state agency to implement the requirements of an environmental regulation.

permit required confined space (PRCS). For a space to be considered a confined space, all of the following must be applicable:

1. It is big enough to bodily enter and perform the assigned task.
2. It has limited means of entry or egress.
3. It is not designed for continuous employee occupancy.

peroxide. 1. An organic hydrocarbon derivative with the general formula R-OO-R', where the R is a hydrocarbon radical or backbone, the R' is either the same hydrocarbon radical or a different one, and the -O-O- is the peroxide radical. 2. An inorganic peroxide is an ionic compound where hydrogen or metals are attached to the peroxide ion (O_2^{-2}). 3. All peroxides are oxidizers.

persistence. Refers to the length of time a compound stays in the environment, once introduced. A compound may persist for less than a second or indefinitely.

persistent pesticides. Pesticides that do not break down chemically or break down very slowly and remain in the environment after a growing season.

personal air sample. An air sample taken with a pump that is directly attached to the worker with the collecting filter and cassette placed in the worker's breathing zone.

personal measurement. A measurement collected from an individual's immediate environment.

personal protective equipment. Clothing and equipment worn by firefighters, hazardous material emergency responders, pesticide mixers, loaders, and applicators, reentry workers, and workers cleaning up Superfund sites, to reduce their exposure to potentially hazardous chemicals and other pollutants.

persulfate. 1. A salt derived from persulfuric acid and contains the persulfate ion ($S_2O_8^{-2}$). 2. Persulfates are strong oxidizers.

pest. An insect, rodent, nematode, fungus, weed or other form of terrestrial or aquatic plant or animal life that is injurious to health or the environment.

pest control operator. Person or company that applies pesticides as a business, usually involves household services, not agricultural applications.

pesticide. 1. Substances or mixture thereof intended for preventing, destroying, repelling, or mitigating any pest. 2. Any substance or mixture intended for use as a plant regulator, defoliant, or desiccant.

pesticide regulation notice. Formal notice to pesticide registrants about important changes in regulatory policy, procedures, and regulations.

Pesticide Safety Team Network (PSTN). Operated by the National Agriculture Chemicals Association (NACA) to minimize environmental damage and injury from accidental pesticide leaks or spills.

pesticide tolerance. The amount of pesticide residue allowed by law to remain in or on a harvested crop. EPA sets these levels well below the point where the compounds might be harmful to consumers.

petitioner. Any person who submits a petition under regulations requesting disclosure of a chemical identity or other information.

petroleum. Crude oil or any fraction thereof that is liquid under normal conditions of temperature and pressure.

petroleum derivatives. Chemicals formed when gasoline breaks down in contact with groundwater.

pH. 1. The negative logarithm of the hydronium ion concentration. 2. A value that represents the acidity or alkalinity of a water solution. 3. Indication of the acidity or alkalinity of a substance in water. 4. An expression of the intensity of the basic or acid condition of a liquid; may range from 0 to 14, where 0 is the most acidic, 7 is neutral, and 14 is the most basic. 5. Natural waters usually have a pH between 6.5 and 8.5.

pharmacokinetics. The study of the way that drugs move through the body after they are swallowed or injected.

pharmacology. The study of drugs, including the determination of biological activity, biological effects, breakdown and synthesis, and delivery.

phenol. A toxic, caustic hydrocarbon derivative (C_6H_5OH) that is very important to the chemical industry. Also called *carbolic acid.*

phenol formaldehyde. *See* **phenolic resin.**

phenolic resin. 1. A thermosetting polymer made from the condensation of phenol and formaldehyde. 2. Also called *phenol formaldehyde resin,* since it is the most important resin in the family.

phenolphthalein alkalinity. The alkalinity in a water sample measured by the amount of standard acid needed to lower the pH to a level of 8.3 as indicated by the change of color of the phenolphthalein from pink to clear.

phenol red. Phenolsulfonphthalein ($C_{19}H_{14}O_5S$), an acid-base indicator that changes from yellow to red as the pH passes through 8.

phenols. Organic compounds that are by-products of petroleum refining, tanning, and textile, dye, and resin manufacturing. Low concentrations cause taste and odor problems in water, and higher concentrations can kill aquatic life and humans.

phenothiazine. 1. An insecticide ($C_{12}H_9NS$). 2. Also a veterinary medicine used to treat intestinal worms.

phenoxy resin. A thermoplastic polymer based on the reaction between bisphenol A and epichlorohydrin.

phenyl. 1. The general name for the benzene radical ($-C_6H_5$). 2. A molecular group or fragment formed by abstracting or substituting one of the hydrogen atoms attached to a benzene ring.

phenyldichloroarsine. A vesicant or blister agent; agent PD.

phosgene. A chemical choking agent; agent PS.

phosgene oxime. A chemical vesicant or blister agent; agent CX.

phosphate. A chemical compound containing the phosphate ion (PO_4^{-3}).

phosphide. A compound made up of a metal and phosphorus.

phosphine. A colorless gas with a garlic-like odor that is air reactive and highly toxic.

phosphogypsum piles. 1. Principal byproduct generated in production of phosphoric acid from phosphate rock. 2. These piles may generate radioactive radon gas. Also called *phosphogypsum stacks.*

phosphogypsum stacks. *See* **phosphogypsum piles**.

phosphorus. 1. A solid nonmetallic element, symbol P, with atomic number 15, and atomic weight 30.97. 2. White phosphorous is pyrophoric. 3. An essential chemical food element that can contribute to the eutrophication of lakes and other water bodies.

phosphorus plants. Facilities using electric furnaces to produce elemental phosphorous for commercial use, such as the manufacture of high-grade phosphoric acid, phosphate-based detergent, and organic chemicals use.

phosphuretted hydrogen. Archaic name for phosphine, PH_3.

photochemical oxidants. Air pollutants formed by the action of sunlight on oxides of nitrogen and hydrocarbons.

photochemical smog. Air pollution caused by chemical reactions of various pollutants emitted from different sources.

photoelectric effect. The ejection of electrons from metals when exposed to UV radiation.

photolysis. The destruction of a molecule by electromagnetic radiation providing energy needed to break the chemical bonds between atoms in the molecule.

photon. 1. A packet of light or electromagnetic radiation. 2. A discrete concentration of energy that moves at the speed of light, has both particle and wave properties, has no rest mass, and can be described only in mathematical terms. 3. The quantum unit of electromagnetic radiation that comprises light waves, gamma rays, and other forms of radiation.

photosynthesis. Plant production of carbohydrates and oxygen from carbon dioxide made possible by the presence of chlorophyll in sunlight.

physical agent. Heat, noise, radiation, or vibration.

physical change. A change that occurs when a substance changes from one physical state to another, such as freezing, evaporation, and melting; no new substances are formed.

physical chemistry. The study of chemical thermodynamics, quantum chemistry, kinetics, spectroscopy, and statistical mechanics.

physical hazard. A hazard of a substance that includes the potential to be combustible or flammable, explosive, an oxidizer, pyrophoric, unstable, or water reactive.

physical property. A property describing only the condition of a substance, not the way it chemically reacts with other substances. Includes size, shape, physical state, hardness, density, ductility, malleability, solubility, heat and electrical conduction, color, and melting and boiling points.

physics. The science of motion, matter, force, and energy, and their relation to each other.

phytoplankton. That portion of the plankton community comprised of tiny plants.

phytoremediation. Low-cost remediation option for sites with widely dispersed contamination at low concentrations.

phytotoxic. Poisonous to plants.

phytotreatment. The treatment of specific areas by using plants that absorb specific contaminants from the soil or water through their roots or foliage.

pickling agent. A corrosive substance that will remove scales, oxides, or other impurities from the surface of metals.

pico-. The prefix used in the SI system that means "multiply by 10^{-12}"; p.

picocuries per liter. A unit of measure for levels of radon gas (pCi/L). The metric equivalent is becquerels (Bq)/m^3.

picogram. One trillionth of a gram (pg); 10^{-12} g.

picrate. A salt produced by the reaction of picric acid with a metal or other compound. Picrates are usually explosive.

piercing nozzle. *See* **puncture nozzle**.

piezometer. 1. A nonpumping well, generally of small diameter, for measuring the elevation of a water table. 2. An instrument used to measure pressure.

pigment. 1. A material that imparts color to a substrate; usually an inorganic or organic compound not soluble in the medium in which it is dispersed. 2. Pigments that are not compounds include carbon black and finely divided metals. 3. *Contrast with* **dyes**.

pigtail. *See* **gooseneck**.

pike pole. A firefighting tool consisting of a sharp prong and hook of metal on a wood, metal, plastic, or fiberglass handle used for pulling, dragging, probing, and other purposes.

pile. A timber, usually round, that is wholly or partly embedded in surface soil or underwater soil as a support for a superstructure such as a bridge, building, trestle, or wharf.

piloted ignition. Initiation of combustion as a result of contact of a material or its vapors with an external high-energy source, such as a flame, spark, electrical arc, or glowing wire (ASTM E 176).

pilot tests. Testing a cleanup technology under actual site conditions to identify potential problems prior to full-scale implementation.

pitot tube. An instrument that is inserted into a stream of water and has a pressure gauge attached that indicates the discharge pressure of the stream.

placard. A sign or symbol designed to be hung on a wall, container, or vehicle containing warning information to convey the level of hazard of the material contained.

plankton. Tiny plants and animals that live in water.

plant-derived pesticide. *See* **botanical pesticide**.

plasma. A gaslike state of matter that exists at extremely high temperatures in which all molecules are dissociated and most atoms are ionized.

plasma-arc reactor. An incinerator that operates at extremely high temperatures; usually for highly toxic wastes that do not burn easily.

plasmid. A circular piece of DNA that exists apart from the chromosome and replicates independently of it.

plaster of paris. Hemihydrated calcium sulfate; $2CaSO_4 \cdot H_2O$.

plastic. A material that contains as an essential ingredient one or more organic polymeric substances of large molecular weight, is solid in its finished state, and, at some stage in its manufacture or processing into finished articles, can be shaped by flow (ASTM D 883).

plastic deformation. The strain at which a solid can no longer regain its original shape.

plasticizer. A material added to a resin or polymer to increase its softness and flexibility.

plastisol. A suspension of resin particles in a liquid plasticizer. The resulting compound is a viscous liquid and is converted into a solid plastic by heat.

plate. A construction member used to form the top and bottom of a frame wall.

plate tower scrubber. An air pollution control device that neutralizes hydrogen chloride gas by bubbling alkaline water through holes in a series of metal plates.

platinum. A silvery white, solid, metallic element, symbol Pt, with atomic number 78, and atomic weight 195.08. It is used in jewelry and as a catalyst.

plug. A fire hydrant.

plug flow. Type of flow that occurs in tanks, basins, or reactors when a slug of water moves through without ever dispersing or mixing with the rest of the water flowing through.

plugging. Act or process of stopping the flow of water, oil, or gas into or out of a formation through a borehole or well penetrating that formation.

plumbum. Latin for "lead," hence the symbol, Pb.

plume. 1. A visible or measurable discharge of a contaminant from a given point of origin, which can be visible in water or air. 2 The area of radiation leaking from a damaged reactor. 3. Area downwind within which a release could be dangerous for those exposed to leaking fumes.

plutonium. A radioactive metallic element; symbol is Pu. Its atomic number is 94, and its atomic weight is 244. It is chemically similar to uranium.

PM2.5. A measure of smaller particles in the air. Particles in the atmosphere with a diameter of less than or equal to 2.5 μm. *Contrast with* **PM10**.

PM10. PM10 is measure of particles in the atmosphere with a diameter of less than 10 or equal to a nominal 10 μm. *Contrast with* **PM2.5**.

pneumoconiosis. Health conditions characterized by permanent deposition of substantial amounts of particulate matter in the lungs and by the tissue reaction to its presence.

point-of-contact measurement of exposure. Estimating exposure by measuring concentrations over time, while the exposure is taking place at or near the place where it is occurring.

point of departure. The dose response point that marks the beginning of a low dose extrapolation.

point-of-disinfectant application. The point where disinfectant is applied and water downstream of that point is not subject to recontamination by surface water runoff.

point-of-use treatment device. Treatment device applied to a single tap to reduce contaminants in the drinking water at the one faucet.

point source. A stationary location or fixed facility from which pollutants are discharged; any single identifiable source of pollution.

poise. The cgs unit of viscosity, equal to 1 dyne-sec/cm^2.

poison. Any substance that causes injury, illness, or death to living tissue, usually in small doses.

poison A. A gas or liquid so toxic that an extremely small amount of the gas or vapor from the liquid is dangerous to life.

poison B. Liquids or solids (including pastes and semisolids), other than class A or irritating materials, that are known to be so toxic to man as to afford a hazard to health during transportation or that, in the absence of adequate data on human toxicity, are presumed to be toxic to man.

poison inhalation hazard (PIH). Term used to describe gases and volatile liquids that are toxic when inhaled. Also called *toxic inhalation hazard (TIH).*

polar. In chemistry, substances having positive and negative ends.

polar bond. A covalent bond in which there is an unsymmetrical distribution of electron density.

polar solvent liquid. A liquid that mixes (is miscible) with water.

pollen. The fertilizing element of flowering plants; background air pollutant.

pollutant. Usually defined as any substance found or introduced into the environment that adversely affects the purity of a resource or the health of humans, animals, or ecosystems.

pollutant pathways. Avenues for distribution of pollutants.

pollutant standards index (PSI). Indicator of one or more pollutants that may be used to inform the public about the potential for adverse health effects from air pollution in major cities. Now called the *air quality index (AQI).*

pollution. 1. Generally, the presence of a substance in the environment that because of its chemical composition or quantity prevents the functioning of natural processes and produces undesirable environmental and health effects. 2. The term has been defined as the man-made or man-induced alteration of the physical, biological, chemical, and radiological integrity of water and other media (Clean Water Act).

pollution prevention. The process of identifying areas, processes, and activities that create excessive waste products or pollutants in order to reduce or prevent them through alteration or by eliminating a process.

polonium. A radioactive metallic element; symbol is Po. Its atomic number is 84, and its atomic weight is 210. It occurs in pitchblende and other uranium-containing ores.

poly-. A prefix meaning "many."

polyacetylene. The polymer of acetylene that has high intrinsic electrical conductivity.

polyacrylamide. A water-soluble polymer used as a thickening agent.

polyacrylate. A family of thermoplastics made from acrylic monomers. Also called *acrylics.*

polyacrylonitrile. A family of thermoplastics based on the acrylonitrile monomer, which contains the cyanide group.

polyallomers. A family of crystalline polymers made from two or more olefin monomers, one of which is usually propylene.

polyamide (PA). A family of polymers in which amide groups link the structural units. Also called **nylon**.

polyarylate. An aromatic engineering thermoplastic.

polybenzimidazole (PBI). A polymer with no melting point. It begins to char at 1,200°F. It can be spun into fibers and made into protective suits.

polybutadiene. An elastomer made from the polymerization of butadiene.

polybutene. *See* **polybutylene**.

polybutylene (PB). A polyolefin thermoplastic made by the polymerization of butylene (butene). Also called *polybutene.*

polybutylene terephthalate (PBT). A thermoplastic polyester.

polycarbonate (PC). A thermoplastic made from the reaction of bisphenol-A with phosgene.

polychlorinated biphenyl (PCB). A colorless liquid used as an insulating liquid in transformers.

polychloroprene. A synthetic rubber also known as Neoprene; $(C_4H_5Cl)_n$.

polycyclic. An organic compound having three or more aromatic rings in its molecular structure.

polyelectrolyte. A synthetic chemical that helps solids to clump together during sewage treatment.

polyene. A compound that contains more than one double bond per molecule.

polyester. A polymer formed by the reaction between dibasic acids and dihydroxy alcohols. Polyesters may be thermoplastic or thermoset resins.

polyethers. A large family of polymers containing the ether group (-C-O-C-).

polyethylene (PE). 1. A thermoplastic polyolefin made by the polymerization of ethylene (ethene). 2. Also called *polyethene.* 3. The largest volume plastic in the world.

polyethylene terephthalate (PET or PETE). A thermoplastic polyester made from the polymerization of ethylene glycol and terephthalic acid.

polyimide (PI). Thermoplastics made by reacting aromatic dianhydrides with aromatic diamines.

polyisobutylene (PIB). The polymer made from the polymerization of isobutylene.

polyisoprene. The base molecule of natural rubber. It may also be synthesized.

polymer. A "giant" molecule made up of up to thousands of monomer molecules that have reacted with themselves in a special type of chemical reaction called polymerization. The name comes from *poly*, which means "many," and *mer*, which means "part."

polymerizable. 1. Capable of polymerizing. 2. A property of all monomers.

polymerization. 1. The process by which monomers combine with themselves to form giant molecules called polymers. The reaction is in a controlled atmosphere (inside a large vat called a reactor). When the reaction is in a runaway (uncontrolled) mode, the result is instant polymerization, which in large quantities is accompanied by a violent and destructive explosion. 2. A unique chemical reaction in which a monomer (a relatively "tiny" molecule) reacts with itself to form a "giant" molecule called a *polymer*. *See also* **polymer**.

polymethyl methacrylate (PMMA). A thermoplastic acrylic polymer made from the polymerization of methyl methacrylate.

polynuclear aromatic hydrocarbons (PAHs). Large ring aromatic hydrocarbons containing carbon and hydrogen. May also contain any elements that may be bonded to the ring, and may be formed by combustion processes.

polyol. An alcohol containing three or more hydroxy groups. A "common" alcohol contains just one hydroxy group and has the general formula R-OH, where the R- is a hydrocarbon radical or backbone.

polyolefin. A polymer made from an alkene (olefin) monomer. The major polyolefins are polyethylene, polypropylene, polybutylene, and polymethylpentene.

polyphenylene oxide (PPO). An engineering thermoplastic polyether.

polypropylene (PP). A polyolefin thermoplastic made by the polymerization of propylene (propene).

polysilyne. A polymer based on silicon.

polystyrene (PS). A hydrocarbon thermoplastic made by the polymerization of styrene.

polytetrafluoroethylene (PTFE). A thermoplastic fluorocarbon polymer made by the polymerization of tetrafluoroethylene. Also known as *Teflon.*

polythene. An alternate name for polyethylene, used in the many countries outside the United States.

polyurethane (PUR). A family of polymers made by reacting a diisocyanate with organic compounds having two free hydrogens. They may be thermoplastic or thermoset resins.

polyvinyl acetal. A family of thermoplastic polymers made by reacting polyvinyl alcohol with an aldehyde.

polyvinyl acetate (PVAc or PVA). A thermoplastic polymer produced by polymerizing vinyl acetate. Used widely in adhesives.

polyvinyl alcohol (PVA, PVOH, or PVAL). A water-soluble thermoplastic; its monomer is vinyl alcohol.

polyvinyl butyral (PVB). A member of the polyvinyl acetal family.

polyvinyl chloride (PVC). A halogenated thermoplastic; its monomer is vinyl chloride. It has more uses than any other plastic in the world. May be rigid, semiflexible, or flexible.

polyvinyl dichloride (PVDC). Chlorinated polyvinyl chloride.

polyvinyl fluoride (PVF). A fluorocarbon thermoplastic made by the polymerization of vinyl fluoride.

polyvinyl formal. A member of the polyvinyl acetal family.

polyvinylidene chloride (PVDC). A halogenated thermoplastic whose trademarked chloride commercial name is Saran.

population. A group of interbreeding organisms occupying a particular space; the number of humans or other living creatures in a designated area.

population at risk. A population subgroup that is more likely to be exposed to a chemical, or is more sensitive to the chemical, than is the general population.

porosity. Degree to which soil, gravel, sediment, or rock is permeated with pores or cavities through which water or air can move.

portal-of-entry effect. A local effect produced in the tissue or organ of first contact between a toxicant and the biological system.

positron. A positively charged particle of antimatter that has the same mass as an electron.

postchlorination. Addition of chlorine to plant effluent for disinfectant purposes after the effluent has been treated.

postclosure. The time period following the shutdown of a waste management or manufacturing facility, usually 30 years.

postconsumer materials. Recovered materials that are diverted from municipal solid waste for the purpose of collection, recycling, and disposition. Also called *postconsumer waste.*

postconsumer recycling. Use of materials generated from residential and consumer waste for new or similar purposes.

postconsumer waste. *See* **postconsumer materials.**

post indicator valve (PIV). A valve that provides a visual means of indicating an "open" or "shut" position and is found on the supply main of installed fire protection systems.

potable water. Water that is safe for drinking and cooking.

potash. Usually potassium hydroxide (KOH), but sometimes potassium carbonate (K_2CO_3), potassium chloride (KCl), potassium sulfate (K_2SO_4), or potassium oxide (K_2O).

potassium. A soft, water-reactive, solid, metallic element, symbol K, with atomic number 19, and atomic weight 39.1. It is a member of the alkali metals group.

potential difference. Work that must be done to move an electric charge between specified points. Electric potential differences are measured in volts.

potential dose. The amount of a compound contained in material swallowed, breathed, or applied to the skin.

potential energy. Energy that matter possesses by virtue of its position, condition, or composition.

potentially responsible party (PRP). Any individual or company that might be responsible for, or contributing to, a spill or other contamination at a Superfund site.

potentiation. The ability of one chemical to increase the effect of another chemical.

potentiometric surface. The surface to which water in an aquifer can rise by hydrostatic pressure.

power. The rate at which energy is consumed. Electrical power is measured in watts. Heating and air power are measured in Btus per hour. Motor power is measured in horsepower.

praseodymium. A soft, solid, ductile, metallic element, symbol Pr, with atomic number 59, and atomic weight 140.91. It is a rare earth metal.

precautionary principle. When information about potential risks is incomplete, basing decisions about the best ways to manage or reduce risks on a preference for avoiding unnecessary health risks instead of unnecessary economic expenditures.

prechlorination. The addition of chlorine at the headworks of a treatment plant prior to other treatment processes.

precipitate. A substance separated from a solution or suspension by chemical or physical change. The precipitate is insoluble in the solution.

precipitation. 1. Removal of hazardous solids from liquid waste to permit safe disposal. 2. Removal of particles from airborne emissions as in rain (e.g., acid precipitation).

precipitator. Pollution control device that collects particles from an airstream.

preconsumer materials. Materials generated in manufacturing and converting processes such as manufacturing scrap and trimmings and cuttings. Also called *preconsumer waste.*

preconsumer waste. *See* **preconsumer materials.**

precursor. In photochemistry, a compound antecedent to a pollutant.

preharvest interval. The time between the last pesticide application and harvest of the treated crops.

prehospital care provider (PHCP). A person with training below that of EMT or paramedic who provides initial care to the sick and injured.

preliminary assessment. The process of collecting and reviewing available information about a known or suspected waste site or release.

premix. A mixture of polyester resin and fillers.

preplan. The result of a prefire inspection that details all hazards, ingress and egress points, alarms, sprinkler systems, water supplies, and any and all information that will prepare the fire department to handle a fire or other emergency at the occupancy.

prepolymer. A polymer of intermediate molecular weight, somewhere between the monomer and final polymer.

prepreg. A mat of reinforcing fibers that have been impregnated with a thermosetting resin that is partially cured.

prescriptive. Water rights that are acquired by diverting water and putting it to use in accordance with specified procedures.

preservative. Any substance applied to wood that is effective in preventing the development and action of wood-destroying fungi and insects.

pressed wood products. Materials used in building and furniture construction that are made from wood veneers, particles, or fibers bonded together with an adhesive under heat and pressure.

pressure. Force per unit area. The SI unit of pressure is the pascal, defined in newtons (N) as 1 N/m^2. Other common pressure units are the atmosphere, the bar, and the Torr.

pressure relief devices. 1. Usually a spring-loaded valve designed to operate at pressures below the failure pressure of the container. 2. May also be a **frangible disc** or a **fusible plug**.

pressure sewers. A system of pipes in which water, wastewater, or other liquid is pumped to a higher elevation.

pressure, total. In flowing air, the sum of the static and velocity pressures.

pressure treating. A process by which preservatives are applied to wood products, usually by forcing the preservative deep into the cellular structure of the wood under pressure in a closed cylinder.

pressure, velocity. In flowing air, the pressure due to velocity and density of air.

pressurized gas. A gas that is still in the gaseous state, but under higher pressure than 14.7 psia.

pretreatment. Processes used to reduce, eliminate, or alter the nature of wastewater pollutants from nondomestic sources before they are discharged into publicly owned treatment works (POTWs).

prevalence. The proportion of disease cases that exist within a population at a specific point in time, relative to the number of individuals within that population at the same point in time.

prevalent levels. Levels of airborne contaminant occurring under normal conditions.

prevalent level samples. Air samples taken under normal conditions. Also called *background samples*.

Prevention of Significant Deterioration (PSD). AN EPA program in which state and/or federal permits are required in order to restrict emissions from new or modified sources in places where air quality already meets or exceeds primary and secondary ambient air quality standards.

Primacord. *See* **pentaerythritol tetranitrate.**

primacy. Having the primary responsibility for administering and enforcing regulations.

primary carbon atom. A carbon atom that is bound to only one other carbon atom by a single covalent bond.

primary drinking water regulation. Applies to public water systems and specifies a contaminant level that, in the judgment of the EPA administrator, will not adversely affect human health.

primary effect. An effect where the stressor acts directly on the ecological component of interest, not on other parts of the ecosystem.

primary explosives. 1. High explosives that explode or detonate by heat or shock with enough brisance to initiate the detonation of the main charge. 2. Also called *initiators* or *detonators*. *See also* **initiator**.

primary standards. National Ambient Air Quality Standards (NAAQS) designed to protect human health with an adequate margin for safety.

primary waste treatment. In the first steps in wastewater treatment, about 30% of carbonaceous biochemical oxygen demand is removed from domestic sewage screens and sedimentation tanks, having settled or floated to the top.

principal organic hazardous constituents (POHCs). Hazardous compounds that have been selected for monitoring due to their high concentration in the waste feed and their difficulty of combustion. Monitored during an incinerator's trial burn.

principal quantum number. A positive integer constant that determines the principal energy level of an electron.

prions. Microscopic particles made of protein that can cause disease.

prior appropriation. A doctrine of water law that allocates the rights to use water on a first-come, first-served basis.

probability of detection. The likelihood, expressed as a percentage, that a test method will correctly identify a leaking tank.

processing equipment (plastics). Those machines and other equipment used to convert plastics resins, compounds, alloys, and blends from the powdered, liquid, cubed, or pelletized state into a finished or semifinished shape. Such equipment includes, but is not limited to, extruders, injection molders, blow molders, blown film towers, calenders, casting lines, mixers, blenders, driers, metering equipment, mills, intensive mixers, dissolvers, presses, and forming equipment.

process (plastics). The method by which plastic resins, compounds, alloys, and blends are converted from the powdered, liquid, cubed, or pelletized state into a finished or semifinished shape. These include extrusion, injection molding, blow molding, calendering, casting, and forming, among others. May also be referred to as *conversion* or *conversion process*.

process (toxic chemicals). The preparation of a toxic chemical (after its manufacture) for distribution in commerce, either:

1. In the same form or physical state as, or in a different form or physical state from, that in which it was received by the person so preparing such substance.
2. As part of an article containing the toxic chemical.

Process also applies to the processing of a toxic chemical contained in the mixture or trade-name product.

process variable. A physical or chemical quantity that is usually measured and controlled in the operation of a water treatment plant or industrial plant.

process verification. Verifying that process raw materials, water usage, waste treatment processes, production rate, and other facts relative to quantity and quality of pollutants contained in discharges are substantially described in the permit application and the issued permit.

process wastewater. Any water that comes into contact with any raw material, product, by-product, or waste.

process weight. Total weight of all materials, including fuel, used in a manufacturing process. Used to calculate the allowable particulate emission rate.

product. A substance that is produced during a chemical change.

product level. The level of a product in a storage tank.

products of incomplete combustion (PICs). Organic compounds formed by combustion, usually generated in small amounts and sometimes toxic. PICs are heat-altered versions of the original material fed into the incinerator.

product water. Water that has passed through a water treatment plant and is ready to be delivered to consumers.

Project XL. An EPA initiative to give states and the regulated community the flexibility to develop comprehensive strategies as alternatives to multiple current regulatory requirements in order to exceed compliance and increase overall environmental benefits.

promethium. A white, solid, metallic element, highly radioactive, symbol Pm, with atomic number 61, and atomic weight 147.

promoter. An agent that is not carcinogenic itself, but when administered after an initiator of carcinogenesis, stimulates the clonal expansion of the initiated cell to produce a **neoplasm**.

propellant. 1. An alternate name for certain low explosives. 2. A liquid in a self-pressurized product that expels the active ingredient from its container. *See also* **low explosives**.

proper name. An agreed-upon system of naming organic compounds according to the longest carbon chain in the compound.

proportionate mortality ratio (PMR). The number of deaths from a specific cause in a specific period of time per 100 deaths compared to all causes in the same time period.

proportioner. A device to introduce the correct amount of additives into streams of water.

proportioning. The occurrence of inter-molecular collisions between oxygen and hydrocarbon molecules.

proposed plan. A plan for a site cleanup that is available to the public for comment.

propyl. The radical ($-C_3H_7$) formed by removing one hydrogen from propane (C_3H_8).

protactinium. A solid, metallic element, symbol Pa, with atomic number 91, and atomic weight 231.

protective clothing. Clothing (with exception of level D) that includes both respiratory and physical protection. These levels were accepted and defined by response organizations such as U.S. Coast Guard, NIOSH, and U.S. EPA:

- *Level A.* SCBA plus totally encapsulating chemical resistant clothing (permeation resistant).
- *Level B.* SCBA plus hooded chemical resistant clothing (splash suit).
- *Level C.* Full or half-face respirator plus hooded chemical resistant clothing (splash suit).
- *Level D.* Coverall with no respiratory protection.

proteins. Complex nitrogenous organic compounds of high molecular weight made of amino acids that are essential for growth and repair of animal tissue.

protocol. A series of formal steps for conducting a test.

proton. A nuclear particle with an atomic weight of 1 and an electrical charge of +1.

protoplast. A membrane-bound cell from which the outer wall has been partially or completely removed. The term often is applied to plant cells.

protozoa. One-celled animals that are larger and more complex than bacteria.

proximity suit. A suit that provides close proximity protection for short periods of time at radiant heat temperatures as high as 2,000°F and may withstand some exposure to water and steam. Respiratory protection must be provided with proximity suits.

Prussian blue. Ferric(III) hexacyano-ferrate(II); $Fe_4[Fe(CN)_6]_3$.

prussic acid. Hydrocyanic acid (HCN).

psig. Pounds per square inch gage. It is the measurement of gas pressure above atmospheric pressure. Psig equals pounds per square inch absolute (psia) plus atmospheric pressure.

psychotomimetic agent. A substance that tends to produce symptoms like those of a psychosis.

public comment period. The time allowed for the public to express its views and concerns regarding an action by EPA.

public health approach. Regulatory and voluntary focus on effective and feasible risk management actions at the national and community level to reduce human exposures and risks, with priority given to reducing exposures with the biggest impacts in terms of the number affected and severity of effect.

public health context. The incidence, prevalence, and severity of diseases in communities or populations and the factors that account for them, including infections, exposure to pollutants, and other exposures or activities.

public hearing. A formal meeting wherein EPA officials hear the public's views and concerns about an EPA action or proposal. EPA is required to consider such comments when evaluating its actions. Public hearings must be held upon request during the public comment period.

public information assistance team (PIAT). Public relations specialists available through an on-scene commander (OSC) to maintain the release of public information.

publicly owned treatment works (POTWs). A waste treatment works owned by a state, unit of local government, or Indian tribe, usually designed to treat domestic wastewaters.

public notice. 1. Notification by EPA informing the public of agency actions, such as the issuance of a draft permit or scheduling of a hearing. EPA is required to ensure proper public notice, including publication in newspapers and broadcast over radio and television stations. 2. In the safe drinking water program, water suppliers are required to publish and broadcast notices when pollution problems are discovered.

public water system. A system that provides piped water for human consumption to at least 15 service connections or regularly serves at least 25 individuals.

public works (PW). The fourth emergency service, with fire, police, and EMS being the first three.

pulmonary edema. Fluid in the lungs.

pulmonary embolism. A blood clot in the lungs.

pulmonary toxin. Toxic to the lungs.

pumping station. Mechanical device installed in sewer or water system or other liquid-carrying pipelines to move the liquids to a higher level. *See also* **lifting station.**

pumping test. A test conducted to determine aquifer or well characteristics.

puncture nozzle. 1. A specially designed nozzle for puncturing and inserting into walls to extinguish hidden fires. 2. Also called a *bayonet* or *piercing nozzle.*

pungent. Biting, penetrating, sharp, or irritating.

pure substance. 1. An element or chemical compound. 2. A substance for which there is a basic unit particle that can be identified as that substance.

purging. Removing stagnant air or water from sampling zone or equipment prior to sample collection.

push technology. *See* **direct push.**

putrefaction. Biological decomposition of organic matter; associated with anaerobic conditions.

putrescible. Able to rot quickly enough to cause odors and attract flies.

pyrite. 1. The name now applies to an iron sulfide or iron-copper sulfide. 2. An archaic name for any "firestone" from which sparks could be struck.

pyrolysis. 1. Decomposition of a chemical by extreme heat. 2. Irreversible chemical decomposition caused by heat, usually without oxidation (ASTM E 176). 3. Breakdown of molecules by heat. Pyrolysis of polymers can produce shorter chain (lower molecular weight) polymers or the original monomer.

pyromania. An uncontrollable impulse to start fires.

pyrometer. A device used to measure temperatures by wavelength or electrical generation.

pyrophoric. The property of a material that ignites spontaneously upon exposure to air (or oxygen) at temperatures below 130°F (some sources quote 86°F).

pyrotechnics. Compounds that include fireworks, signal flares, and warning devices.

Q

quad. A four-way combination fire apparatus, sometimes referred to as *quadruple combination.* A quad combines the water tank, pump, and hose of a pumper with the ground ladder complement of a truck company.

quadruple combination. *See* **quad.**

qualitative analysis. Chemical analysis that detects the presence of a substance in a sample.

qualitative fit test. A method of measuring the effectiveness of a respirator by exposing wearer to a test atmosphere containing an irritating or smelly substance. The wearer should not be able to detect the substance.

qualitative use assessment. Report summarizing the major uses of a pesticide, including the percentage of crop treated and the amount of pesticide used on a site.

quality assurance/quality control. A system of procedures, checks, audits, and corrective actions to ensure that all EPA research design and performance, environmental monitoring and sampling, and other technical and reporting activities are of the highest achievable quality.

quantitative analysis. Chemical analysis that determines what is in a sample, and how much of each substance is present.

quantitative fit test. A method of measuring the effectiveness of a respirator in preventing a substance from entering the facepiece while the wearer is in a test chamber. The actual amount of the concentration of the substance is measured inside the facepiece of the respirator.

quantum. The smallest amount of physical energy that can exist independently, especially a finite amount of electromagnetic radiation.

quantum mechanics. The branch of physics that describes mathematically the wave properties of subatomic particles. Also called *wave mechanics.*

quantum number. 1. The basic unit of electromagnetic energy. 2. The quantum number defines the wave properties of electrons, separate from their properties as particles, and determines the principle energy level of an electron. 3. The quantum number describes the distance, shape, and orientation of the electronic orbitals.

quaternary carbon atom. A carbon atom attached to four other carbon atoms with single covalent bonds.

quench. To extinguish a fire by cooling.

quenchant. Any substance that absorbs another substance.

quench tank. A water-filled tank used to cool incinerator residues or hot materials during industrial processes.

quicklime. Calcium oxide, CaO.

quicksilver. An older name for mercury. *See also* **mercury**.

quint. Fire apparatus, the same as a quad, but with an aerial ladder added. *See also* **quad.**

R

rad. The unit of radiation absorbed dose.

radiant. The emission of light, heat, or other form of energy in the form of rays or waves.

radiant energy. *See* **radiation**.

radiant heat flux. The amount of heat flowing through a given area in a given time.

radiation. 1. Energy in the form of electromagnetic waves. 2. Transmission of energy though space. 3. Some types of radiation associated with radioactivity are alpha and beta particles and gamma rays and X-rays. 4. Also known as *radiant energy.* 5. Pertaining to heat, it is the transfer of heat without use of a medium. 6. Energy traveling through space.

radiation authority. The radiation authority is either a federal or state/provincial agency or a state- or province-designated official. The responsibilities of this authority include evaluating radiological hazard conditions during normal operations and during emergencies.

radiation flux. The radiation arrival rate per the unit of area of the surface.

radiation standards. Regulations that set maximum exposure limits for protection of the public from radioactive materials.

radical. 1. A highly reactive molecular fragment that, when attached to another molecular fragment or a hydrocarbon backbone, will impart specific properties to the new compound. 2. An atom or group of atoms bound together chemically that will impart a particular set of chemical properties to a compound. 3. Also called **functional group** and **free radical**.

radioactive decay. 1. Spontaneous change in an atom by the emission of charged particles and/or gamma rays. 2. Also known as *radioactive disintegration* and *radioactivity*. *See also* **radioactivity**.

radioactive disintegration. *See* **radioactive decay.**

radioactive substance. A substance that emits ionizing radiation.

radioactive waste. Hazardous materials resulting from nuclear reactions.

radioactivity. 1. The property of some substances to emit invisible and potentially harmful radiation. 2. The spontaneous emission of radiation from the nucleus of an unstable atom. As a result of this emission, the radioactive atom is converted, or decays, into an atom of a different element that might or might not be radioactive.

radio frequency radiation. *See* **nonionizing electromagnetic radiation**.

radioisotope. A chemical variant of a radioactive element with potentially oncogenic, teratogenic, and mutagenic effects on the human body.

radiological material. Any material that spontaneously emits ionizing radiation [National Fire Protection Association (NFPA) Standard # 472].

radionuclide. Radioactive particle, man-made (anthropogenic) or natural, with a distinct atomic weight number. Can have a long life as soil or water pollutant.

radium. A white, solid, metallic element, highly radioactive, symbol Ra, with atomic number 88, and atomic weight 226.

radius of influence. 1. The radial distance from the center of a wellbore to the point where there is no lowering of the water table or potentiometric surface (the edge of the cone of depression). 2. The radial distance from an extraction well that has adequate air flow for effective removal of contaminants when a vacuum is applied to the extraction well.

radius of vulnerability zone. The maximum distance from the point of release of a hazardous substance in which the airborne concentration could reach the level of concern under specified weather conditions.

radon. A radioactive, nonflammable, gaseous, nonmetallic element, symbol Rn, with atomic number 86, and atomic weight 222. It is a member of group VIII on the periodic table of the elements (the inert, or "noble," gases). It is formed by the radioactive decay of radium atoms in soil or rocks.

radon daughters. Short-lived radioactive decay products of radon that decay into longer-lived lead isotopes that can attach themselves to airborne dust and other particles, and if inhaled, damage the linings of the lungs. Also called *radon progeny*.

radon decay products. A term used to refer collectively to the immediate products of the radon decay chain. These include Po-218, Pb-214, Bi-214, and Po-214, which have an average combined half-life of about 30 minutes.

radon progeny. *See* **radon daughters.**

rainbow report. Comprehensive document giving the status of all pesticides now or ever in registration or special reviews. Known as the "rainbow report" because chapters are printed on different colors of paper; its actual title is *Status of Pesticides in Registration, Registration, and Special Review.*

Rankine scale. An absolute temperature scale (i.e., one in which absolute zero is assigned the value of zero) named after the 19th-century Scottish engineer William Rankine, and denoted by °R. One Rankine degree is the same size as a Fahrenheit degree, so absolute zero (–460°F) is 0°R, the normal freezing point of water (32°F) is 492°R and the normal boiling point (212°F) is 672°R. *Contrast with* **Celsius scale**, **Fahrenheit scale**, and **Kelvin scale**.

rappel. A method of descending by means of a rope and descending friction device.

rare earth metal. A metallic element that belongs to the lanthanide series on the periodic table of the elements.

rasp. A machine that grinds waste into a manageable material and helps prevent odor.

rate of explosion. The rate of decomposition of the exploding material is measured in feet per second in relation to the speed of sound. If subsonic, the rate is described as a *deflagration.* If supersonic, the rate of decomposition is defined as a *detonation. See also* **detonation** and **deflagration**.

rate of flame spread. 1. The measure of the speed of propagation of the flame away from the source of ignition across the surface of a liquid or solid.

rate of heat release. The amount of heat released (over time) by a material as it burns. The rate must be high for the material to spread flame to adjoining material.

raw agricultural commodity. An unprocessed human food or animal feed crop.

raw sewage. Untreated wastewater and its contents.

raw water. Intake water prior to any treatment or use.

rayon. Originally a name for yarns made from regenerated cellulose, but now may include cellulose acetate or cellulose triacetate.

reactant. 1. Any substance that takes part in a chemical reaction. 2. Any chemical compounds that are brought together in a chemical reaction. 3. Any substance that is consumed during a chemical change.

reactivity. The ease with which a substance enters into chemical reactions.

reactor. A pressurized vessel used to carry out certain chemical reactions, especially polymerization.

reaeration. Introduction of air into the lower layers of a reservoir to regenerate dissolved oxygen.

reagent. A grade of chemical of known purity and concentration used in laboratories for performing chemical reactions.

reasonable further progress. Annual incremental reductions in air pollutant emissions as reflected in a state implementation plan that EPA deems sufficient to provide for the attainment of the applicable National Ambient Air Quality Standards by the statutory deadline.

reasonable maximum exposure. The maximum exposure reasonably expected to occur in a population.

reasonable worst case. An estimate of the individual dose, exposure, or risk level received by an individual in a defined population that is greater than the 90th percentile but less than that received by anyone in the 98th percentile in the same population.

reasonably available control measures (RACM). A broadly defined term referring to technological and other measures for pollution control.

reasonably available control technology (RACT). Control technology that is reasonably available, and both technologically and economically feasible.

rebuttable presumption against registration (RPAR). *See* **special review**.

recarbonization. Process in which carbon dioxide is bubbled into water that is being treated to lower the pH.

receiving waters. A river, lake, ocean, stream, or other watercourse into which wastewater or treated effluent is discharged.

receptor. Ecological entity exposed to a stressor. Compare with **stressors**.

recharge. The process by which water is added to a zone of saturation, usually by percolation from the soil surface; e.g., the recharge of an aquifer.

recharge area. A land area in which water reaches the zone of saturation from surface infiltration, e.g., where rainwater soaks through the ground to reach an aquifer.

recharge rate. The quantity of water per unit of time that replenishes or refills an aquifer.

reclamation (in recycling). Restoration of materials found in the waste stream to a beneficial use that may be for purposes other than the original use.

recombinant bacteria. A microorganism with its genetic makeup altered by deliberate introduction of new genetic elements.

recombinant DNA. The new DNA that is formed by combining pieces of DNA from different organisms or cells.

recommended exposure limit (REL). The maximum recommended exposure limit. Usually only suggested industry practices and not enforced by legal regulations, as are permissible exposure limits (PELs). *See also* **permissible exposure limit**.

recommended maximum contaminant level (RMCL). The maximum level of a contaminant in drinking water at which no known or anticipated adverse effect on human health would occur, and that includes an adequate margin of safety.

reconstruction of dose. Estimating exposure after it has occurred by using evidence within an organism such as chemical levels in tissue or fluids.

record of decision (ROD). A public document that explains which cleanup alternative(s) will be used at National Priorities List sites where, under CERCLA, trust funds pay for the cleanup.

recovery rate. Percentage of usable recycled materials that have been removed from the total amount of municipal solid waste generated in a specific area or by a specific business.

recycling. The minimization of waste generation by recovering and reprocessing usable products that might otherwise become waste. Also called *reuse*.

recycling and reuse business assistance centers. Centers located in state solid waste or economic development agencies that provide recycling businesses with customized and targeted assistance.

recycling mill. A facility where recovered materials are remanufactured into new products.

Recycling Technical Assistance Partnership National Network. A national information-sharing resource designed to help businesses and manufacturers increase their use of recovered materials.

red bag waste. *See* **infectious waste**.

red border. An EPA document undergoing review before being submitted for final management decision making.

redemption program. Program in which consumers are monetarily compensated for the collection of recyclable materials, generally through prepaid deposits or taxes on beverage containers.

redox reaction. An oxidation-reduction chemical reaction.

red tide. A proliferation of a marine plankton toxic and often fatal to fish, perhaps stimulated by the addition of nutrients.

reducing agent. Any substance that removes oxygen from a compound, thereby reducing it. 2. Any substance that donates electrons to another substance. 3. *Contrast with* an **oxidizer**, which is a substance that contains oxygen and gives it up readily, or accepts electrons from another substance.

reduction. The addition of hydrogen, removal of oxygen, or addition of electrons to an element or compound. *Contrast with* **oxidation**, its opposite.

red vitriol. An archaic name for cobalt(II) sulfate; $CoSO_4{\cdot}7H_2O$. Also called *rose vitriol.*

reentry. In reference to an indoor air program, the air exhausted from a building that is immediately brought back into the system through the air intake and other openings.

reentry interval. The period of time immediately following the application of a pesticide during which unprotected workers should not enter a field.

reference group. A group used as the baseline for comparison in epidemiologic studies or laboratory studies. This group is selected because it either lacks the disease of interest (case-control group) or lacks the exposure of concern (cohort study). *See also* **control group**.

reformulated gasoline. Gasoline with a different composition from conventional gasoline (e.g., lower aromatics content) that cuts air pollutants.

refraction. The change in direction of light as it passes between two objects of differing densities.

refrigerated liquid. *See* **cryogenic liquid**.

refueling emissions. Emissions released during vehicle refueling.

refuse. *See* **solid waste**.

refuse reclamation. The conversion of solid waste into useful products.

regeneration. Manipulation of cells to cause them to develop into whole plants.

regional gas dose. The gas dose calculated for the region of interest as related to the observed effect for respiratory effects.

regional gas dose ratio (RGDR). The ratio of the regional gas dose calculated for a given exposure in the animal species of interest to the regional gas dose of the same exposure in humans.

regional response plan (RRP). A plan developed to meet the needs of the region involved.

regional response team (RRT). Representatives of federal, state, and local agencies who may assist in coordination of activities at the request of the on-scene coordinator (OSC) before and during a significant pollution incident such as an oil spill, major chemical release, or Superfund response.

registrant. Any manufacturer or formulator who obtains registration for a pesticide active ingredient or product.

registration. Formal listing with EPA of a new pesticide before it can be sold or distributed.

registration standards. Published documents that include summary reviews of the data available on a pesticide's active ingredient, data gaps, and the EPA's existing regulatory position on the pesticide.

Registry of Toxic Effects of Chemical Substances (RTECS). A database of toxicity information on many substances, created by the National Institute for Occupational Safety and Health (NIOSH). Sometimes referred to as the *NIOSH designation*.

regrind. Rejected or recycled plastic parts and any other parts of the finished molding that are removed from the item being manufactured (or anything classified as scrap) and then ground up into small particles to be reprocessed with virgin (unused) material.

regulated asbestos-containing material (RACM). Friable asbestos material or nonfriable asbestos-containing material that will be or has been subjected to sanding, grinding, cutting, or abrading, or that has crumbled or been pulverized or reduced to powder in the course of demolition or renovation operations.

regulated medical waste. Under the Medical Waste Tracking Act of 1988, any solid waste generated in the diagnosis, treatment, or immunization of human beings or animals, in research pertaining thereto, or in the production or testing of biologicals. Included are: cultures and stocks of infectious agents; human blood and blood products; human pathological body wastes from surgery and autopsy; contaminated animal carcasses from medical research; waste from patients with communicable diseases; and all used sharp implements, such as needles and scalpels, and certain unused "sharps."

reinforced plastic. A plastic resin or compound into which fillers are added to greatly increase the strength or other physical properties of the finished part.

reinforced response. Resources needed in addition to the initial response.

rekindle. The reignition of a fire because of latent heat, sparks, or smoldering embers.

relative ecological sustainability. Ability of an ecosystem to maintain relative ecological integrity indefinitely.

relative humidity. The ratio between the actual water vapor content of the atmosphere and the maximum water vapor content possible at that given temperature, expressed as a percentage.

relative permeability. The permeability of a rock to gas, nonaqueous phase liquid (NAPL), or water, when any two or more are present.

relative risk. 1. The relative measure of the difference in risk between the exposed and unexposed populations in a cohort study. 2. The relative risk is defined as the rate of disease among the exposed divided by the rate of the disease among the unexposed. Also called *risk ratio*.

relative risk assessment. Estimating the risks associated with different stressors or management actions.

relay. The use of two or more pumpers to move water distances that would require excessive pressures if only one pumper were employed.

release. Any spilling, leaking, pumping, pouring, emitting, emptying, discharging, injecting, escaping, leaching, dumping, or disposing into the environment of a hazardous or toxic chemical or extremely hazardous substance.

release inventory. Form for annual release reporting.

rem. A measure of radiation dose related to biological effect.

remedial action (RA). The actual construction or implementation phase of a Superfund site cleanup that follows remedial design.

remedial design. A phase of remedial action that follows the remedial investigation/feasibility study and includes development of engineering drawings and specifications for a site cleanup.

remedial investigation. An in-depth study designed to gather data needed to determine the nature and extent of contamination at a Superfund site, establish site cleanup criteria, identify preliminary alternatives for remedial action, and support technical and cost analyses of alternatives.

remedial project manager (RPM). The EPA or state official responsible for overseeing on-site remedial action.

remedial response. Long-term action that stops or substantially reduces a release or threat of a release of hazardous substances that pose a serious but not an immediate threat to public health.

remediation. 1. Cleanup or other methods used to remove or contain a toxic spill or hazardous materials from a Superfund site. 2. For the Asbestos Hazard Emergency Response Act program, abatement methods including evaluation, repair, enclosure, encapsulation, or removal of greater than 3 ft (linear) or 3 ft^2 of asbestos-containing materials from a building.

remote sensing. The collection and interpretation of information about an object without physical contact with the object.

remote storage sites (RSS). Sites located in the Caribbean and Pacific to ensure readiness and "just in time" logistics for disaster responders. *Contrast with* **territory logistics centers**.

removal action. Short-term immediate actions taken to address releases of hazardous substances that require expedited response.

renal. Pertaining to the kidney.

Renewable Energy Production Incentive (REPI). Incentive established by the Energy Policy Act available to renewable energy power projects owned by a state or local government or nonprofit electric cooperative.

repeat compliance period. Any subsequent compliance period after the initial one.

repeating unit. The identifiable fragment of the monomer(s) that formed the polymer. When monomers combine with themselves to form a polymer, they line up in clearly distinguishable units that repeat throughout the polymer.

reportable quantity (RQ). 1. Quantity of a hazardous substance that triggers reports under CERCLA. If a substance exceeds its RQ, the release must be reported to the National Response Center, the SERC, and community emergency coordinators for areas likely to be affected. 2. That amount of a CERCLA hazardous substance or extremely hazardous substance listed in 40 CFR 355, appendix A, which when exceeded as a release, requires reporting.

repowering. Rebuilding and replacing major components of a power plant instead of building a new one.

representative elements. The chemical elements of the long groups in the periodic table. Also called the **main group elements**.

representative sample. A portion of material or water that is as nearly identical in content and consistency as possible to that in the larger body of material or water being sampled.

reproductive toxins. Chemicals that affect the reproductive capabilities, including chromosomal damage (mutations) and effects on fetuses (teratogenesis).

reregistration. The reevaluation and relicensing of existing pesticides originally registered prior to current scientific and regulatory standards.

rescue. To access, stabilize, and remove endangered or injured individuals by whatever means necessary to ensure their timely transfer to appropriate care or to a place of safety.

reserve capacity. Extra treatment capacity built into solid waste and wastewater treatment plants and interceptor sewers to accommodate flow increases due to future population growth.

reserve volume. The volume of air remaining in the lungs after a maximal expiration.

reservoir. Any natural or artificial holding area used to store, regulate, or control water.

residential use. Pesticide application in and around houses, office buildings, apartment buildings, motels, and other living or working areas.

residential waste. Waste generated in single-family and multifamily homes, including newspapers, clothing, disposable tableware, food packaging, cans, bottles, food scraps, and yard trimmings, other than those that are diverted to backyard composting. *See also* **household hazardous waste**.

residual. Amount of a pollutant remaining in the environment after a natural or technological process has taken place.

residual risk. The extent of health risk from air pollutants remaining after application of the maximum achievable control technology (MACT).

residual saturation. Saturation level below which fluid drainage will not occur.

residual volume (RV). The lung volume after maximal expiration. Residual volume (RV) equals total lung capacity (TLC) minus vital capacity (VC); RV = TLC – VC.

residue. The dry solids remaining after the evaporation of a sample of water or sludge.

resin (natural). A solid or semisolid viscous substance secreted by certain plants and trees.

resin (synthetic). A solid, semisolid, or pseudosolid organic material that has an indefinite and often high molecular weight, exhibits a tendency to flow when subjected to stress, usually has a softening or melting range, and usually fractures conchoidally (ASTM D 883).

resistance. The ability of plants and animals to withstand poor environmental conditions or attacks by chemicals or disease.

resonance. 1. A molecular structure that is fluctuating (resonating) back and forth between alternate forms. 2. A theory used to explain molecular structure that cannot be explained by the rules of conventional covalent bonding.

Resource Conservation and Recovery Act (RCRA). An Environmental Protection Agency regulation that describes "cradle-to-grave" management of hazardous waste, whereby the generator of the waste is ultimately responsible for its proper handling, packaging, transport, and disposal. Its purpose is to protect human health and the environment from improperly managed hazardous waste. Also called the *Solid Waste Disposal Act*.

resource identification and analysis (RIA). A two-step process involving identification of available resources and determination of their capabilities.

resource recovery. The process of obtaining matter or energy from materials formerly discarded.

respirator. A device worn over the nose and mouth to prevent a person from inhaling harmful substances in contaminated air.

respiratory asphyxiant. A material that prevents or reduces the available oxygen necessary for normal breathing. Divided into *simple asphyxiants* and *chemical asphyxiants*. *See also* **simple asphyxiants**.

response. That portion of incident management in which personnel are involved in controlling a hazardous materials incident (ANSI/NFPA 471).

response action. 1. Generic term for actions taken in response to actual or potential health-threatening environmental events such as spills, sudden releases, and asbestos abatement/management problems. 2. A CERCLA-authorized action involving either a short-term removal action or a long-term removal response. This may include but is not limited to: removing hazardous materials from a site to an EPA-approved hazardous waste facility for treatment; containment or treatment of the waste on-site; identifying and removing the sources of groundwater contamination; and halting further migration of contaminants. 3. Any of the following actions taken in school buildings in response to AHERA to reduce the risk of exposure to asbestos: removal, encapsulation, enclosure, repair, and operations and maintenance. *See also* **cleanup**.

response team. Shortened form of National Response Team. Responds to emergency situations at the direction of EPA regional offices.

responsiveness summary. A summary of oral and/or written public comments received by EPA during a comment period on key EPA documents, and EPA's response to those comments.

restoration. Measures taken to return a site to previolation conditions.

restricted entry interval. The time after a pesticide application during which entry into the treated area is restricted.

restricted use. A pesticide may be classified (under FIFRA regulations) for restricted use if it requires special handling because of its toxicity, and, if so, it may be applied only by trained, certified applicators or those under their direct supervision.

restriction enzyme. An enzyme that recognizes specific regions of a DNA molecule and cuts it at those points.

retarder. Anything that inhibits a process.

retention level. 1. Refers to the amount of a particular preservative remaining in 1 ft^3 of wood after being treated. For instance, a 0.25 retention level means that about 0.25 lb of preservative is in every cubic foot of wood fiber. 2. Preservative retention levels vary, based on the type of lumber and its intended use.

retrofit. Addition of a pollution control device on an existing facility without making major changes to the generating plant. Also called *backfit.*

reuse. Using a product or component of municipal solid waste in its original form more than once.

reverse osmosis. A treatment process used in water systems by adding pressure to force water through a semipermeable membrane. Reverse osmosis removes most drinking water contaminants. Also used in wastewater treatment.

reversible effect. An effect that is not permanent; especially adverse effects that diminish when exposure to a toxic chemical stops.

rhenium. A heavy, silvery white, solid, metallic element, symbol Re, with atomic number 75, and atomic weight 186.2.

rhodium. A hard, silvery white, solid metallic element, symbol Rh, with atomic number 45, and atomic weight 102.905.

RHYTHM. Registered trademark for the Du Pont Company Safe Distribution Program: Remember How You Treat Hazardous Materials.

ribonucleic acid (RNA). A molecule that carries the genetic message from DNA to a cellular protein-producing mechanism.

ricin. A poison made from the common castor bean that can be inhaled, injected, or ingested. It is stable, easy to produce, and can be dispersed via chemical agent munitions.

rig. Any piece of fire apparatus.

rill. A small channel eroded into the soil by surface runoff; can be easily smoothed out or obliterated by normal tillage.

Ringelmann chart. A series of shaded illustrations used to measure the opacity of air pollution emissions, ranging from light grey through black; used to set and enforce emissions standards.

rings. The paths around the nucleus in which the orbiting electrons travel. Also called **orbitals**.

riot control agent (RCA). Any chemical that can be used to produce irritating or disabling effects on personnel that last a short time.

riparian habitat. Areas adjacent to rivers and streams with a differing density, diversity, and productivity of plant and animal species relative to nearby uplands.

riparian rights. Entitlement of a land owner to certain uses of water on or bordering the property, including the right to prevent diversion or misuse of upstream waters.

risk. 1. A measure of the probability that damage to life, health, property, and/or the environment will occur as a result of a given hazard. 2. Exposure to the chance of injury or loss. 3. In the context of human health, the probability of injury, disease, or death from exposure to a chemical agent or a mixture of chemicals. In quantitative terms, risk is expressed in values ranging from zero (representing the certainty that harm will not occur) to one (representing the certainty that harm will occur).

risk (adverse) for endangered species. Risk to aquatic species if anticipated pesticide residue levels equal 20% of LD_{10} or 10% of LC_{50}; risk to terrestrial species if anticipated pesticide residue levels equal 20% of LC_{10} or 10% of LC_{50}.

risk analysis. A process by which the probability can be determined that harm may occur to life, property, and the environment, and to note the risks to be taken to identify the incident objectives.

risk assessment. Qualitative and quantitative evaluation of the risk posed to human health and/or the environment by the actual or potential presence and/or use of specific pollutants.

risk-based targeting. The direction of resources to those areas that have been identified as having the highest potential of actual adverse effect on human health and/or the environment.

risk characterization. The last phase of the risk assessment process that estimates the potential for adverse health or ecological effects to occur from exposure to a stressor and evaluates the uncertainty involved.

risk communication. The exchange of information about health or environmental risks among risk assessors and managers, the general public, news media, and interest groups, etc.

risk difference. *See* **additional risk**.

risk estimate. A description of the probability that organisms exposed to a specific dose of a chemical or other pollutant will develop an adverse response; e.g., cancer.

risk factor. Characteristics (e.g., race, sex, age, or obesity) or variables (e.g., smoking or occupational exposure level) associated with increased probability of a toxic effect.

risk for nonendangered species. Risk to species if anticipated pesticide residue levels are equal to or greater than LC_{50}.

risk management. 1. The process of evaluating and selecting alternative regulatory and nonregulatory responses to risk. 2. A decision-making process that accounts for political, social, economic, and engineering implications together with risk-related information in order to develop, analyze, and compare management options and select the appropriate managerial response to a potential chronic health hazard.

risk management plan (RMP). The amendments to the Chemical Accident Prevention Rule that were published in the Federal Register on April 9, 2004. Requires businesses handling certain toxic or flammable chemicals to create specific plans related to their safe use, storage, and handling.

risk ratio (RR). *See* **relative risk**.

risk-specific dose. The dose associated with a specified risk level.

river basin. The land area drained by a river and its tributaries.

rodenticide. A chemical or agent used to destroy rats or other rodent pests, or to prevent them from damaging food, crops, etc.

roentgen. The unit of exposure from X-rays or gamma rays (*see* exposure). One roentgen (R) = 2.58×10^{-4} C/kg (where C = couloumbs).

Roman vitriol. An archaic name for copper sulfate, $CuSO_4 \cdot 5H_2O$.

rope rescue. The act of rescuing through the use of rigging techniques, anchor systems, belays, mechanical advantages, subject extrication techniques, and low- and high-angle rescue techniques. Also known as *high-angle rescue, low-angle rescue,* and *technical rescue.*

rose vitriol. An archaic name for cobalt(II) sulfate, $CoSO_4{\cdot}7H_2O$. Also called *red vitriol.*

rotary kiln incinerator. An incinerator with a rotating combustion chamber that keeps waste moving through its interior while it operates, thereby allowing it to vaporize for easier burning.

rotational casting. The forming of plastic articles by adding to a rotating mold a fluid plastic material and rotating the mold so the fluid is distributed on the mold walls, and then heating until the plastic material has hardened.

rotational molding. Same as rotational casting, except that a dry powdered plastic is used.

route of entry. The process by which a chemical comes into contact with an organism, e.g., inhalation, ingestion, dermal contact, or injection. Also called *route of exposure.*

route of exposure. *See* **route of entry.**

rubber. A high polymer, either natural or synthetic, that becomes a thermosetting elastomer after vulcanization. A thermoplastic rubber is produced by using certain block copolymers.

rubbing alcohol. Isopropyl alcohol (IPA); i-C_3H_7OH.

rubbish. Solid waste, excluding food waste and ashes, from homes, institutions, and workplaces.

rubidium. A soft, silvery white, radioactive, water-reactive, solid, metallic element, symbol Rb, with atomic number 37, and atomic weight 85.47. It is a member of the alkali metal family.

ruby. A precious stone made of aluminum oxide (Al_2O_3).

run. A response to a fire or alarm.

runaway polymerization. The almost instantaneous, uncontrolled conversion of monomers to polymers, with a great release of heat energy. If the release of the energy is instantaneous, the result is an explosion.

running losses. Evaporation of motor vehicle fuel from the fuel tank while the vehicle is in use.

run-off. 1. Excess water produced during firefighting efforts or from rain. 2. That part of precipitation, snow melt, or irrigation water that runs off the land into streams or other surface water. It can carry pollutants from the air and land into receiving waters.

rupture disc. A safety relief device in the form of a metal disc that closes the relief channel under normal conditions. It will burst at a set pressure to permit the escape of all the gas. *See also* **frangible disc.**

rust. A reddish corrosion product (Fe_2O_3) formed by the oxidation of iron. Rusting is increased in the presence of water.

ruthenium. A brittle, white, solid, metallic element, symbol Ru, with atomic number 44, and atomic weight 101.07.

rutherfordium. A solid, radioactive, metallic element, symbol Rf, with atomic number 104, and atomic weight 261.

S

sacrificial anode. An easily corroded material deliberately installed in a pipe or intake with the intent of giving it up (sacrificing it) to corrosion, while the rest of the water supply facility remains relatively corrosion free.

SADT. *See* **self-accelerating decomposition temperature**.

safe. Condition of exposure under which there is a practical certainty that no harm will result to exposed individuals.

safety relief device. Any device that relieves internal pressure before the design strength of the container is reached.

safe water. Water that does not contain harmful bacteria, toxic materials, or chemicals, and is considered safe for drinking even if it may have taste, odor, color, and certain mineral problems.

safe yield. The annual amount of water that can be taken from a source of supply over a period of years without depleting that source beyond its ability to be replenished naturally in wet years with greater rainfall.

safener. A chemical added to a pesticide to keep it from injuring plants.

safety relief device. Any device that relieves internal pressure before the design strength of the container is reached.

safe zone. An area beyond the warm zone where there is no suspected product contamination. Often referred to as the *cold zone* or the *outermost zone*. *See also* **cold zone**.

saline solution. A blood volume substitute made of salt and water; a temporary substitute for lost blood.

salinity. The percentage of salt in water.

salt. 1. The ionic compound formed by the replacement of hydrogen in an acid by a metal or a complex cation. 2. An ionic compound formed by a metal and a nonmetal.

salt of vitriol. Archaic term for zinc sulfate ($ZnSO_4{\cdot}7H_2O$).

saltpeter. Potassium nitrate, KNO_3. Also called *nitre*.

salts. Ionic compounds that water picks up as it passes through the air, over and under the ground, or from households and industry.

saltwater intrusion. The invasion of fresh surface water or groundwater by salt water. If it comes from the ocean, it may be called a *seawater intrusion*.

salvage. 1. The utilization of waste materials. 2. In firefighting, the process of protecting the contents of a building from fire, smoke, and water damage.

samarium. A solid metallic element, symbol Sm, with atomic number 62, and atomic weight 150.4.

sampling frequency. The interval between the collection of successive samples.

sanctions. Actions taken by the federal government for failure to provide or implement a state implementation plan (SIP).

sand filter. A device that removes some suspended solids from sewage. Air and bacteria decompose additional wastes filtering through the sand so that cleaner water drains from the bed.

sanitary landfill. *See* **landfills**.

sanitary sewers. Underground pipes that carry off only domestic or industrial waste, not storm water.

sanitary survey. An on-site review of the water sources, facilities, equipment, operation, and maintenance of a public water system to evaluate the adequacy of those elements for producing and distributing safe drinking water.

sanitary water. Water discharged from sinks, showers, kitchens, or other nonindustrial operations, but not from commodes. Also known as **gray water**.

sanitation. Control of physical factors in the human environment that could harm development, health, or survival.

sanitized. A version of a document from which information claimed as a trade secret or as confidential has been omitted or withheld.

saprolite. A soft, clay-rich, thoroughly decomposed rock formed in place by chemical weathering of igneous or metamorphic rock. Forms in humid, tropical, or subtropical climates.

saprophytes. Organisms living on dead or decaying organic matter that help natural decomposition of organic matter in water.

sapwood. The outer, light-colored wood of the tree trunk, which is more susceptible to attack by decay than the heartwood.

SARA. *See* **Superfund Amendments and Reauthorization Act of 1986**.

sarin. 1. A highly toxic cholinesterase inhibitor. 2. A chemical nerve gas (GB). 3. Chemical names include isopropyl methylphospha nofluoridate, methylphosphonofluoridic acid, and isopropyl ester (of methyphos-phonofluoridic acid).

saturated. Referring to hydrocarbon compounds that contain only single covalent bonds between the carbon atoms. They are "saturated" with hydrogen atoms.

saturated solution. A solution in which no more solute will dissolve.

saturated zone. The area below the water table in which all open spaces are filled with water under pressure equal to or greater than that of the atmosphere.

saturation. The condition of a liquid when it has taken into solution the maximum possible quantity of a given substance at a given temperature and pressure.

scandium. A silvery white, solid, metallic element, symbol Sc, with atomic number 21, and atomic weight 44.956.

Science Advisory Board (SAB). A group of external scientists who advise EPA on science and policy.

SCBA. *See* **self-contained breathing apparatus**.

scientific support coordinators (SSC). Members of the on-scene coordinator's staff who act as technical and scientific advisors and as contacts for the scientific community.

scrap. Materials discarded from manufacturing operations that may be suitable for reprocessing.

scrap metal processor. Intermediate operating facility where recovered metal is sorted, cleaned of contaminants, and prepared for recycling.

screening. Use of screens to remove coarse floating and suspended solids from sewage.

screening risk assessment. A risk assessment process performed with relatively little data and many assumptions to identify exposures that should be evaluated more carefully for potential risk.

scrubber. An air pollution device that uses a spray of water or reactant, or a dry process, to trap pollutants in emissions.

seaborgium. A solid, radioactive, metallic element, symbol Sg, with atomic number 106, and atomic weight 263.

sealed source. A radioactive source, sealed in an impervious container that has sufficient mechanical strength to prevent contact with and dispersion of the radioactive material under the conditions of use and wear for which it was designed.

search suit. A protective suit made of Kevlar and Nomex 3, often used by (but not limited to) bomb squad personnel; significantly lighter than bomb suits. Allows user to conduct search with increased mobility.

seawater intrusion. *See* **saltwater intrusion**.

secondary. A particular arrangement of elements within a chemical molecule.

secondary carbon atom. 1. A carbon atom attached to two other carbon atoms with single covalent bonds. 2. When a functional group is attached to a secondary carbon, the name of the compound starts with "s-," "sec-", or "secondary."

secondary contamination. Contamination by emergency response personnel of medical or related personnel outside of the hot zone.

secondary decontamination. Decontamination between the primary (gross) and tertiary stages, usually used after gross decontamination removes the major portion of the product.

secondary drinking water regulations. Nonenforceable regulations applying to public water systems and specifying the maximum contamination levels that, in the judgment of EPA, are required to protect the public welfare. These regulations apply to any contaminants that may adversely affect the odor or appearance of such water and consequently may cause people served by the system to discontinue its use.

secondary effect. Action of a stressor on supporting components of the ecosystem, which in turn impacts the ecological component of concern.

secondary explosive. High explosive used to build up the relatively weak shock of the primary explosive sufficient to detonate the main charge, which is also made up of high explosives.

secondary materials. Materials that have been manufactured and used at least once and are to be used again.

secondary standards. National Ambient Air Quality Standards designed to protect welfare, including effects on soils, water, crops, vegetation, man-made materials, animals, wildlife, weather, visibility, and climate; also designed to protect from damage to property, economic values, and personal comfort and well-being, as well as from dangers related to transportation hazards.

secondary treatment. The second step in most publicly owned waste treatment systems in which bacteria consume the organic parts of the waste. It is accomplished by bringing together waste, bacteria, and oxygen in trickling filters or in the activated sludge process. This treatment removes floating and settleable solids and about 90% of the oxygen-demanding substances and suspended solids. Disinfection is the final stage of secondary treatment.

secondhand smoke. Inhalation of other smokers' tobacco smoke. Also called *passive smoking*.

secure chemical landfill. *See* **landfills**.

secure maximum contaminant level. Maximum permissible level of a contaminant in water delivered to the free flowing outlet of the ultimate user, or of contamination resulting from corrosion of piping and plumbing caused by water quality.

sedimentation. Letting solids settle out of wastewater by gravity during treatment.

sedimentation tank. A wastewater tank in which floating wastes are skimmed off, and settled solids are removed for disposal.

sediments. Soil, sand, and minerals washed from land into water, usually after rain.

sediment yield. The quantity of sediment arriving at a specific location.

seed protectant. A chemical applied before planting to protect seeds and seedlings from disease or insects.

seepage. Percolation of water through the soil from unlined canals, ditches, laterals, watercourses, or water storage facilities.

selective pesticide. A chemical designed to affect only certain types of pests, leaving other plants and animals unharmed.

selenium. A steel gray, toxic, solid, nonmetallic element, symbol Se, with atomic number 34, and atomic weight 78.96.

selenium oxide fume. A chemical choking agent.

self-accelerating decomposition temperature (SADT). A property of most organic peroxides. The temperature at which the molecule begins to decompose, liberating enough energy to increase the speed of the decomposition until it becomes self-feeding and irreversible.

self-contained breathing apparatus (SCBA). Breathing apparatus with full facepiece and an independent supply of air; usually a seal-tested mask, positive pressure regulator, and a pressurized air supply.

self-heating. An exothermic reaction within a material resulting in a rise in temperature in the material (ISO/IEC Guide 52.1989).

self-ignition. Ignition resulting from self-heating (ISO/IEC Guide 52.1989).

semiconductor. 1. Elements (usually all are considered nonmetals) with properties intermediate between metals and nonmetals: boron, silicon, germanium, arsenic, antimony, tellurium, and polonium. 2. Formerly called *metalloids.* Some lists include carbon, selenium, and phosphorous. 3. A substance that has conductivity between a conductor and an insulator. 4. *See also* **metalloids**.

semiconfined aquifer. An aquifer partially confined by soil layers of low permeability through which recharge and discharge can still occur.

semipermeable membrane. A thin film between two solutions through which certain molecules can pass but others cannot.

semivolatile organic compounds. Organic compounds that volatilize slowly at standard temperature (20°C) and 1 atm pressure.

senescence. The aging process that is sometimes used to describe lakes or other bodies of water in advanced stages of eutrophication. Also used to describe plants and animals.

sensitization. A reaction in which exposure to a particular chemical will cause reactions to future exposures to be much more severe, and/or will cause adverse reactions to chemicals that previously caused no problems to the now-sensitized individual.

sensitizer. A chemical that causes a substantial proportion of exposed people or animals to develop an allergic reaction in normal tissue after repeated exposure to the chemical. Repeated exposure may cause a marked response not necessarily limited to the contact site.

septic system. An on-site system designed to treat and dispose of domestic sewage.

septic tank. An underground storage tank for wastes from homes not connected to a sewer line. Waste goes directly from the home to the tank.

service connector. The pipe that carries tap water from a public water main to a building.

service line sample. A 1-L sample of water that has been standing for at least six hours in a service pipeline and is collected according to federal regulations.

service pipe. The pipeline extending from the water main to the building served or to the consumer's system.

sesqui-. A prefix meaning "one and one-half."

sesquimustard. A vesicant or blister agent; agent Q.

set. To change from an uncured state to a cured state. *See* **cure**.

setback. 1. Setting a thermometer to a lower temperature when the building is unoccupied to reduce consumption of heating energy. 2. Also refers to setting the thermometer to a higher temperature during unoccupied periods in the cooling season.

settleable solid. An insoluble material heavy enough to sink to the bottom of a wastewater treatment tank.

settling chamber. A series of screens placed in the way of flue gases to slow the stream of air, thus helping gravity to pull particles into a collection device.

settling tank. A holding area for wastewater, where heavier particles sink to the bottom for removal and disposal.

seven planets, seven metals. In astrological and alchemical thought, the seven heavenly bodies known to the ancients were associated with seven metals also known in antiquity. The associations were:

- Sun gold (*aurum*)
- Mercury mercury (quicksilver, *hydrargyrum*)
- Venus copper (*cuprum*)
- Moon silver (*argentum*)
- Mars iron (*ferrum*)
- Jupiter tin (*stannum*)
- Saturn lead (*plumbum*)

7Q10. Seven-day, consecutive low flow with a 10-year return frequency; the lowest stream flow for seven consecutive days that would be expected to occur once in 10 years.

sewage. The waste and wastewater produced by residential and commercial sources and discharged into sewers.

sewage lagoon. *See* **lagoon**.

sewage sludge. Sludge produced at a publicly owned treatment works, the disposal of which is regulated under the Clean Water Act.

sewer. A channel or conduit that carries wastewater and stormwater runoff from the source to a treatment plant or receiving stream. *Sanitary sewers* carry household, industrial, and commercial waste. *Storm sewers* carry runoff from rain or snow. *Combined sewers* handle both.

sewerage. The entire system of sewage collection, treatment, and disposal.

shading coefficient. The amount of the Sun's heat transmitted through a given window compared with that of a standard 1/8-in.-thick single pane of glass under the same conditions.

shell. Electron orbitals with the same quantum number.

shelter-in-place. A method to protect people in a hazardous materials incident without evacuating by keeping them inside a building with windows and doors closed and external ventilation systems shut off until the hazardous situation has resolved.

shipper's declaration for dangerous goods. Regarding International Air Transport Association (IATA) certification, a declaration form completed by the shipper for every shipment containing dangerous goods so defined or classified in the IATA regulation.

shipping papers. Documents such as shipping orders, bills of lading, manifests, or other shipping documents serving a similar purpose and containing hazardous materials descriptions and shipper's certification.

shock load. The arrival at a water treatment plant of raw water containing unusual amounts of algae, colloidal matter, color, suspended solids, turbidity, or other pollutants.

short-circuiting. When some of the water in tanks or basins flows faster than the rest. This may result in shorter contact, reaction, or settling times than calculated or presumed.

short-term exposure. Multiple or continuous exposure to an agent for a short period of time, usually one week.

short-term exposure limit (STEL). Usually a 15-minute time-weighted average exposure that should not be exceeded at any time during a workday, even if the eight-hour time-weighted average is within the TLV-TWA.

short ton. A unit of weight equivalent to 2,000 pounds.

Siamese. A hose appliance that has two or more female inlets and one male outlet.

sick building syndrome (SBS). A building's occupants experience acute health and/or comfort effects that appear to be linked to time spent therein, but no specific illness or cause can be identified.

side chain. A functional group, usually made up of carbon and hydrogen, that is connected to a carbon atom on the main chain and branch off to the side.

sievert. The SI unit of dose equivalent; 1 sievert (Sv) = 100 rem.

sigma G. Geometric standard deviation; sg. *See also* **mass median aerodynamic diameter**.

signal. The volume or product-level change produced by a leak in a tank.

signal words. The words used on a pesticide label—Danger, Warning, Caution—to indicate level of toxicity.

significant deterioration. Pollution resulting from a new source in previously "clean" areas. *See* **prevention of significant deterioration**.

significant municipal facilities. Those publicly owned sewage treatment plants that discharge 1 million gallons per day or more and are therefore considered by states to have the potential to substantially affect the quality of receiving waters.

significant noncompliance. *See* **significant violations**.

significant potential source of contamination. A facility or activity that stores, uses, or produces compounds with potential for significant contaminating impact if released into the source water of a public water supply.

significant violations. Violations by point source dischargers of sufficient magnitude or duration to be a regulatory priority.

silica. Silicon dioxide.

silicate. A negatively charged ion containing silicon and oxygen.

siliceous earth. Silicon dioxide, SiO_2.

silicon. A dark brown, solid, nonmetallic element, symbol Si, with atomic number 14, and atomic weight 28.086. It is used in alloys and in semiconductors.

silt. Sedimentary materials composed of fine or intermediate-sized mineral particles.

silver. A shiny, white, solid, metallic element, symbol Ag, with atomic number 47, and atomic weight 107.87. It has the highest electrical conductivity of any metal and is used in photographic chemicals, coinage, and jewelry.

silviculture. Management of forest land for timber.

simple asphyxiant. A substance that will replace the oxygen in the air to a level below that required to sustain life. *See also* **respiratory asphyxiant**; *Contrast with* **chemical asphyxiant**.

single-breath canister. Small 1-L canister designed to capture a single breath. Used in air pollutant ingestion research.

single covalent bond. A covalent bond resulting from the sharing of two electrons (one pair) between two atoms.

sink. Place in the environment where a compound or material collects.

sinking. Controlling oil spills by using an agent to trap the oil and sink it to the bottom of the body of water, where the agent and the oil are biodegraded.

SIP call. EPA action requiring a state to resubmit all or part of its state implementation plan to demonstrate attainment of the required National Ambient Air Quality Standards within the statutory deadline.

site. An area or place within the jurisdiction of the EPA and/or a state.

site assessment program. A means of evaluating hazardous waste sites through preliminary assessments and site inspections to develop a hazard ranking system score.

site inspection. The collection of information from a Superfund site to determine the extent and severity of hazards posed by the site.

site safety plan. A crucial element in all removal actions that includes information on equipment being used, precautions to be taken, and steps to take in the event of an on-site emergency.

siting. The process of choosing a location for a facility.

size-up. The process of evaluating all of the influencing factors at an emergency scene before committing personnel and equipment to a course of action.

skimming. Using a machine to remove oil or scum from the surface of the water.

slaked lime. Calcium hydroxide, $Ca(OH)_2$.

slow sand filtration. Passage of raw water through a bed of sand at low velocity, resulting in substantial removal of chemical and biological contaminants.

sludge. A semisolid residue from any of a number of air or water treatment processes; can be a hazardous waste.

sludge digester. Tank in which complex organic substances like sewage sludge are biologically dredged. During these reactions, energy is released, and much of the sewage is converted to methane, carbon dioxide, and water.

slurry. A watery mixture of insoluble matter resulting from some pollution control techniques.

small quantity generator (SQG). Persons or enterprises that produce 220 to 2,200 lb/month of hazardous waste. They are required to keep more records than conditionally exempt generators. *Contrast with* **conditionally exempt generators**.

smelter. A facility that melts or fuses ore, often with an accompanying chemical change, to separate its metal content. Emissions cause pollution; *smelting* is the process involved.

smog. 1. Air pollution typically associated with oxidants. 2. A mixture of smoke and fog.

smoke. 1. Particles suspended in air after incomplete combustion. 2. The airborne solid and liquid particulates and gases evolved when a material undergoes pyrolysis or combustion (ASTM E 176).

smokeless powder. Nitrocellulose containing a specified amount of nitrogen.

smoldering. 1. Combustion of a solid without flame, often evidenced by visible smoke (ASTM E 176). 2. The third stage of burning in which flames cease to exist because the area of confinement is airtight and lacks enough oxygen to support flaming combustion.

soap. A salt of a fatty acid. Commercial soaps are mixtures of fatty acid salts.

soda ash. Anhydrous sodium carbonate (Na_2CO_3).

sodium. A soft, solid, water-reactive, metallic element, symbol Na, with atomic number 11, and atomic weight 22.9898. It is a member of the alkali metal family and is very reactive.

soft detergents. Cleaning agents that break down in nature.

soft water. Any water that does not contain a significant amount of dissolved minerals such as the salts of calcium or magnesium.

soil adsorption field. A subsurface area containing a trench or bed with clean stones and a system of piping through which treated sewage may seep into the surrounding soil for further treatment and disposal.

soil and water conservation practices. Control measures consisting of managerial, vegetative, and structural practices to reduce the loss of soil and water.

soil conditioner. An organic material like humus or compost that helps soil absorb water, build a bacterial community, and take up mineral nutrients.

soil erodibility. An indicator of a soil's susceptibility to raindrop impact, runoff, and other erosive processes.

soil gas. Gaseous elements and compounds in the small spaces between particles of soil that can be moved or driven out under pressure.

soil moisture. The water contained in the pore space of the unsaturated zone.

soil sterilant. A chemical that temporarily or permanently prevents the growth of all plants and animals.

solar wind. The somewhat steady flow of charged particles from the solar corona into space.

solder. A metallic alloy that is used to seal joints between pipes. Formerly contained 50% lead, a level that is now prohibited.

sole-source aquifer. An aquifer that supplies 50% or more of the drinking water of an area.

solid. A state of matter having definite volume and rigid shapes, either crystalline or amorphous.

solid casting. The pouring of a liquid resin into a mold and curing the resin to a solid part.

solidification and stabilization. Removal of wastewater from a waste or changing it chemically to make it less permeable and susceptible to transport by water.

solid waste. Nonliquid, nonsoluble materials ranging from municipal garbage to industrial wastes that contain complex and sometimes hazardous substances. Solid wastes also include sewage sludge, agricultural refuse, demolition wastes, and mining residues. Technically, solid waste also refers to liquids and gases in containers. Also called *refuse*. *See also* **other solid waste**.

solid waste disposal. The final placement of refuse that is not salvaged or recycled.

Solid Waste Disposal Act. *See* **Resource Conservation and Recovery Act**.

solid waste management. Supervised handling of waste materials from their source through recovery processes to disposal.

solubility. 1. The amount of mass of a compound that will dissolve in a unit volume of solution. 2. Aqueous solubility is the maximum concentration of a chemical that will dissolve in pure water at a reference temperature.

soluble glass. *See* **water glass**.

soluble P. *See* **total dissolved phosphorous**.

soluble preservatives. Soluble substances, such as the preservatives used in wood treatment, may dissolve in particular liquids. However, when certain preservatives (such as inorganic arsenicals) are applied to wood under pressure, the preservatives become fixed to the wood cells and then are insoluble.

solute. A substance that is dissolved in a solvent.

solution. A uniformly dispersed mixture of one material dissolved in another. The usual solutions are solids, liquids, or gases dissolved in water, but they may be any substance dissolved in another substance.

solvating power. The ability of one material to dissolve another material.

solvent. A substance capable of dissolving another substance to form a uniformly dispersed mixture called a solution.

soman. A chemical nerve gas; agent GD.

soot. Carbonaceous material, usually very finely divided particles, produced by the incomplete combustion of carbon-containing materials.

sorption. 1. The action of soaking up or attracting substances. 2. The process used in many pollution control systems. *See also* **absorption** and **adsorption**.

source area. The location of liquid hydrocarbons or the zone of highest soil or groundwater concentrations, or both, of the chemical of concern.

source characterization measurements. Measurements made to estimate the rate of release of pollutants into the environment from a source such as an incinerator, landfill, etc.

source reduction. 1. Reducing the amount of materials entering the waste stream from a specific source by redesigning products or patterns of production or consumption (e.g., using returnable beverage containers). 2. Synonymous with *waste reduction*.

source separation. Segregating various wastes at the point of generation (e.g., separation of paper, metal, and glass from other wastes to make recycling simpler and more efficient).

source water protection area. The area delineated by a state for a public water supply, or including numerous such suppliers, whether the source is groundwater or surface water, or both.

space burning. 1. A phenomenon of combustion that occurs when a flame exists. 2. Flames are present when fuel mixes with the air during combustion, releasing heat and light. 3. Also called *flaming combustion*. 4. *Contrast with* **surface burning**.

sparging. 1. Injection of air below the water table to strip dissolved volatile organic compounds and/or oxygenate groundwater to facilitate aerobic biodegradation of organic compounds. 2. A process by which air or other gas is bubbled through a liquid, solid, or gas to remove a contaminant.

spark. 1. A small particle of burning material that is released from a fire. 2. A discharge of electricity. 3. A small piece of metal thrown off a larger piece by friction.

spark arrester. A device installed in a chimney, flue, or exhaust pipe to stop the emission of sparks and burning fragments.

special local-needs registration. Registration of a pesticide product by a state agency for a specific use that is not federally registered.

special-needs shelter. A refuge specifically designed to accommodate individuals with special medical needs who are not ill enough to require hospitalization.

special review. Formerly known as *rebuttable presumption against registration (RPAR)*, this is the regulatory process through which existing pesticides suspected of posing unreasonable risks to human health, nontarget organisms, or the environment are referred for review by EPA.

special waste. Items such as household hazardous waste, bulky wastes (refrigerators, pieces of furniture, etc.), tires, and used oil.

special weapons and tactics (SWAT) teams. Teams that are specially trained to handle high-risk situations and specialized tactical needs. Team members have advanced skills beyond that of typical patrol officers.

species. 1. A reproductively isolated aggregate of interbreeding organisms having common attributes and usually designated by a common name. 2. An organism belonging to such a category.

specific activity. Referring to radioactivity, it is the measurement of the amount of radioactivity (activity) per unit weight of the substance.

specific chemical identity. 1. The chemical name, Chemical Abstracts Service (CAS) registry number, or any other information that reveals the precise chemical designation of the substance. 2. Where the trade name is reported in lieu of the specific chemical identity, the trade name will be treated as the specific chemical identity for purposes of trade secrecy claims.

specific conductance. Rapid method of estimating the dissolved solid content of a water supply by testing its capacity to carry an electrical current.

specific gravity. The weight of a solid or liquid as compared to the weight of an equal volume of pure water, whose specific gravity is 1.0 by definition. A water-insoluble material with a specific gravity greater than 1.0 will sink in water, while a water-insoluble material with a specific gravity equal to or less than 1.0 will float on water.

specific heat. 1. The ratio between the amount of heat necessary to raise the temperature of a substance and the amount of heat necessary to raise the same weight of water the same number of degrees. 2. The amount of heat energy required to raise 1 g of material 1°C. 3. The ratio of the heat capacity of a substance to that of water.

specific volume. The volume of a specified weight of a substance.

specific yield. The amount of water a unit volume of saturated permeable rock will yield when drained by gravity.

spectrophotometer. An instrument for measuring the amount of light absorbed by the substance being examined.

spectrophotometry. A technique used to measure the relative intensities of wavelengths in a spectrum and to determine the concentration of a material in a sample by measurement of the amount of light the sample absorbs.

spectroscopy. 1. The study of spectra to determine the chemical composition of a material. 2. The analysis of the lines of light emitted from excited atoms as the electrons drop back to their original orbitals.

spectrum. The display of the component wavelengths of electromagnetic radiation.

spent. 1. As in *spent acid,* those acids that have been "used" in a chemical reaction; some of the acidity is lost. 2. An acid now contaminated because of the reaction in which it has just participated.

spill prevention, control, and countermeasure (SPCC) plan. Plan covering the release of hazardous substances as defined in the Clean Water Act.

spirit of alum. Sulfuric acid, H_2SO_4.

spirit of nitre. Nitric acid, HNO_3.

spirit of salt. Hydrochloric acid, HCl.

spirit of vitriol. Archaic term for sulfuric acid, H_2SO_4.

spirit of wine. Concentrated aqueous ethanol, C_2H_5OH, typically prepared by distilling wine.

spirit of wood. Methanol (methyl alcohol), CH_3OH.

splash suit. *See* **level of protection**.

splitting. Separation of the wood through the piece to the opposite surface or to an adjoining surface, caused by the tearing apart of wood cells.

spoil. Dirt or rock removed from its original location, destroying the composition of the soil in the process, as in strip mining, dredging, or construction.

spontaneous combustion. The original name for the phenomenon now known as *spontaneous ignition. See* **spontaneous ignition**.

spontaneous heating. Heating resulting from chemical or bacterial action in combustible materials that may lead to **spontaneous ignition**.

spontaneous ignition. 1. The process by which oxygen combines slowly with a fuel, usually on its surface, with the slow evolution of heat energy. The heat energy is absorbed by the fuel, raising its temperature slowly, until the fuel's ignition temperature is reached, and it breaks into flame. 2. Its older name is *spontaneous combustion.*

sprawl. Unplanned development of open land.

spray tower scrubber. A device that sprays alkaline water into a chamber where acid gases are present to aid in neutralizing the gas.

spray-up. The application of resin and reinforcement into a mold by use of a spray gun.

spring. Groundwater seeping out of the Earth where the water table intersects the ground surface.

spring loaded valve. A valve that is held in place by a spring with a built-in design strength, usually one-fourth that of the container it is protecting. When internal pressure surpasses the strength of the spring, the valve opens and relieves the pressure by venting gas or vapor. When the internal pressure drops below the design strength of the spring, the valve reseats itself, and the container is resealed.

spring melt. The process whereby warm temperatures melt winter snow and ice. Because various forms of acid deposition may have been stored in the frozen water, the melt can result in abnormally large amounts of acidity entering streams and rivers, sometimes causing fish kills. Also called *spring thaw*.

spring thaw. *See* **spring melt**.

stability. 1. An expression of the ability of a material to remain unchanged. 2. For MSDS purposes, a material is stable if it remains in the same form under expected and reasonable conditions of storage or use. 3. Conditions that may cause instability (dangerous change) are stated. Examples are temperatures above 150°F or shock from dropping.

stabilization. Conversion of the active organic matter in sludge into inert, harmless material.

stabilization ponds. *See* **lagoon**.

stabilized. A substance containing a small amount of stabilizer.

stabilizer. 1. A chemical added to another material that will keep an unwanted reaction from occurring (thus allowing it to remain stable). 2. In monomers, a stabilizer prevents premature polymerization. 3. Also called an **inhibitor**. 4. In plastics compounding, it will allow the plastic to be processed without degradation, or will protect it against oxidation or UV exposure.

stable air. A motionless mass of air that holds, instead of disperses, pollutants.

stack. A chimney, smokestack, or vertical pipe that discharges used air.

stack effect. 1. Air, as in a chimney, that moves upward because it is warmer than the ambient atmosphere. 2. Flow of air resulting from warm air rising, creating a positive pressure area at the top of a building and negative pressure area at the bottom. This effect can overpower the mechanical system and disrupt building ventilation and air circulation.

stack gas. *See* **flue gas**.

staging area. Locations set up at an incident where resources can be placed while awaiting a tactical assignment.

stagnation. Lack of motion in a mass of air or water that holds pollutants in place.

stakeholder. Any organization, governmental entity, or individual who has a stake or interest in, or may be impacted by, a given approach to environmental regulation, pollution prevention, or energy conservation, etc.

Standard Industrial Classification (SIC) Code. A system of identification codes, beginning with numbers 20 through 39, that includes all manufacturing facilities.

standardized mortality ratio (SMR). The relative measure of the difference in risk between the exposed and unexposed populations in a cohort study. The SMR is similar to the relative risk in both definition and interpretation. *See also* **relative risk**.

standard molar volume. The volume (22.4 L) occupied by 1 mole of an ideal gas under standard temperature and pressure.

standard operating procedures (SOP). The written descriptions of tasks and activities to be followed during work.

standard pressure. Standard pressure is a pressure of 1 bar; P°.

standard sample. The part of finished drinking water that is examined for the presence of coliform bacteria.

standard state. A reference value used in thermodynamic measurements to reflect the state of the system in question.

standard temperature and pressure (STP). Standard conditions of 273.15 K and 1 atm (0°C at sea level). Used as a baseline for calculations involving quantities that vary with temperature and pressure.

standard transportation commodity code (STCC). A code used by railroads. It is a seven-digit number beginning with "49-" for hazardous materials. Also called the *STCC number*.

stannum. Latin for "tin," hence the symbol, Sn.

starter. *See* **initiator**.

start of a response action. The point in time when there is a guarantee or set aside of funding by EPA, other federal agencies, states, or principal responsible parties in order to begin response actions at a Superfund site.

state. Any state of the United States, the District of Columbia, the Commonwealth of Puerto Rico, Guam, American Samoa, the United States Virgin Islands, the Northern Mariana Islands, and any other territory or possession over which the United States has jurisdiction.

state emergency response commission (SERC). 1. Commission appointed by each state governor according to the requirements of SARA Title III. The SERCs designate emergency planning districts, appoint local emergency planning committees, and supervise and coordinate their activities. 2. The planning commission, or, for the purpose of emergency planning, the governor, if there is no commission, for the state in which the facility is located.

State Environmental Goals and Indication Project. A program to assist state environmental agencies by providing technical and financial assistance in the development of environmental goals and indicators.

state implementation plans (SIP). EPA-approved state plans for the establishment, regulation, and enforcement of air pollution standards.

state management plan. Under FIFRA, a state management plan required by EPA to allow states, tribes, and U.S. territories the flexibility to design and implement ways to protect groundwater from the use of certain pesticides.

states of matter. The possible physical states of matter of substances are solid, liquid, and gas. A fourth state of matter is plasma. Mixtures of these are possible.

static pressure. In flowing air, the total pressure minus velocity pressure, pushing equally in all directions.

static water depth. The vertical distance from the centerline of the pump discharge down to the surface level of the free pool while no water is being drawn from the pool or water table.

static water level. 1. Elevation or level of the water table in a well when the pump is not operating. 2. The level or elevation to which water would rise in a tube connected to an artesian aquifer or basin in a conduit under pressure.

stationary source. A fixed-site producer of pollution, mainly power plants and other facilities using industrial combustion processes. *See also* **point source**.

statistical significance. The probability that a result is likely to be due to chance alone. By convention, a difference between two groups is usually considered statistically significant if chance could explain it only 5% of the time or less. Study design considerations may influence the a priori choice of a different statistical significance level.

steel. An alloy of iron and a small amount of carbon, and in some cases, another element.

sterilization. The removal or destruction of all microorganisms, including pathogenic and other bacteria, vegetative forms, and spores.

sterilizer. One of three groups of antimicrobials registered by EPA for public health uses. EPA considers an antimicrobial to be a sterilizer when it destroys or eliminates all forms of bacteria, viruses, and fungi and their spores.

stoichiometry. 1. The branch of chemistry that studies the quantitative relationship between chemical substances in a reaction. 2. It measures the proportions of elements that combine during chemical reactions.

storage. Temporary holding of waste pending treatment or disposal, as in containers, tanks, waste piles, and surface impoundments.

storm sewer. A system of pipes (separate from sanitary sewers) that carries water runoff from buildings and land surfaces.

straight chain. The configuration of the molecule of a hydrocarbon when a carbon atom attaches itself to another carbon atom that has only one other carbon atom already attached to it. A chain of carbon atoms (and perhaps other atoms) that has an open-ended structure. That is, a drawing of the structure will show its ends.

straight (solid) stream. A firefighting method used to apply or distribute water from the end of a hose. The water is delivered under pressure for maximum penetration.

strategy. A carefully devised overall plan of action to handle emergencies.

stratification. Separating into layers.

stratigraphy. Study of the formation, composition, and sequence of sediments, whether consolidated or not.

stratosphere. 1. The portion of the atmosphere 10 to 25 miles above the Earth's surface. 2. The region of the atmosphere between the troposphere and the mesosphere.

strength. Referring to an acid, it is the degree to which the acid ionizes when dissolved in water. Some inorganic acids are strong acids, while organic acids are weak acids.

stressor. A physical, chemical, or biological entity that can induce adverse effects on systems, ecosystems, or human health. *Contrast with* **receptor**.

strike team. A special team made up of members with the same skill and training that can handle specialized responses.

strip cropping. Growing crops in a systematic arrangement of strips or bands that serve as barriers to wind and water erosion.

strip mining. A process that uses machines to scrape soil or rock away from mineral deposits just under the Earth's surface.

strong acid. 1. A strong acid is an acid that completely dissociates into hydrogen ions and anions in solution. Strong acids are strong electrolytes. 2. There are only six common strong acids: hydrochloric acid (HCl), hydrobromic acid (HBr), hydroiodic acid (HI), sulfuric acid (H_2SO_4), perchloric acid ($HClO_4$), and nitric acid (HNO_3).

strong base. 1. A strong base is a base that completely dissociates into ions in solution. 2. Strong bases are strong electrolytes. 3. The most common strong bases are alkali metal and alkaline earth metal hydroxides.

strong electrolyte. 1. A substance that conducts electricity well in a dilute water solution. 2. Strong acids and bases.

strontium. A silvery white, solid, metallic element, symbol Sr, with atomic number 38, and atomic weight 87.62. It is a member of the alkaline earth metals.

structural deformation. Distortion in walls of a tank after liquid has been added or removed.

structural effect. 1. The effect upon certain properties of an analogous series of compounds by branching. 2. Properties such as boiling point, flash point, ignition temperature, and others change as branches are added to compounds, including isomers. 3. An additional structure effect is the effect of molecular weight, which, as it increases or decreases within an analogous family of covalent compounds, will have an effect on these same properties.

structural firefighting clothing. *See* **full turnouts**.

structural formula. A drawing of the molecule using the dash method, which shows all the atoms present and their bonding to each other. *See also* **chemical formula** and **molecular formula**.

structure fire. A fire originating in and/or burning any part or all of any building, shelter, or other structure.

styrene. Technically, the monomer of polystyrene ($CH_2{=}CHC_6H_5$), but polystyrene (PS) is often referred to as styrene.

styrene acrylonitrile (SAN). A thermoplastic made from the copolymerization of styrene and acrylonitrile.

styrene butadiene (SB). An elastomer made from the copolymerization of styrene and butadiene.

subacute exposure. Exposure less than acute.

subatomic particles. The nucleus and orbiting electrons.

subchronic. Of intermediate duration, usually used to describe studies or periods of exposure lasting between 5 and 90 days.

subchronic exposure. Multiple or continuous exposures lasting for approximately 10% of an experimental species lifetime, usually over a three-month period. Exposure to a substance spanning approximately 10% of the lifetime of an organism.

subchronic study. A toxicity study designed to measure effects from subchronic exposure to a chemical.

subcutaneous. Refers to being below the skin (as in a penetrating injury, injection, or intravenous line).

subdural. Beneath the dura matter of the brain and spinal cord.

sublimation. The act of changing physical state from solid directly to vapor.

sublime. To pass from the solid phase to the vapor stage, bypassing the liquid phase.

sublingual. 1. A medication that is taken by dissolving under the tongue. 2. Under the tongue.

submerged aquatic vegetation. Vegetation that lives at or below the water surface; an important habitat for young fish and other aquatic organisms.

submitter. A person filing a required report or making a claim of trade secrecy to EPA under Sections 303(d)(2) and (d)(3), 311, 312, and 313 of Title III.

substantiation. The written answers submitted to EPA by a submitter to the specific questions set forth in this regulation in support of a claim that chemical identity is a trade secret.

substituted. A compound that has had one or more of its atoms removed and replaced by atoms of other elements.

subwatershed. Topographic perimeter of the catchment area of a stream tributary.

suction. The admission of fresh air into an interior space by lowering the pressure outside of the space, thereby drawing the contaminated air outward. *See also* **ventilation**.

sufficient evidence. A term used in evaluating study data for the classification of a carcinogen under the 1986 U.S. EPA guidelines for carcinogen risk assessment. This classification indicates that there is a causal relationship between the agent or agents and human cancer.

sugar. A carbohydrate with a characteristically sweet taste. Sugars are classified as monosaccharides, disaccharides, or trisaccharides. Common table sugar is sucrose.

sugar of lead. Lead acetate; $Pb(CH_3CO_2)_2{\cdot}3H_2O$.

sulfate. A salt of sulfuric acid (H_2SO_4) when combined with a metallic ion; SO_4^{-2}.

sulfide. 1. A binary chemical compound where sulfur is bound to metal ions. 2. May also be an organic compound where sulfur is bonded to hydrocarbon backbones.

sulfite. A salt of sulfurous acid (H_2SO_3), when combined with a metallic ion; SO_3^{-2}.

sulfur. A solid, yellow, nonmetallic element, symbol S, with atomic number 16, and atomic weight 32.065.

sulfur dioxide. A pungent, colorless gas formed primarily by the combustion of fossil fuels; becomes a pollutant when present in large amounts; SO_2.

sulfuretted. Combined with or impregnated with sulfur.

sulfuretted hydrogen. Hydrogen sulfide, H_2S.

sulfuric acid. 1. A strong acid; H_2SO_4. It is also a moderately strong oxidizing agent and a powerful dehydrating agent. 2. The number one volume chemical in the world.

sump. A pit or tank that catches liquid runoff for drainage or disposal.

superchlorination. Chlorination with doses that are deliberately selected to produce water free of combined residuals so large as to require dechlorination.

superconductive. The ability to conduct electricity with no electrical resistance.

supercooled. The condition of a liquid cooled below its usual freezing point without solidifying, usually under pressure.

supercooled liquid. A liquid that, when cooled, appears to solidify, but actually continues to flow very slowly under the influence of gravity.

supercritical fluid. A substance at temperature above its critical temperature and critical pressure.

supercritical water. A thermal treatment that uses moderate temperatures and high pressures to enhance the ability of water to break down large organic molecules into smaller ones, after which oxygen is injected during this process, oxidizing those simple organic compounds into carbon dioxide and water.

Superfund. The program operated under the legislative authority of CERCLA and SARA that funds and carries out EPA solid waste emergency and long-term removal and remedial activities.

Superfund Amendments and Reauthorization Act of 1986 (SARA). The Superfund Amendments and Reauthorization Act of 1986, et seq. Title III is the Emergency Planning Community Right-to-Know Act (EPCRA).

Superfund Innovative Technology Evaluation (SITE) Program. An EPA program to promote development and use of innovative treatment and site characterization technologies in Superfund site cleanups.

superheated. When a substance is heated to an abnormally high temperature, or when a liquid is heated above its normal boiling point without causing vaporization (under pressure).

superoxide. A binary compound containing oxygen in the –½ oxidation state. For example, KO_2 is potassium superoxide, an ionic compound containing the superoxide ion, O_2^{-1}.

supersaturated solution. A solution containing a higher-than-saturation concentration of solute; slight disturbance or seeding causes crystallization of excess solute.

supplemental registration. An arrangement whereby a registrant licenses another company to market its pesticide product under the second company's registration.

supplier of water. Any person who owns or operates a public water supply.

supporting study. A study that contains information useful for providing insight and support for conclusions.

support zone. The area where administrative and support functions not requiring respiratory protective equipment are performed. Also called the **cold zone**.

suppressant. An agent, such as water or foam, used to restrain production of gases or vapors, or to extinguish the flaming and glowing phases of combustion when it is applied to burning fuels.

suppression. Control, inhibition, or reduction of hazards, particularly in incidents that involve fire, production of dangerous gases, or the release of hazardous materials.

surface burning. 1. A phenomenon of combustion that occurs when oxygen combines (with the release of heat and light) with the fuel on the surface of the fuel rather than mixing in the air. 2. Also called **glowing combustion**.

surface impoundment. Treatment, storage, or disposal of liquid hazardous wastes in ponds.

surface runoff. Precipitation, snow melt, or irrigation water in excess of what can infiltrate the soil surface and be stored in small surface depressions; a major transporter of nonpoint source pollutants in rivers, streams, and lakes.

surface tension. 1. The property of liquids that imparts a slight elasticity to its surface. 2. It also allows liquids to form separate drops.

surface uranium mines. Strip mining operations for removal of uranium-bearing ore.

surface water. All water naturally open to the atmosphere (rivers, lakes, reservoirs, ponds, streams, impoundments, seas, and estuaries, etc.).

Surface-Water Treatment Rule. The rule that specifies maximum contaminant level goals for *Giardia lamblia*, viruses, and *Legionella pneumophila*, and promulgates filtration and disinfection requirements for public water systems using surface water or groundwater sources under the direct influence of surface water.

surfacing asbestos-containing material (ACM). Asbestos-containing material that is sprayed or troweled on or otherwise applied to surfaces, such as acoustical plaster on ceilings and fireproofing materials on structural members.

surfacing material. Material sprayed or troweled onto structural members (beams, columns, or decking) for fire protection; or on ceilings or walls for fireproofing, acoustical, or decorative purposes. Includes textured plaster and other textured wall and ceiling surfaces.

surfactant. Any substance that changes the properties of the surface of another material.

surrogate data. Data from studies of test organisms or a test substance that are used to estimate the characteristics or effects on another organism or substance.

surveillance system. A series of monitoring devices designed to check on environmental conditions.

surveying. *See* **monitoring**.

susceptibility analysis. An analysis to determine whether a public water supply is subject to significant pollution from known potential sources.

suspected human carcinogen. A material that has caused cancer in laboratory animals, but such studies do not permit a definitive evaluation of carcinogenic risks to humans. The conservative approach is to consider it a possible human carcinogen.

suspect material. Building material suspected of containing asbestos; e.g., surfacing material, floor tile, ceiling tile, and thermal system insulation.

suspended loads. Specific sediment particles maintained in the water column by turbulence and carried with the flow of water.

suspended solids. Small particles of solid pollutants that float on the surface of, or are suspended in, sewage or other liquids. They resist removal by conventional means.

suspension. 1. Suspending the use of a pesticide when EPA deems it necessary to prevent an imminent hazard resulting from its continued use. An emergency suspension takes effect immediately. Under an ordinary suspension, a registrant can request a hearing before the suspension goes into effect. 2. The dispersion of a fine solid in a liquid.

suspension culture. Cells growing in a liquid nutrient medium.

swamp. A type of wetland dominated by woody vegetation but without appreciable peat deposits. Swamps may be fresh or salt water and tidal or nontidal. *See* **wetlands.**

swarf. Waste material from metal grinding processes.

sweet salt. Sodium chlorite, $NaClO_2$.

sym. An abbreviation for "symmetrical," referring to a particular arrangement of elements within a chemical molecule.

symbol. *See* **chemical symbol**.

synapse. A junction between two nerve cells close enough so that an electrical impulse may jump from one nerve cell to the other.

synergism. 1. An interaction of two or more chemicals that results in an effect greater than the sum of their separate effects. 2. A phenomenon in which the chemical effect of two materials added together is greater than the effect that would be produced by both materials acting individually with the effects added together. 3. Also known as *synergistic effect.*

synergist. A substance that, when added to a compound in conjunction with another substance, causes an enhancement of the properties of the other substance. It is said to cause **synergism**.

synergistic effect. *See* **synergism**.

synfuel. A liquid fuel synthesized from a source other than petroleum.

synthesis. The chemical reaction by which a molecule or compound that exists in nature is made by man.

synthesize. To make a molecule (man-made) duplicating a molecule made in nature.

synthetic. Made by man, as opposed to being made in nature.

synthetic organic chemicals (SOCs). Man-made (anthropogenic) organic chemicals. Some SOCs are volatile; others tend to stay dissolved in water instead of evaporating.

synthetic polymer. A polymer made by man, as opposed to a natural polymer. Rubber and plastics are synthetic polymers.

systemic effects. *See* **systemic toxicity**.

systemic pesticide. A chemical absorbed by an organism that interacts with the organism and makes the organism toxic to pests.

systemic poison. Any poison that interferes with any vital bodily process.

systemic toxicity. Toxic effects as a result of absorption and distribution of a toxicant to a site distant from its entry point, at which point effects are produced. Not all chemicals that produce systemic effects cause the same degree of toxicity in all organs.

system with a single service connection. A system that supplies drinking water to consumers via a single service line.

T

table salt. Sodium chloride (NaCl).

table sugar. Sucrose ($C_{12}H_{11}O_{22}$).

tabun. 1. Dimethylphosphoramidocyanidic acid, ethyl ester. 2. Highly toxic cholinesterase inhibitor. 3. A chemical nerve gas; agent GA.

tailings. Residue of raw material or waste separated out during the processing of crops or mineral ores.

tailpipe standards. Emissions limitations applicable to mobile source engine exhausts.

tailwater. The runoff of irrigation water from the lower end of an irrigated field.

tampering. Adjusting, negating, or removing pollution control equipment on a motor vehicle.

tantalum. A dense, blue gray, solid, metallic element, symbol Ta, with atomic number 73, and atomic weight 180.948.

target organ. The biological organ (or organs) most adversely affected by exposure to a chemical substance.

target tissue. The tissue to which specific chemicals cause harm.

technetium. A silvery gray, solid, radioactive, metallic element, symbol Tc, with atomic number 43, and atomic weight 98.

technical assistance grant (TAG). As part of the Superfund program, technical assistance grants of up to $50,000 are provided to citizens' groups to obtain assistance in interpreting information related to cleanups at Superfund sites or those proposed for the National Priorities List. Grants are used by such groups to hire technical advisors to help them understand the site-related technical information for the duration of response activities.

technical-grade active ingredient (TGA or TGAI). A pesticide chemical in pure form as it is manufactured prior to being formulated into an end-use product (e.g., wettable powders, granules, or emulsifiable concentrates). Registered manufactured products composed of such chemicals are known as *technical grade products.*

technical grade products. *See* **technical-grade active ingredient**.

technical name. The recognized chemical name currently used in scientific and technical handbooks, journals, and texts for a substance.

technical rescue. *See* **rope rescue**.

technology-based limitations. Industry-specific effluent limitations based on best available preventive technology applied to a discharge when it will not cause a violation of water quality standards at low stream flows. Usually applied to discharges into large rivers.

technology-based standards. Industry-specific effluent limitations applicable to direct and indirect sources that are developed on a category-by-category basis using statutory factors, not including water-quality effects.

Teflon. *See* **polytetrafluoroethylene**.

tellurium. A solid metallic element, symbol Te, with atomic number 52, and atomic weight 127.60.

temperature. A measure of how fast a group of molecules is moving.

temperature inversion. The abnormal reversal of temperature in the troposphere caused by the entrapment of urban air pollution.

tensile. 1. Pertaining to tension. 2. Capable of being stretched.

tensile strength. 1. The pulling stress required to break a specimen, measured in pounds per square inch. 2. Resistance of a material to a force tending to tear it by stretching. 3. The maximum stress sustained by a specimen during a tension test.

tera-. The prefix meaning "10^{12}."

teratogen. Material that affects the offspring when a developing embryo or fetus is exposed to that material.

teratogenesis. The introduction of non-hereditary birth defects in a developing fetus by exogenous factors such as physical or chemical agents acting in the womb to interfere with normal embryonic development.

teratogenic. Structural developmental defects due to exposure to a chemical agent during formation of individual organs, causing a fetus to develop unnaturally.

terbium. A solid, silvery gray, metallic element, symbol Tb, with atomic number 65, and atomic weight 158.925. A rare earth element that is used in lasers, TV tubes, and X-ray tubes.

ternary acid. A ternary compound containing hydrogen, oxygen, and another element, often a nonmetal.

ternary compound. An ionic or covalent compound consisting of three elements.

terpolymer. A polymer that is a product of the copolymerization of three different monomers, such as those in acrylonitrile-butadiene-styrene (ABS), even though the three monomers were not polymerized together.

terracing. Dikes built along the contour of sloping farm land that hold runoff and sediment to reduce erosion.

territory logistics centers (TLC). Centers located in continental United States to ensure readiness and "just in time" logistics for disaster responders. Remote storage sites (RSS) are in the Caribbean and Pacific. *Contrast with* **remote storage sites**.

tert. Abbreviation for *tertiary*.

tertiary. 1. Primarily used in reference to alcohols based on methanol, containing one hydroxyl (-OH) radical. 2. A tertiary alcohol has three alkyl radicals attached to the carbon atom. 3. A tertiary amine is where all three hydrogen atoms are replaced by alkyl radicals. 4. When a functional group is attached to this carbon, the name of the compound starts with "t-," "tert-," or "tertiary."

tertiary carbon atom. A carbon atom attached to three other carbon atoms with single covalent bonds.

tertiary decontamination. A third phase of decontamination usually accomplished at a medical facility to remove remaining minute quantities of contaminant.

tertiary treatment. Advanced cleaning of wastewater that goes beyond the secondary or biological stage, removing nutrients such as phosphorus, nitrogen, and most biochemical oxygen demand (BOD) and suspended solids.

test assembly. The wall or floor into which the test samples are mounted or installed (ASTM E 800).

tetra-. The prefix that means "four."

tetrahedron of fire. A theory of fire that states that there are four elements necessary to have a fire: fuel, energy, an oxidizer, and the chain reaction of burning.

tetryl. An explosive used as a detonator for high explosives; trinitrophenylmethylnitramine.

thallium. A soft, solid, toxic, metallic element, symbol Tl, with atomic number 81, and atomic weight 204.38.

Thénard's blue. Blue cobalt aluminate, $Co(AlO_2)_2$, named for Louis-Jacques Thénard.

theoretical maximum residue contribution (TMRC). The theoretical maximum amount of a pesticide in the daily diet of an average person. It assumes that the diet is composed of all food items for which there are tolerance-level residues of the pesticide. The TMRC is expressed as milligrams of pesticide/kilograms of body weight/day.

therapeutic index. The ratio of the dose required to produce toxic or lethal effects to the dose required to produce nonadverse or therapeutic responses.

thermal column. 1. The rising column of heated air or gases above a continuing heat or fire source. 2. Also known as a *convection column*.

thermal cracking. A refining process that, through the breaking of covalent bonds, decomposes, rearranges, or combines hydrocarbon molecules by the application of heat without the aid of catalysts.

thermal pollution. Discharge of heated water from industrial processes that can kill or injure aquatic organisms.

thermal stratification. The formation of layers of different temperatures in a lake or reservoir.

thermal stressor. Any system or condition that may cause a container to fail through heat, coldness, or pressure.

thermal system insulation (TSI). Asbestos-containing material applied to pipes, fittings, boilers, breeching, tanks, ducts, or other interior structural components to prevent heat loss or gain or water condensation.

thermal treatment. Use of elevated temperatures to treat hazardous wastes.

thermocline. The middle layer of a thermally stratified lake or reservoir in which there is a rapid decrease in temperatures in a lake or reservoir. *See also* **metalimnion**.

thermodynamics. 1. The branch of physics that deals with the energy transfers accompanying physical and chemical processes. 2. The science that deals with the conversion of heat into mechanical, electrical, or chemical energy.

thermoforming. A plastic sheet that is formed into a finished part by clamping it onto a frame over a mold, softening it with heat, and then applying pressure to make it conform to the mold.

thermogravimetric analysis (TGA). A method of analysis to observe weight changes, such as studying the loss of waters of hydration or carbon dioxide (CO_2).

thermonuclear energy. Energy from nuclear fusion reactions.

thermoplastic. 1. A class of plastics that can be subjected to heat and pressure more than once without degradation. 2. Depending on the particular thermoplastic, it may be "ground up" and resubmitted to heat and pressure many times. 3. *Contrast with* **thermoset**.

thermoset. A class of plastics that can be subjected to heat and pressure only once. Any further exposure to heat and/or pressure will cause the material to grade and/or decompose. *Contrast with* **thermoplastic**, which can be subjected to heat and pressure more than once without degradation.

thermosphere. 1. The area of the atmosphere between the mesosphere and outer space. 2. The outermost shell of the atmosphere.

thia-. Prefix used to indicate the presence of sulfur in a cyclic compound.

thickened agent. An agent that has had a substance added to it to make it less volatile.

thio-. 1. Prefix used to indicate the presence of sulfur in a compound. 2. It usually means "replace an oxygen with sulfur." For example, the cyanate ion is OCN^{-1}, and the thiocyanate ion is SCN^{-1}.

thioether. Sulfur has replaced the oxygen in an ether molecule (R-S-R').

thiol. 1. A class of chemicals resembling alcohols, but having the oxygen in the hydroxyl radical replaced by sulfur. 2. The general formula is R-SH, where the R- is a hydrocarbon radical. 3. Also called **mercaptans**. 4. Most members of this chemical class are flammable, toxic, and have strong odors.

thorium. A soft, silvery white, solid, radioactive, metallic element, symbol Th, with atomic number 90, and atomic weight 232.

threshold. 1. The lowest dose of a chemical at which a specified measurable effect is observed and below which it is not observed. 2. The dose or exposure level below which a significant adverse effect is not expected.

threshold amount. The annual amount of a toxic chemical manufactured, processed, or otherwise used that, when exceeded, subjects the facility to toxic chemical release inventory (TCRI) reporting.

threshold level. 1. Time-weighted average pollutant concentration values, exposure beyond which is likely to adversely affect human health. 2. The amount of a hazardous chemical present in a facility at any one time, which when exceeded subjects the facility to hazardous chemical reporting.

threshold limit value (TLV). The concentration of an airborne substance to which an average person can be repeatedly exposed without adverse effects. TLVs may be expressed in three ways:

1. TLV-TWA (time-weighted average), based on an allowable exposure averaged over a normal 8-hour workday or 40-hour work week.
2. TLV-STEL (short-term exposure limit), or maximum concentration for a brief specified period of time, depending on a specific chemical. (TWA must still be met.)
3. TLV-C (ceiling exposure limit), or maximum exposure concentration not to be exceeded under any circumstances. (TWA must still be met.)

threshold limit value-ceiling (TLV-C). Also known as the *ceiling limit,* above which the concentration of the substance in question must not rise at any time. Set by the American Conference of Governmental Industrial Hygienists (ACGIH).

threshold limit value–short-term exposure limit (TLV-STEL). 1. Maximum concentration for a brief specified period of time, depending on a specific chemical (TWA must still be met). 2. The short-term exposure limit, or maximum concentration for a continuous 15-minute exposure period (maximum of four such periods a day, with at least 60 minutes between exposure periods, and provided that the daily TLV-TWA is not exceeded).

threshold limit value–time-weighted average (TLV-TWA). 1. The average (weighted over time) maximum amount of gas, vapor, dust or fumes to which a person may be exposed for 8 hours a day, five days a week, without harm. 2. The time-weighted average concentration for a normal 8-hour workday and a 40-hour work week, to which nearly all workers may be repeatedly exposed, day after day, without adverse effect (ACGIH). 3. The OSHA term is permissible exposure limit (PEL). *See* **permissible exposure limit**.

threshold odor. *See* **odor threshold**.

threshold planning quantity (TPQ). 1. A quantity designated for each chemical on the list of extremely hazardous substances that triggers notification by facilities to the state emergency response commission that such facilities are subject to emergency planning requirements under SARA Title III. 2. The amount of an extremely hazardous substance present in a facility at any one time that, when exceeded, subjects the facility to the emergency planning requirements.

threshold reportable quantity (TRQ). Specific quantities of substances, above which a facility must report. The two types are: *inventory forms* and *routine release forms.* Inventory forms represent the quantity of material a facility has present; reports to SERC, LEPC, and FD. Routine release reporting concerns quantities of toxic substances used at a facility above which the facility is required to provide routine release information to EPA.

thropic levels. A functional classification of species that is based on feeding relationships (e.g., generally aquatic and terrestrial green plants comprise the first thropic level, and herbivores comprise the second).

thulium. A solid metallic element, symbol Tm, with atomic number 69, and atomic weight 168.934. It is a rare earth element.

thymol blue. A common name for thymolsulphonphthalein, $C_{27}H_{30}O_5S$, an acid-base indicator that changes from pink to yellow as the pH is raised through 2.2, and then to blue as the pH is raised through 8.8.

tidal marsh. Low, flat marshlands traversed by channels and tidal hollows, subject to tidal inundation. Normally, the only vegetation present is salt-tolerant bushes and grasses. *See* **wetlands**.

tidal volume (TV). The volume of air inhaled/exhaled during normal breathing.

tier I/tier II. Inventory forms for reporting hazardous chemicals.

tillage. Plowing, seedbed preparation, and cultivation practices.

timber. A size classification of lumber in which the smallest dimension is at least 5 in.

time-weighted average (TWA). 1. In air sampling, the average air concentration of contaminants during a given period. 2. A measurement to determine the worker's average exposure to a substance over a typical eight-hour work shift. The actual exposure is then compared to OSHA standards or other professional guidelines.

tin. A silvery, solid, metallic element, symbol Sn, with atomic number 50, and atomic weight 118.71.

tire processor. Intermediate operating facility where recovered tires are processed in preparation for recycling.

tires. As used in recycling, passenger car and truck tires (excludes airplane, bus, motorcycle, and special service military, agricultural, off-the-road, and slow-speed industrial tires). Car and truck tires are recycled into rubber products such as trash cans, storage containers, or rubberized asphalt, or are used whole for playground and reef construction.

tissue asphyxiant. A substance that replaces oxygen in the red blood cell and poisons the body cell to which it is transferred.

titanium. A silvery, solid, metallic element, symbol Ti, with atomic number 22, and atomic weight 47.87. It is used in making alloys.

Title III. A section of SARA known as The Emergency Planning and Community Right-to-Know Act (EPCRA).

tolerance petition. A formal request to establish a new tolerance or modify an existing one.

tolerances. Permissible residue levels for pesticides in raw agricultural produce and processed foods.

ton. A unit of weight equal to 2,000 pounds. Also called a *short ton* or a *net ton.*

tonnage. 1. The amount of waste that a landfill accepts, usually expressed in tons per month. 2. The rate at which a landfill accepts waste is limited by the landfill's permit.

topography. The physical features of a surface area, including relative elevations and the position of natural and man-made (anthropogenic) features.

torr. The unit of pressure equivalent to the amount of pressure that will support a column of mercury (Hg) 1 millimeter (mm) high; 760 torr (760 mm Hg) is equal to atmospheric pressure at sea level or 14.7 psi. One torr = 1 mm of mercury.

total containment vessel (TCV). A total containment vessel is designed to transport explosive or chemical devices, fully enclosed. Used for explosive and hazardous materials.

total dissolved phosphorous. The total phosphorous content of all material that will pass through a filter, which is determined as orthophosphate without prior digestion or hydrolysis. Also called *soluble P* or *ortho P*.

total dissolved solids (TDS). All material that passes the standard glass river filter; now called *total filterable residue*. The term is used to reflect salinity.

total filterable residue. *See* **total dissolved solids.**

total flux meter. The instrument used to measure the level of radiant heat energy incident on the specimen plane at any point (ASTM E 648).

total lung capacity. (TLC) The maximum amount of air that can be exhaled (vital capacity) plus the amount of air left in the lungs (residual volume).

total lung volume (TLV). The lung volume at maximal inspiration.

total petroleum hydrocarbons (TPH). Measure of the concentration or mass of petroleum hydrocarbon constituents present in a given amount of soil or water.

total recovered petroleum hydrocarbon. A method for measuring petroleum hydrocarbons in samples of soil or water.

total suspended particulates (TSP). A method of monitoring airborne particulate matter by total weight.

total suspended solids (TSS). A measure of the suspended solids in wastewater, effluent, or water bodies, determined by tests for total suspended nonfilterable solids.

toxaphene. Chemical that causes adverse health effects in domestic water supplies and is toxic to freshwater and marine aquatic life.

toxic. 1. Anything harmful, destructive, poisonous, or deadly to the body. 2. A chemical falling within any of the following categories:

A. A chemical that has a median lethal dose (LD_{50}) of more than 50 milligrams (mg) per kilogram (kg) of body weight, but not more than 500 mg/kg of body weight when administered orally to albino rats weighing between 200 and 300 grams (g) each.

B. A chemical that has an LD_{50} of more than 200 mg/kg of body weight, but not more than 1,000 mg/kg of body weight when administered by continuous contact for 24 hours (or less if death occurs within 24 hours), with the bare skin of albino rabbits weighing between 200 g and 300 g each.

C. A chemical that has a median lethal concentration (LC_{50}) in air of more than 200 parts per million (ppm), but not more than 2,000 ppm by volume of gas or vapor, or more than 2 mg per liter (mg/L), but not more than 20 mg/L of mist, fume, or dust, when administered by continuous inhalation for 1 hour (or less if death occurs within 1 hour) to albino rats weighing between 200 g and 300 g each.

toxicant. A harmful substance or agent that may injure an exposed organism.

toxic chemical. Any chemical listed in EPA rules as "Toxic Chemicals Subject to Section 313 of the Emergency Planning and Community Right-to-Know Act of 1986."

toxic chemical release form. Information form required of facilities that manufacture, process, or use (in quantities above a specific amount) chemicals listed under SARA Title III.

toxic chemical use substitution. Replacing toxic chemicals with less harmful chemicals in industrial processes.

toxic cloud. Airborne plume of gases, vapors, fumes, or aerosols containing toxic materials.

toxic concentration. The concentration at which a substance produces a toxic effect.

toxic dose. The dose level at which a substance produces a toxic effect.

toxic inhalation hazard (TIH). Term used to describe gases and volatile liquids that are toxic when inhaled. Also called *poison inhalation hazard (PIH).*

toxicity. 1. The ability of a chemical substance to produce injury once it reaches a susceptible site in or near the body. 2. The harmful effects of a chemical on some biologic mechanism. 3. The degree to which a substance or mixture of substances can harm humans or animals.

toxicity assessment. Characterization of the toxicological properties and effects of a chemical, with special emphasis on establishment of dose-response characteristics.

toxicity testing. Biological testing (usually with an invertebrate, fish, or small mammal) to determine the adverse effects of a compound or effluent.

toxicological profile. An examination, summary, and interpretation of a hazardous substance to determine levels of exposure and associated health effects.

toxicology. The study of the harmful effects of chemicals on living tissue.

toxic pollutants. Materials that cause death, disease, or birth defects in organisms that ingest or absorb them.

Toxic Release Inventory. The database containing the annual toxic chemical release reports submitted by certain manufacturing facilities, specified in Section 313 of SARA, Title III.

toxic substance. A chemical or mixture that may present an unreasonable risk of injury to health or the environment.

Toxic Substances Control Act (TSCA). A list of reviewed harmful substances that require precautions and safe work practices by the community and industry (40 CFR 700–799).

toxic waste. 1. A waste that can produce injury if inhaled, swallowed, or absorbed through the skin. 2. A hazardous waste that meets the characteristics of extraction procedure (EP) toxicity as defined in the RCRA regulations by the EPA (40 CFR).

toxin. Poison produced by a living organism; also, its synthetic equivalent (e.g., ricin or botulinum toxin).

trace gases. Gases in the atmosphere that occur in very small quantities but are important to life on Earth or are necessary components of the chemical cycles in the atmosphere.

trade name product. A chemical or mixture of chemicals that is distributed to other persons and that incorporates a toxic chemical component that is not identified by the applicable chemical name or Chemical Abstracts Service registry number listed in Section 372.65.

trade secrecy claim. A submittal under sections 303(d)(2) or (d)(3), or 311, 312 or 313 of Title III, in which a chemical identity is claimed as trade secret and is accompanied by a substantiation in support of the claim of trade secrecy for chemical identity.

trade secret. Any confidential formula, pattern, process, device, information, or compilation of information that is used in a submitter's business, and that gives the submitter an opportunity to obtain an advantage over competitors who do not know or use it. EPA intends to be guided by the Restatement of Torts, Section 757, Comment b.

training levels, first responder. The training levels include awareness level, operations level, hazardous materials technician, and hazardous materials specialist. OSHA regulations [OSHA 1910.120 (q)(6)] specify the following:

First responder awareness level. First responders at the awareness level are individuals who are likely to witness or discover a hazardous substance release and who have been trained to initiate an emergency response sequence by notifying the authorities of the release. First responders at the awareness level shall have sufficient training or have had sufficient experience to objectively demonstrate competency in the following areas:

A. An understanding of what hazardous substances are, and the risks associated with them in an incident.

B. An understanding of the potential outcomes associated with an emergency created when hazardous substances are present.

C. The ability to recognize the presence of hazardous substances in an emergency.

D. The ability to identify the hazardous substances, if possible.

E. An understanding of the role of the first responder awareness individual in the employer's emergency response plan, including site security and control and the U.S. Department of Transportation's *Emergency Response Guidebook.*

F. The ability to realize the need for additional resources, and to make appropriate notifications to the communication center.

First responder operations level. First responders at the operations level are individuals who respond to releases or potential releases of hazardous substances as part of the initial response to the site for the purpose of protecting nearby persons, property, or the environment from the effects of the release. They are trained to respond in a defensive fashion without actually trying to stop the release. Their function is to contain the release from a safe distance, keep it from spreading, and prevent exposures. First responders at the operations level shall have received at least eight hours of training or have had sufficient experience to objectively demonstrate competency in the following areas in addition to those listed for the awareness level, and the employer shall so certify:

A. Knowledge of the basic hazard and risk assessment techniques.

B. Know how to select and use proper personal protective equipment provided to the first responder operational level.

C. An understanding of basic hazardous materials terms.

D. Know how to perform basic control, containment, and/or confinement operations within the capabilities of the resources and personal protective equipment available with their unit.

E. Know how to implement basic decontamination procedures.

F. An understanding of the relevant standard operating procedures and termination procedures.

Hazardous materials technician. Hazardous materials technicians are individuals who respond to releases or potential releases for the purpose of stopping the release. They assume a more aggressive role than a first responder at the operations level does, in that they will approach the point of release in order to plug, patch, or otherwise stop the release of a hazardous substance. Hazardous materials technicians shall have received at least 24 hours of training equal to the first responder operations level and in addition have competency in the following areas, and the employer shall so certify:

A. Know how to implement the employer's emergency response plan.

B. Know the classification, identification, and verification of known and unknown materials by using field survey instruments and equipment.

C. Be able to function within an assigned role in the incident command system.

D. Know how to select and use proper specialized chemical personal protective equipment provided to the hazardous materials technician.

E. Understand hazard and risk assessment techniques.

F. Be able to perform advance control, containment, and/or confinement operations within the capabilities of the resources and personal protective equipment available with the unit.

G. Understand and implement decontamination procedures.

H. Understand termination procedures.

I. Understand basic chemical and toxicological terminology and behavior.

Hazardous materials specialist. Hazardous materials specialists are individuals who respond with and provide support to hazardous materials technicians. Their duties parallel those of the hazardous materials technician; however, their duties require a more directed or specific knowledge of the various substances they may be called upon to contain. The hazardous materials specialist would also act as the site liaison with federal, state, local, and other government authorities in regards to site activities. Hazardous materials specialists shall have received at least 24 hours of training equal to the technician level and in addition have competency in the following areas, and the employer shall so certify:

A. Know how to implement the local emergency response plan.

B. Understand classification, identification, and verification of known and unknown materials by using advanced survey instruments and equipment.

C. Know of the state emergency response plan.

D. Be able to select and use proper specialized chemical personal protective equipment provided to the hazardous materials specialist.

E. Understand in-depth hazard and risk techniques.

F. Be able to perform specialized control, containment, and/or confinement operations within the capabilities of the resources and personal protective equipment available.

G. Be able to determine and implement decontamination procedures.

H. Have the ability to develop a site safety and control plan.

I. Understand chemical, radiological, and toxicological terminology and behavior.

trans-. Referring to a particular arrangement of elements within a chemical molecule.

transboundary pollutants. Air pollution that travels from one jurisdiction to another, often crossing state or international boundaries. Also applies to water pollution.

transfer molding. Resins or plastic compounds are placed in a heated vessel above the mold, and once fluxed, can be forced into the mold by the pressure of a ram or plunger. Usually used for thermosetting plastics.

transfer station. Facility where solid waste is transferred from collection vehicles to larger trucks or rail cars for longer distance transport.

transformer. A device that changes the voltage of electrical energy in transmission lines either up or down.

transient water system. A noncommunity water system that does not serve 25 of the same nonresidents per day for more than six months per year.

transition elements. The elements of the short groups in the periodic table. They all have an incomplete d subshell; that is, the first shell in from the outermost shell begins filling to 18 or 32 electrons before the outer shell fills.

transmission lines. Pipelines that transport raw water from its source to a water treatment plant, then to the distribution grid system.

transmissivity. The ability of an aquifer to transmit water.

transpiration. 1. The process by which water vapor is lost to the atmosphere from living plants. 2. The term can also be applied to the quantity of water thus dissipated.

transportation control measures (TCMs). Steps taken by a locality to reduce vehicular emissions and improve air quality by reducing or changing the flow of traffic.

transporter. Hauling firm that picks up properly packaged and labeled hazardous waste from generators and transports it to designated facilities for treatment, storage, or disposal. Transporters are subject to EPA and DOT hazardous waste regulations.

Transport of Dangerous Goods. *See* **Orange Book**.

trash. 1. Material considered worthless or offensive that is thrown away. 2. Generally defined as dry waste material, but in common usage, it is a synonym for garbage, rubbish, or refuse.

trash-to-energy plan. A program that involves burning trash to produce energy.

treatability studies. Tests of potential cleanup technologies conducted in a laboratory.

treated regulated medical waste. Medical waste treated to substantially reduce or eliminate its pathogenicity, but that has not yet been destroyed.

treated wastewater. Wastewater that has been subjected to one or more physical, chemical, and biological processes to reduce its potential of being a health hazard.

treatment. 1. Any method, technique, or process designed to remove solids and/or pollutants from solid waste, waste streams, effluents, and air emissions. 2. Methods used to change the biological character or composition of any regulated medical waste so as to substantially reduce or eliminate its potential for causing disease.

treatment plant. A structure built to treat wastewater before discharging it into the environment.

treatment, storage, and disposal (TSD) facility. Site where a hazardous substance is treated, stored, or disposed of. TSD facilities (also called TSDF) are regulated by EPA and states under RCRA.

tremie. Device used to place concrete or grout under water.

tri-. The prefix that means "three."

triage. The procedure of prioritizing patients according to the need of medical attention in an emergency situation in which there are a large number of injured or ill.

trial burn. An incinerator test in which emissions are monitored for the presence of specific organic compounds, particulates, and hydrogen chloride.

tribasic. Concerning acids, those having three displaceable hydrogen atoms for each molecule of the acid.

trichloroethylene (TCE). A stable, low boiling-point colorless liquid, toxic if inhaled. Used as a solvent or metal degreasing agent, and in other industrial applications.

trickle irrigation. Method in which water drips to the soil from perforated tubes or emitters.

trickling filter. A coarse treatment system in which wastewater is trickled over a bed of stones or other material covered with bacteria that break down the organic waste and produce clean water.

trihalomethane (THM). One of a family of organic methane-derived compounds. THMs are generally by-products of chlorination of drinking water that contains organic material.

trimer. A molecule formed from three molecules of the same monomer.

trinitrotoluene (TNT). A high explosive made by nitrating toluene.

triple covalent bond. Three covalent bonds between two atoms. The sharing of three pairs of electrons between certain atoms. In a structural formula, it is represented as -C≡C-.

triple point. The temperature and pressure at which the solid, liquid, and gaseous forms of a substance are at equilibrium.

tritium. Radioactive isotope of hydrogen with an atomic weight of 3.

trona. Natural sodium carbonate/bicarbonate, $Na_2CO_3 \cdot NaHCO_3 \cdot 2H_2O$.

troposphere. The layer of the atmosphere from the Earth's surface to the base of the stratosphere, with an altitude of six to nine miles.

trust fund. A fund set up under the Comprehensive Environmental Response, Compensation, and Liability Act (CERCLA) to help pay for cleanup of hazardous waste sites and for legal action to force those responsible for the sites to clean them up.

tuberculation. Development or formation of small mounds of corrosion products on the inside of iron pipe. These tubercles roughen the inside of the pipe, increasing its resistance to water flow.

tube settler. Device using bundles of tubes to let solids in water settle to the bottom for removal by conventional sludge collection means; sometimes used in sedimentation basins and clarifiers to improve particle removal.

tularemia. Also know as rabbit or deerfly fever, it is one of the most infectious pathogenic bacteria known. Symptoms include: fever, chills, headache, shortness of breath, sweating, joint stiffness, muscle pains, enlarged lymph nodes, conjunctivitis, weight loss, and red spots or ulcers on the skin.

tumor. An abnormal, uncontrolled growth of cells. Also called a *neoplasm*.

tumor progression. Under the Armitage-Doll multistage theory of cancer development, the transition of a cell line between the stages that lead to cancer.

tundra. 1. A type of treeless ecosystem dominated by lichens, mosses, grasses, and woody plants. 2. Tundra is found at high latitudes (arctic tundra) and high altitudes (alpine tundra). 3. Arctic tundra is underlain by permafrost and is usually water saturated.

tungsten. A lustrous, gray, solid, metallic element, symbol W, with atomic number 74, and atomic weight 183.84. It is used as lamp filaments, among other uses.

turbidimeter. A device that measures the cloudiness of suspended solids in a liquid.

turbidity. 1. Haziness in air caused by the presence of particles and pollutants. 2. A cloudy condition in water due to suspended silt or organic matter.

Turnbull's blue. Ferroferricyanide, $Fe_3[Fe(CN)_6]_2$; also known as *insoluble Prussian blue.*

turnout gear. An entire set of firefighter's protective clothing that includes helmet, coat, pants, boots, and gloves. Also known as **bunker gear**.

U

ullage. The amount of product by which a packaging falls short of being liquid full. Also called *outage.*

ultra clean coal (UCC). Coal that is washed, ground into fine particles, and then chemically treated to remove sulfur, ash, silicone, and other substances; usually briquetted and coated with a sealant made from coal.

ultrahigh pressure. A container designed to withstand pressures from 3,000 to 6,000 psi.

ultrahigh vacuum (UHV) ultraviolet (UV). Ultraviolet of higher frequency than vacuum ultraviolet.

ultrasonic. Sound waves that have frequency higher than humans can hear (20,000 Hz).

ultrasound. A test similar to an X-ray, but which uses sound waves.

ultraviolet rays (UV). 1. Radiation from the Sun that can be useful or potentially harmful. 2. UV rays from one part of the spectrum (UV-A) enhance plant life, while UV rays from other parts of the spectrum (UV-B) can cause skin cancer or other tissue damage. UV-C light is the shortest wavelength and has the highest energy, and therefore is the most dangerous. 3. The ozone layer in the atmosphere acts as a barrier preventing a great deal of ultraviolet rays from reaching the Earth's surface.

umbilical air respirator. A device whereby air or oxygen is supplied (in an unlimited amount) by a remote compressor or supply tank through a hose connection.

uncertainty factor (UF). One of several, generally 10-fold factors, used in operationally deriving the reference dose (RfD) and reference concentration (RfC) from experimental data.

unconfined aquifer. An aquifer containing water that is not under pressure. The water level in a well is the same as the water table outside the well.

uncontrolled polymerization. A rapid chemical reaction in which the polymerization occurs without an opportunity for the heat to be dissipated. The result may be an explosion.

underburn. A fire that consumes surface fuels but not trees or shrubs.

Underground Injection Control (UIC) Program. The program under the Safe Drinking Water Act that regulates the use of wells to pump fluids into the ground.

underground injection wells. Steel- and concrete-encased shafts into which hazardous waste is deposited by force and under pressure.

underground sources of drinking water. Aquifers currently being used as a source of drinking water or those capable of supplying a public water system. They have a total dissolved solids content of 10,000 mg/L or less, and are not "exempted aquifers."

underground storage tank (UST). A tank located at least partially underground and designed to hold gasoline or other petroleum products or chemicals.

UN identification number. A serial number assigned to the article or substance under the United Nations classification symbol. It must be prefixed by the letters "UN." It identifies a substance or particular group of substances.

uninhibited. 1. A term that usually refers to a monomer that has not had an inhibitor added to it in order to stabilize it. 2. May also refer to a monomer in which the inhibitor has been driven out of solution.

unit. A molecular fragment that repeats itself in a series.

unit-based pricing. *See* **pay-as-you-throw**.

***United States Pharmacopeia-National Formulary* (USP-NF).** The official publication of drug product standards.

unit of issue (UI). A standard or basic quantity that is expressed as a unit and indicated in a requisition, contract, or order as the minimum quantity issued [e.g., bottle (BT), can (CN), each (EA), pair (PR), bag (BG), box (BX), or drum (DR)].

unit risk. The upper bound excess lifetime cancer risk estimated to result from continuous exposure to an agent at a concentration of 1 µg/L in water, or 1 µg/m^3 in air. The interpretation of unit risk would be as follows: if unit risk = 1.5 x 10^{-6} µg/L, 1.5 excess tumors are expected to develop per 1,000,000 people if exposed daily for a lifetime to 1 μg of the chemical in 1 L of drinking water.

unity of command. A concept that states that each individual within an organization will report to one and only one designated person.

UN/NA number. A four-digit number representing a particular chemical or group of chemicals. These numbers are assigned by the United Nations (UN numbers), the U.S. Department of Transportation (NA numbers), or Transport Canada (NA numbers).

unpaired electrons. The electrons that are ready to react or pair up with electrons of another atom to form a covalent bond.

unreasonable risk. Under the Federal Insecticide, Fungicide, and Rodenticide Act (FIFRA), "unreasonable adverse effects" means any unreasonable risk to man or the environment, taking into account the medical, economic, social, and environmental costs and benefits of any pesticide.

unsanitized. A version of a document from which information claimed as a trade secret or confidential has not been withheld or omitted.

unsaturated compound. Referring to hydrocarbon compounds that contain at least one multiple covalent bond between two carbon atoms.

unsaturated zone. The area above the water table where soil pores are not fully saturated, although some water may be present. Also called **vadose zone**.

unstable material. Any substance that will decompose spontaneously, polymerize, or otherwise self-react.

UN standard packaging. Packaging that conforms to standards in the UN modal regulations on the transportation of dangerous goods.

upper bound. An plausible upper limit to the true value of a quantity. This is usually not a true statistical confidence limit.

upper detection limit. The largest concentration that an instrument can reliably detect.

upper explosive limit (UEL). 1. The maximum percentage of gas or vapor in air above which ignition will not occur (the mixture is too rich). 2. Also called the **upper flammable limit**.

upper flammable limit (UFL). *See* **upper explosive limit**.

uranium. A silvery white, highly toxic, solid, radioactive, metallic element, symbol U, with atomic number 92, and atomic weight 238.03. It is used in nuclear fuel and to produce uranium-235 and plutonium.

uranium mill tailings pile. A former uranium ore processing site that contains leftover radioactive materials (wastes), including radium and unrecovered uranium.

uranium mill tailings waste piles. Licensed active mills with tailings piles and evaporation ponds created by acid or alkaline leaching processes.

uranvitriol. Archaic term for a uranium sulfate.

urban runoff. Storm water from city streets and adjacent domestic or commercial properties that carries pollutants of various kinds into the sewer systems and receiving waters.

urea formaldehyde. A thermosetting polymer made from the reaction of urea and formaldehyde.

urea-formaldehyde foam insulation. A material once used to conserve energy by sealing crawl spaces and attics, etc. It is no longer used because emissions from the foam were found to be a health hazard.

use cluster. A set of competing chemicals, processes, and/or technologies that can substitute for one another in performing a particular function.

used oil. Spent motor oil from passenger cars and trucks collected at specified locations for recycling.

user fee. Fee collected from only those persons who use a particular service, as compared to one collected from the public in general.

utility load. The total electricity demand for a utility district.

UV stabilizer. An additive that protects materials from the harmful effects of ultraviolet rays by selectively absorbing them.

V

vacuum forming. In thermoforming, where the pressure applied is that of a vacuum.

vacuum ultraviolet (VUV). Ultraviolet radiation of high enough frequency that air will absorb it.

vadose zone. The zone between land surface and the water table within which the moisture content is less than saturation (except in the capillary fringe), and pressure is less than atmospheric. Also known as the **unsaturated zone**.

V-agents. 1. The second-generation, post–World War II nerve agents, which include VX-gas. 2. The V-agents are all organophosphates and are significantly more potent than sarin and the first-generation nerve gases.

valence. The combining power of an element. *See also* **oxidation number**.

valence bond theory. The theory that states that a covalent bond is formed when atomic orbitals on different atoms overlap, and electrons are shared by those atoms.

valence electron. An electron in the outermost ring or orbital of an atom, which is usually involved in bonding. The chemistry of each element is due to the configuration of this outer ring, i.e., the number of unpaired electrons in the valence ring.

valence orbital. *See* **valence ring**.

valence ring. The outermost ring or orbit in which electrons are held around the nucleus. Also called *valence shell* and *valence orbital*.

valence shell. *See* **valence ring**.

valves. Movable parts that control the flow of a liquid or gas through a pipe or out of an enclosed space by opening or closing the passage.

vanadium. A silvery white, toxic, solid, metallic element, symbol V, with atomic number 23, and atomic weight 50.94.

van der Waals force. 1. A force acting between nonbonded atoms or molecules, about 1% as strong as the covalent bond. 2. Van der Waals forces influence melting and boiling points, which occur when these forces between molecules are overcome.

vapor. The gaseous form of a substance that is solid or liquid under ordinary conditions.

vapor capture system. Any combination of hoods and ventilation system that captures or contains organic vapors so they may be directed to an abatement or recovery device.

vapor density. 1. The relative density of a vapor or gas (with no air present) as compared to clean, dry air. 2. The vapor density of clean, dry air is 1.0. 3. Any gas or vapor with a vapor density greater than 1.0 will sink in air, while any gas or vapor with a vapor density less than 1.0 will rise in air. 4. It may be calculated by dividing the average molecular weight of air (29) into the molecular weight of the vapor or gas.

vapor dispersion. The movement of vapor clouds in air due to wind, thermal action, gravity spreading, and mixing.

vaporization. 1. The process by which a liquid converts to a vapor. 2. Also known as **evaporation**.

vapor plumes. Flue gases visible because they contain water droplets.

vapor pressure. 1. The pressure exerted by a gas or vapor on the sides of its container, at equilibrium. Equilibrium is reached when the vapor pressure of the vapor in the container has stabilized. 2. The force per unit area exerted by vapor in an equilibrium state with surroundings at a given pressure. It increases dramatically as the temperature increases. 3. A relative measure of chemical volatility, the tendency of a material to evaporate.

vapor protective ensemble. A vapor protective ensemble or garment that is intended for use in an unknown threat atmosphere or for known high health risk atmospheres. It is vapor tight and is in compliance with National Fire Protection Association (NFPA) Standard #1991, "Standard on Vapor-Protective Ensembles for Hazardous Materials Emergencies."

vapor recovery. A system that removes the vapors coming off liquids and draws them back into the feed tank (as seen at a gasoline pump).

vapor valve. Valves used to remove vapor from the tank or to the pressurized tank. On the pressure cars, it is called the *vapor valve*, but on nonpressure tank cars, it is called the *air inlet* or *air valve*.

variance. Government permission for a delay or exception in the application of a given law, ordinance, or regulation.

vector. 1. An organism or any other carrier, often an insect or rodent, that carries disease. Vectors may also be letters or packages, or contaminated clothing, food, or water. 2. Plasmids, viruses, or bacteria used to transport genes into a host cell. A gene is placed in the vector; the vector then "infects" the bacterium.

vegetative controls. Nonpoint source pollution control practices that involve vegetative cover to reduce erosion and minimize loss of pollutants.

vehicle miles traveled (VMT). A measure of the extent of motor vehicle operation; the total number of vehicle miles traveled within a specific geographic area over a given period of time.

ventilation. 1. Creation of an opening in a burning building or container to allow the release of heat and smoke. 2. A form of engineering control that removes airborne contaminants. 3. The act of admitting fresh air into a space in order to replace stale or contaminated air; achieved by blowing air into the space. *See also* **suction**.

ventilation rate. The rate at which indoor air enters and leaves a building. Expressed as the number of changes of outdoor air per unit of time [air changes per hour (ACH)], or the rate at which a volume of outdoor air enters in cubic feet per minute (CFM).

vent pipe. Any opening leading out of or into some enclosed space, designed especially for the safe passage of air or liquid; an escape outlet.

venturi scrubber. An air pollution control device that uses water to remove particulate matter from emissions.

verdigris. Basic copper acetate, used as a pigment from green to blue.

vermilion. Mercury(II) sulfide (HgS), a red pigment. Also known as **cinnabar**.

vesicant. A substance that will cause blisters to form on contact with the skin. *See also* **blister agents**.

vessel manifest. The vessel manifest lists various details about each shipment by bill of lading (B/L) number. The international carrier is obligated to make declarations of the ship's crew and contents at both the port of departure and port of arrival.

V-gas. A chemical nerve agent.

vinegar. Dilute acetic acid.

vinyl. 1. The general name for the radical ($-C_2H_3$) formed when one hydrogen is removed from the ethylene (or ethene) molecule (C_2H_4). 2. Also, a generic term for vinyl polymers, or for polyvinyl chloride alone.

vinyl chloride. A chemical compound, used in producing some plastics, that is believed to be oncogenic.

vinyl resins. Any polymer made from a monomer containing the vinyl group (CH_2=CH-), but usually restricted to polyvinyl acetate, alcohol, butyral, chloride, and formal resins.

violent reaction. The action whereby a chemical changes its composition near or exceeding the speed of sound, often releasing heat and gases.

virgin materials. Resources extracted from nature in their raw form, such as timber or metal ore.

viscosity. 1. A measure of a liquid's internal resistance to flow. 2. The molecular friction within a fluid that produces flow resistance.

visible light. The electromagnetic radiation with a wavelength between 400 and 750 nm. Also called the *visible spectrum.*

visible spectrum. *See* **visible light**.

vital capacity (VC). The maximum volume that can be exhaled in a single breath [VC = total lung capacity (TLC) – residual capacity (RC)].

vitamin. An organic substance essential in small quantities to the normal health of an animal. Vitamins must typically be supplied to the animal through diet.

vitamin A. Retinol, $C_{20}H_{30}O$, a fat-soluble vitamin derived from carotenes.

vitamin B. In general use, a group of water-soluble, heat-labile compounds that typically serve as coenzymes. They include many examples that contain amine groups (as in "vital amine").

vitamin B$_1$. Thiamine, $C_{12}H_{17}N_4OSCl$.

vitamin B$_2$. Riboflavin, $C_{17}H_{20}N_4O_6$.

vitamin B$_3$. Niacin (or nicotinic acid), $C_6H_5NO_2$.

vitamin B$_6$. Pyridoxine, $C_8H_{11}NO_3$.

vitamin B$_{12}$. Cyanocobalamin (or cyanocobalamine), $C_{63}H_{82}CoN_{14}O_{14}P$.

vitamin Bc. Folic acid, $C_{19}H_{19}N_7O_6$.

vitamin C. Ascorbic acid, $C_6H_8O_6$, a water-soluble vitamin found in many fruits and green vegetables.

vitamin D. This fat-soluble vitamin consists of steroid derivatives including ergocalciferol (vitamin D$_2$, $C_{28}H_{44}O$), and cholecalciferol (vitamin D$_3$, $C_{27}H_{44}O$).

vitamin E. This vitamin occurs in four naturally occurring forms, called α-tocopherol, β- tocopherol, γ- tocopherol, and δ-tocopherol. The α-tocopherol form, $C_{29}H_{50}O_2$, has the greatest activity. The β-tocopherol and γ-tocopherol forms have one fewer methyl group, and the δ-tocopherol form has two fewer methyl groups.

vitamin H. Emergency room shorthand for Haldol.

Viton. A trademarked fluoroelastomer copolymer used in chemical protective clothing and container materials such as gaskets and linings.

vitriol. Archaic term for a sulfate, especially iron sulfate.

vitriolic acid. Archaic term for sulfuric acid, H_2SO_4.

vitriolic acid air. Archaic term for sulfur dioxide, SO_2, also known as sulfurous acid or sulfurous gas.

volatile. 1. Any substance that evaporates readily. 2. To cause to be evaporated. 3. The capability of evaporating rapidly at normal temperatures and pressures.

volatile alkali. Aqueous ammonia, NH_3; also called *spirit of hartshorn.*

volatile liquids. Liquids that easily vaporize or evaporate at room temperature.

volatile organic compound (VOC). Any organic compound that participates in atmospheric photochemical reactions except those designated by EPA as having negligible photochemical reactivity.

volatile solids. Those solids in water or other liquids that are lost on ignition of the dry solids at 550°C.

volatile synthetic organic chemicals. Chemicals that tend to volatilize or evaporate.

volatility. The tendency of a liquid to evaporate at a given temperature. The higher a liquid's volatility, the faster it will evaporate.

volatilization. The act of changing of a liquid to a vapor.

volt. 1. The unit of pressure that is available to move electrons. 2. One volt (V) equals 1 joule per coulomb.

voltage. The difference in potential between two electrodes.

voltaic cell. An electrochemical cell in which spontaneous chemical reactions produce electricity; also called a **galvanic cell**.

voltammeter. An instrument for measuring voltages and amperages.

volt-ohm meter (VOM). A multimeter that measures voltage, current, and resistance.

volume. The measurement of anything in 3-D (cubic magnitude).

volume percentage. Volume percentages [(v/v)%] express the concentration of a component in a mixture or an element in a compound. For example, 95% ethanol by volume contains 95 ml of ethanol in 100 ml of solution (not in 100 ml of water!).

volume reduction. Processing waste materials to decrease the amount of space they occupy, usually by compacting, shredding, incinerating, or composting.

volumetric tank test. One of several tests to determine the physical integrity of a storage tank; the volume of fluid in the tank is measured directly or calculated from product-level changes. A marked drop in volume indicates a leak.

vulcanization. The cross-linking of the unsaturated hydrocarbon chain in rubber.

vulnerability analysis. Assessment of elements in the community that are susceptible to damage if hazardous materials are released.

vulnerable zone. An area over which the airborne concentration of a chemical accidentally released could reach the level of concern.

VX-gas. One of the V-agents. It is far more persistent than the first-generation nerve agents.

W

warm zone. The controlled and well-marked area between hot and cold zones where personnel and equipment decontamination and hot zone support take place. It includes control points for the access corridor and thus assists in reducing the spread of contamination. Also referred to as the *contamination reduction corridor (CRC)*, *contamination reduction zone (CRZ)*, *yellow zone*, or *limited access zone* in other documents (EPA Standard Operating Safety Guidelines, OSHA 29 CFR 1910.120, and NFPA 472).

waste. 1. Unwanted materials left over from a manufacturing process. 2. Refuse from places of human or animal habitation.

waste characterization. Identification of chemical and microbiological constituents of a waste material.

waste exchange. Arrangement in which companies exchange their wastes for the benefit of both parties.

waste feed. The continuous or intermittent flow of wastes into an incinerator.

waste generation. The weight or volume of materials and products that enter the waste stream before recycling, composting, deposition in a landfill, or combustion takes place. Also can represent the amount of waste generated by a given source or category of sources.

waste-heat recovery. Recovering heat discharged as a by-product of one process to provide heat needed by a second process.

waste load allocation. 1. The maximum load of pollutants each discharger of waste is allowed to release into a particular waterway. Discharge limits are usually required for each specific water quality criterion being, or expected to be, violated. 2. The portion of a stream's total assimilative capacity assigned to an individual discharge.

waste minimization. Measures or techniques that reduce the amount of wastes generated during industrial production processes; term is also applied to recycling and other efforts to reduce the amount of waste going into the waste stream.

waste piles. Noncontainerized, lined or unlined, accumulations of solid, nonflowing waste.

waste profile sheet. The document that is provided by the laboratory that conducted the analysis of the hazardous waste and provides a description of the physical and chemical properties of the waste sample.

waste reduction. Using source reduction, recycling, or composting to prevent or reduce waste generation. *See also* **source reduction**.

waste stream. 1. The total flow of solid waste from homes, businesses, institutions, and manufacturing plants that is recycled, burned, or disposed of in landfills. 2. Certain segments of the waste stream, such as the residential waste stream or the recyclable waste stream.

waste-to-energy facility. Facility where recovered municipal solid waste is converted into a usable form of energy, usually via combustion. Also called a *municipal waste combustor*.

waste treatment lagoon. Impoundment made by excavation or earth fill for biological treatment of wastewater.

waste treatment plant. A facility containing a series of tanks, screens, filters, and other processes by which pollutants are removed from water.

waste treatment stream. The continuous movement of waste from generator to treater and disposer.

wastewater. The spent or used water from a home, community, farm, or industry that contains dissolved or suspended matter.

wastewater infrastructure. The plan or network for the collection, treatment, and disposal of sewage in a community.

wastewater operations and maintenance. Actions taken after construction to ensure that facilities constructed to treat wastewater will be operated, maintained, and managed to reach prescribed effluent levels in an optimum manner.

water. A colorless, tasteless liquid with some extremely important properties that stem from the bent H-O-H structure of its molecules; H_2O.

waterborne disease outbreak. The significant occurrence of acute illness associated with drinking water from a public water system that is deficient in treatment, as determined by appropriate local or state agencies.

water cycle. The process by which water is evaporated from the land and bodies of water, condensed in the clouds, and precipitated back again onto the Earth.

water glass. A hydrated sodium silicate, $Na_2Si_4O_9{\cdot}xH_2O$, either an amorphous solid or in thick aqueous solution, used as a binder or adhesive. Also called **soluble glass**.

water hardness. When water contains compounds of calcium and magnesium (and sometimes iron, manganese, and strontium), the water is considered "hard," and must be treated with water softeners. Hard water produces scale in hot water pipes and boilers and lowers the effectiveness of detergents.

water of crystallization. Water that is stoichiometrically bound in a crystal; for example, the waters in copper sulfate pentahydrate. Also called *water of hydration*.

water of hydration. *See* **water of crystallization.**

water pollution. The presence in water of enough harmful or objectionable material to damage the water's quality.

water purveyor. A public utility, mutual water company, county water district, or municipality that delivers drinking water to customers.

Water Quality Act. The amended Clean Water Act.

water quality–based limitations. Effluent limitations applied to dischargers when mere technology-based limitations would cause violations of water quality standards. Usually applied to discharges into small streams.

water quality–based permit. A permit with an effluent limit more stringent than one based on technology performance. Such limits may be necessary to protect the designated use of receiving waters (e.g., recreation, irrigation, industry, or water supply).

water quality criteria. Levels of water quality expected to render a body of water suitable for its designated use. Criteria are based on specific levels of pollutants that would make the water harmful if used for drinking, swimming, farming, fish production, or industrial processes.

Water Quality Standards. State-adopted and EPA-approved ambient standards for water bodies. The standards prescribe the use of the water body and establish the water quality criteria that must be met to protect designated uses.

water reactive material. Any material that, when it contacts water, will enter into a reaction, chemical or physical. This includes the evolution of other hazardous materials, the production of large amounts of heat, or violent spattering.

water repellent treated wood. Lumber impregnated with water repellent and preservatives.

water-sensitive materials. Substances that may produce flammable and/or toxic decomposition products upon contact with water.

watershed. The land area that drains into a stream; the watershed for a major river may encompass a number of smaller watersheds that ultimately combine at a common point.

watershed approach. A coordinated framework for environmental management that focuses public and private efforts on the highest priority problems within hydrologically-defined geographic areas, taking into consideration both groundwater and surface water flow.

watershed area. A topographic area within a line drawn connecting the highest points uphill of a drinking water intake into which overland flow drains.

water softener. A material that lowers water hardness when dissolved in water, usually by precipitating out calcium and/or magnesium compounds.

water solubility. The maximum possible concentration of a chemical compound dissolved in water. If a substance is water soluble, it can very readily disperse through the environment.

water-soluble packaging. Packaging that dissolves in water; used to reduce exposure risks to pesticide mixers and loaders.

water source heat pump. Heat pump that uses wells or heat exchangers to transfer heat from water to the inside of a building. Most such units use groundwater. *See* **ground source heat pump** and **heat pump**.

water spray. A method or way to apply or distribute water. The water is finely divided to provide for high heat absorption. It is particularly effective on fires of flammable liquids and volatile solids having flash points above 37.8°C (100°F). With proper training and care, water spray can be used successfully on flammable liquids with low flash points. Also called *firefighting fog.*

water storage pond. An impound for liquid wastes designed to accomplish some degree of biochemical treatment.

water supplier. One who owns or operates a public water system.

water supply system. The collection, treatment, storage, and distribution of potable water from source to consumer.

water table. The level of groundwater.

water treatment lagoon. An impound for liquid wastes designed to accomplish some degree of biochemical treatment.

watertube boiler. A boiler in which the water passes through tubes around which combustion gases are passed. *Contrast with* **firetube boiler**.

water vapor. Water in its gaseous form. In the atmosphere, it is the source of all forms of condensation and precipitation.

water well. An excavation where the intended use is for location, acquisition, development, or artificial recharge of groundwater.

watt. A unit used to measure electric power. Watts are equal to volts multiplied by amperes.

wave mechanics. *See* **quantum mechanics**.

way bill. A railroad document describing a shipment for materials being transported by rail showing the shipper, consignee, routing, and weights. Used by the carrier for internal record and control, especially when the shipment is in transit.

weak acid. An acid that only partially dissociates into hydrogen ions and anions in solution. Weak acids are weak electrolytes.

weak base. A base that only partially dissociates into ions in solution. Weak bases are weak electrolytes. Ammonia is an example of a weak base.

weak electrolyte. A substance that conducts electricity poorly in a dilute water solution. Weak acid and/or base.

weapons of mass destruction (WMD). 1. Any destructive device as defined in section 921 of the U.S. Code, Title 18. ("Destructive device" is defined as any explosive, incendiary, or poison gas, bomb, grenade, rocket having a propellant charge of more than 4 oz, missile having an explosive or incendiary charge of more than 0.25 oz, mine, or device similar to the above.) 2. Any weapon that is designed or intended to cause serious bodily injury through the release, dissemination, or impact of toxic or poisonous chemicals, or their precursors. 3. Any weapon involving a disease organism. 4. Any weapon that is designed to release radiation or radioactivity at a level dangerous to human life. United States Code, Title 18, "Crimes and Criminal Procedure," Part I, "Crimes," ch. 113B, "Terrorism," Sec. 2332a.)

weapons of mass destruction, chemical/biological (WMD chem/bio). In reference to those substances that were developed by military institutions to create widespread injury, illness, or death.

weatherometer. A device that simulates, in one manner or another, conditions to which a finished article would be exposed when used outdoors.

weight. Weight is the force exerted by an object due to gravity. The weight of an object (w) arises from its mass (m); $w = mg$, where g is the acceleration due to gravity (about 9.8 m/s^2 on Earth).

weight effect. The change produced in certain properties, including flash point, boiling point, and water solubility, as the molecular weight (calculated by adding the atomic weights of all the atoms in the molecule) of compounds in an analogous series is increased or decreased.

weight-of-evidence (WOE) for carcinogenicity. A system used by the EPA for characterizing the extent to which the available data support the hypothesis that an agent causes cancer in humans.

weight of scientific evidence. Considerations in assessing the interpretation of published information about toxicity.

weir. 1. A wall or plate placed in an open channel to measure the flow of water. 2. A wall or obstruction used to control flow from settling tanks and clarifiers to ensure a uniform flow rate and avoid short-circuiting.

well. A bored, drilled, or driven shaft, or a dug hole with a depth greater than the largest surface dimension, the purpose of which is to reach underground water supplies or hydrocarbons, or to store or bury fluids below ground.

well field. Area containing one or more wells that produce usable amounts of water or oil.

wellhead. The top of a structure built over a well. In hazardous materials, it usually occurs over the top of an oil well.

wellhead protection area. A protected surface and subsurface zone surrounding a well or well field supplying a public water system to keep contaminants from reaching the well water.

well injection. The subsurface emplacement of fluids into a well.

well monitoring. Measurement by on-site instruments or laboratory methods of well water quality.

well plug. A watertight, gastight seal installed in a borehole or well to prevent movement of fluids.

well point. A hollow vertical tube, rod, or pipe terminating in a perforated pointed shoe and fitted with a fine-mesh screen.

wetlands. An area that is saturated by surface water or groundwater, with vegetation adapted for life under those soil conditions, such as swamps, bogs, fens, marshes, and estuaries. *See also* **swamp**.

wettability. The relative degree to which a fluid will spread into or coat a solid surface in the presence of other immiscible fluids.

wettable powder. Dry formulation that must be mixed with water or other liquid before it is applied.

wheeling. The transmission of electricity owned by one entity through the facilities owned by another (usually a utility).

white caustic. Archaic term for sodium hydroxide.

white vitriol. Archaic term for zinc sulfate, $ZnSO_4{\cdot}7H_2O$.

white wood. Lumber intended for treating that has not yet been treated.

whole effluent toxicity (WET) tests. Tests to determine the toxicity levels of the total effluent from a single source as opposed to a series of tests for individual contaminants.

wildlife refuge. An area designated for the protection of wild animals, within which hunting and fishing are either prohibited or strictly controlled.

wire-to-wire efficiency. The efficiency of a pump and motor together.

wolfram. The Germanic word for the element tungsten, hence the symbol, W.

wood alcohol. Methyl alcohol (methanol), CH_3OH.

wood-burning stove pollution. Air pollution caused by emissions of particulate matter, carbon monoxide, total suspended particulates, and polycyclic organic matter from wood-burning stoves.

wood packaging. Wood products such as pallets, crates, and barrels.

wood treatment facility. An industrial facility that treats lumber and other wood products for outdoor use. The process employs chromated copper arsenate, which is regulated as a hazardous material.

work. Work is the energy required to move an object against an opposing force. Work (W) is usually expressed as a force (F) times a displacement (d); $W = F x d$.

worker right-to-know. Legislation communicating chemical information to employees.

working level (WL). A unit of measure for documenting exposure to radon decay products, the so-called "daughters." One working level is equal to approximately 200 picocuries per liter (pCi/L).

working level month (WLM). A unit of measure used to determine cumulative exposure to radon.

X

xenobiota. Any biota displaced from their normal habitat. Also, chemicals foreign to a biological system.

xenon. A nonflammable, gaseous, nonmetallic element, symbol Xe, with atomic number 54, and atomic weight 131.3. It is a member of group VIII on the periodic table of the elements (the inert, or "noble," gases). It is used to fill cathode ray tubes.

X-rays. Penetrating electromagnetic radiation with wavelengths shorter than those of visible light.

X-ray tube. A cathode ray tube that focuses energetic streams of electrons on a metal target, causing the metal to emit X-rays.

xylenol blue. 1,4-dimethyl-5-hydroxybenzenesulfonphthalein, an acid-base indicator that changes from red to yellow as the pH is raised through 2, and then to blue as the pH is raised through 8.8.

Y

yard waste. The part of solid waste composed of grass clippings, leaves, twigs, branches, and other garden refuse.

yellow-boy. Iron oxide flocculant (clumps of solids in waste or water). Usually observed as orange-yellow deposits in surface streams with excess iron content. *See also* **floc** and **flocculation**.

yellow zone. *See* **warm zone**.

yield. 1. The amount of product actually obtained in a chemical reaction. 2. The quantity of water (expressed as a rate of flow or total quantity per year) that can be collected for a given use from surface or groundwater sources.

ytterbium. A solid metallic element, very rare, with symbol Yb, atomic number 70, and atomic weight 173.04.

yttrium. A solid metallic element, symbol Y, with atomic number 39, and atomic weight 88.9.

Z

zero air. Atmospheric air purified to contain less than 0.1 ppm total hydrocarbons.

zeolite. Microscopic particles of silicate- or aluminosilicate-structured minerals that may be used as an absorbing filter or sieve on a molecular level. Used by the petroleum industry in the cracking of petroleum.

zinc. A solid, bluish white, metallic element, symbol Zn, with atomic number 30, and atomic weight 65.41. It is a reactive metal, releasing hydrogen in contact with dilute acids. It is used in galvanizing and in many alloys.

zirconium. A solid, grayish white, metallic element, symbol Zr, with atomic number 40, and atomic weight 91.22. It is used in steel manufacture and as a coating for fuel rods in nuclear reactors.

zones. The separation of hot, warm, and cold zones during an incident. The separation can be physical (barriers), geographical, or by the use of temporary isolation barriers (colored tape).

zooplankton. Small (often microscopic), free-floating aquatic plants or animals.

GENERAL ABBREVIATIONS and ACRONYMS

A

a	acceleration
Å	angstrom
A	ampere
A	mass number
A	absolute temperature
AA	Alcoholics Anonymous
AA	The Aluminum Association
AA	atomic absorption
AAA	American Automobile Association
AAAS	American Association for Advancement of Science
AAC	alkyl ammonium compound (wood preservative)
AADPA	assistant associate director for public and intergovernmental affairs (FEMA)
AAMA	American Architectural Manufacturers Association
AAOHN	American Association of Occupational Health Nurses
AAOM	American Academy of Occupational Medicine (merged with AOMA in 1988 to form American College of Occupational Medicine)
AAR	Association of American Railroads
AARP	American Association of Retired People
AAS	American Association of Suicidology
AAS	American Academy of Sciences
AASHTO	American Association of State Highway and Transportation Officials
AASW	American Association of Scientific Workers
AATCC	American Association of Textile Chemists and Colorists
ABA	acrylonitrile-butadiene-acrylate

ABC	atomic, biological, and chemical
ABC	Association of Boards of Certification
ABCHS	American Board for Certification in Homeland Security
ABECI	American Board of Examiners in Crisis Intervention
ABFA	American Board of Forensic Accounting
ABFC	American Board of Forensic Counselors
ABFE	American Board of Forensic Examiners
ABFET	American Board of Forensic Engineering and Technology
ABFM	American Board of Forensic Medicine
ABFN	American Board of Forensic Nursing
ABG	arterial blood gas
ABL	atmospheric boundary layer
ABOHN	American Board for Occupational Health Nurses
abs	absolute
ABS	acrylonitrile-butadiene-styrene
ABS	alkyl benzene sulfonate (a detergent)
ABS	antilock braking system
abstr	abstract
Ac	acetyl (-CH_3CO)
Ac	actinium
AC	hydrogen cyanide (a chemical blood agent)
AC	allyl chloride
AC	alternating current
AC	advisory circulars
ACA	ammoniacal copper arsenate (wood preservative)
ACAA	automatic chemical agent alarm
ACADA	automatic chemical agent detection alarm
ACAMS	automatic continuous agent monitoring system
ACC	acid copper chromate (wood preservative)
ACC	American Chemistry Council (formerly CMA)
ACC	acceptable container condition
ACerS	American Ceramic Society
ACF	activated carbon fibers
ACFEI	American College of Forensic Examiners Institute
acfm	actual cubic feet per minute
ACGIH	American Conference of Governmental Industrial Hygienists

ACh	acetylcholine
ACH	air changes per hour
AChE	acetylcholinesterase
ACHMM	Academy of Certified Hazardous Materials Managers
ACHP	Advisory Council on Historic Preservation
ACI	American Concrete Institute
ACI	activated carbon injection
ACL	a trademark for a group of solid organic compounds that liberate chlorine
ACL	alternate concentration limit
ACLS	advanced cardiac life support
ACLU	American Civil Liberties Union
ACM	asbestos-containing material
ACMI	Art and Craft Materials Institute
ACOM	American College of Occupational Medicine
ACPE	American Council on Pharmaceutical Education
ACQ	alkaline copper quat (wood preservative)
ACR	American College of Radiology
ACS	American Ceramic Society (*also* **ACerS**)
ACS	American Chemical Society
ACT	asbestos control technology
ACTS	Arts, Crafts, and Theatre Safety
ACWM	asbestos-containing waste materials
ACZA	ammoniacal copper zinc arsenate (wood preservative)
AD	airworthiness directives
ADA	acetonedicarboxylic acid
ADA	Americans with Disabilities Act
ADAMHA	alcohol, drug abuse, and mental health association
ADAMS	Automated Disaster Assistance Management System
ADAT	air-dried after treatment
ADD	average daily dose
ADF	advanced disposal fee
ADI	acceptable daily intake
ADNR	dangerous goods by water (European regulations; Règlement pour le Transport des Matières Dangereuses sur le Rhin)
ADP	AHERA designated person
ADP	ammonium dihydrogen phosphate

ADP	adenosine diphosphate
ADP	automated data processing
ADR	dangerous goods by road (European regulations; Accord Européan Relatif au Transport International des Marchandises Dangereuses par Voies de Navigation Intérieures)
ADRS	automated disaster recovery system
AE	aeromedical evacuation
AEC	agency emergency coordinators
AEC	Atomic Energy Commission
AECE	aeromedical evacuation control element
AEGL	acute exposure guideline level
AENOR	Asociación Española de Normalización y Certificación
AEROS	Aerometric and Emissions Reporting System
AES	aeromedical evacuation system
AES	auger electron spectroscopy
AESF	American Electroplaters and Surface Finishers Society
af	atomic formula
AFB	Air Force base
AFFF	aqueous film forming foam (*also called* "A triple F")
AFIA	American Feed Industry Association
AFL-CIO	American Federation of Labor- Congress of Industrial Organizations
AFMAN	Air Force Joint Manual
AFNOR	Association Française de Normalisation
AFPR	Association of Foam Packaging Recyclers
AFRCC	Air Force Rescue Coordination Center
AFS	American Foundrymen's Society
Ag	silver
AG	attorney general
AGA	American Gas Association
AGAUS	Adjutants General Association of the United States
AHA	activity hazard analysis
AHCM	Academy of Hazard Control Management
AHCPR	Agency for Health Care Policy and Research
AHERA	Asbestos Hazard Emergency Response Act of 1986 (Title II of TSCA)
AHIMA	American Health Information Management Association
AHJ	authority having jurisdiction

AHLS	advanced hazmat life support
AHP	accountable health plan
AHU	air handling unit
AI	artificial intelligence
AI	active ingredient
AI	Asphalt Institute
AIA	American Institute of Architects
AIA	American Insurance Association
AIA/NAS	Aerospace Industries Association of America/National Aerospace Standards
AIC	American Institute of Chemists
AIChE	American Institute of Chemical Engineers
AIChE–CCPS	American Institute of Chemical Engineers–Center for Chemical Process Safety
AIDS	acquired immune deficiency syndrome
AIF	Atomic Industrial Forum, Inc.
AIHA	American Industrial Hygiene Association
AIHC	American Industrial Health Council
AIP	autoignition point
AIRS	Aerometric Information Reporting System
AISC	American Institute of Steel Construction
AISE	Association of Iron and Steel Engineers
AISI	American Iron and Steel Institute
AK	Alaska
a.k.a.	*also* known as
Al	aluminum
AL	acceptable level
AL	Alabama
ALA	American Lung Association
ALA	delta-amino levulinic acid
ALA-O	delta-amino levulinic acid dehydrates
ALARA	as low as reasonably achievable
alc	alcohol
ALCA	American Leather Chemists Association
ALCC	airlift control center
alk	alkaline
ALOC	acute loss of consciousness

ALOHA	area locations of hazardous atmospheres
ALPA	Air Line Pilots Association
ALR	allergenic effects
ALS	advanced life support
ALSTTL	advanced LSTTL
Am	americium
AMA	American Medical Association
AMA	American Management Association
AMAD	automatic mustard agent detector
AMBER	America's Missing: Broadcast Emergency Response
ambi-	prefix meaning "both"
AMC	Air Mobility Command, U.S. Air Force
amorph	amorphous
amp	ampere
AMRA	American Medical Records Association
AMS	Aerial Measuring System (National Nuclear Security Administration)
amu	atomic mass unit (*also* **AMU**)
AMU	atomic mass unit (*also* **amu**)
AN	ammonium nitrate
AN	acrylonitrile
ANFI	Association of the Nonwoven Fabrics Industry
ANFO	ammonium nitrate/fuel oil (a blasting agent)
ANG	Air National Guard
anhy	anhydrous
ANPRM	advanced notice of proposed rule making
ANRC	American National Red Cross
ANSI	American National Standards Institute
ANSIR	Awareness of National Security Issues and Response Program (FBI)
AOA	airfield operating area
AOA	American Osteopathic Association
AOAC	Association of Official Analytical Chemists
AOC	Army Operations Center (Pentagon)
AOCS	American Oil Chemists' Society
AOMA	American Occupational Medical Association (merged with AAOM in 1988 to form American College of Occupational Medicine)

AOR	area of responsibility
AP	ammonium perchlorate (*also* **APC**)
APA	Allied Pilots Association
APA	Airline Plywood Association
APA	American Psychiatric Association
APA	American Pyrotechnics Association
APAP	acetaminophen
APC	American Plastics Council
APC	ammonium perchlorate (*see also* **AP**)
APhA	American Pharmaceutical Association
APHA	American Public Health Association
APHIS	Animal and Plant Health Inspection Service
API	American Petroleum Institute
APO	triethylenephosphoramide
APP	atactic polypropylene
approx	approximate
APPS	Act to Prevent Pollution from Ships
APR	air purification respirator
aq	aqueous
AQCR	air quality control regions
AQI	air quality index (EPA)
AQM	air quality model
AQTX	aquatic toxicity (*also* **TLm**)
Ar	argon
Ar	aryl group
AR	Arkansas
AR	added risk
AR	analytical reagent
ARAR	applicable or relevant and appropriate requirements
ARC	American Red Cross
ARCHIE	Automated Resource for Chemical Hazard Incident Evaluation
ARD	acute respiratory disease
ARES	Automated Residential Energy Standard (DOE)
ARES	Amateur Radio Emergency Service
ARI	Air-Conditioning and Refrigeration Institute
ARIP	Accidental Release Information Program

ARM	Association of Rotational Molders
ARMA	Asphalt Roofing Manufacturers Association
ARPES	angle-resolved photoemission spectroscopy
ARRL	American Radio Relay League
ARS	acute radiation syndrome
ARTCC	air route traffic control centers
as-	prefix meaning "asymmetrical"
As	arsenic
ASA	acrylic-styrene-acrylonitrile
ASA	acetylsalicylic acid (aspirin)
ASA	American Standards Association (now **ANSI**)
ASCE	American Society of Civil Engineers
ASCII	American Standard Code for Information Interchange
ASEP	American Society of Electroplated Plastics
ASHRAE	American Society of Heating, Refrigerating and Air-Conditioning Engineers
ASM	American Society for Metals International
ASME	American Society of Mechanical Engineers
asn	*Aspergillus nidulans*
ASNT	American Society for Nondestructive Testing
ASP	American Society for Plasticulture
ASPET	American Society of Pharmacology and Experimental Therapeutics
ASQ	American Society for Quality (formerly American Society for Quality Control)
ASQC	American Society for Quality Control (now known as American Society for Quality)
ASR	atmosphere-supplying respirator
ASSE	American Society of Safety Engineers
ast	ascites tumor
AST	aboveground storage tank
AST	advanced secondary (wastewater) treatment
ASTM	American Society for Testing and Materials
asym	asymmetrical (or unsymmetrical)
at	atomic
At	astatine
ATA	Air Transport Association
ATA	American Trucking Associations

ATC	Applied Technology Council
-ate	the suffix of a salt whose metal or radical is in its highest oxidation state
ATE	aluminum triethyl
ATF	Bureau of Alcohol, Tobacco, Firearms and Explosives
atm	atmosphere
ATM	aluminum trimethyl
ATM	automatic (or automated) teller machine
atmos	atmosphere
at no	atomic number (*also* **Z**)
ATP	adenosine triphosphate
ATS	air traffic services
ATSDR	Agency for Toxic Substances and Disease Registry
atto-	prefix meaning "10^{-18}"
at wt	atomic weight
au	astronomical unit (*also* **AU**)
Au	gold
AU	astronomical unit (*also* **au**)
AUTODIN	Automatic Digital Network (Department of Defense)
autoign	autoignition
autoign temp	autoignition temperature
AUTOVON	Automatic Voice Network (Department of Defense)
AW	atomic weight
AWMA	Air & Waste Management Association
AWPA	American Wood-Preservers' Association
AWPI	American Wood Preservers Institute
AWS	American Welding Society
AWT	advanced wastewater treatment
AWWA	American Water Works Association
AZ	Arizona
aza-	prefix indicating the presence of nitrogen in the heterocyclic ring
AZERC	Arizona Emergency Response Commission

B

B	boron

Ba	barium
BAC	biological activated carbon
BAC	blood alcohol content
BACM	best available control measures
BACT	best available control technology
BAL	British anti-lewisite
BAN	British approved name
BaP	benzo(a)pyrene
bar	100 kPa (14.5 psi)
BASIS	Battelle's Automated Search Information System
BAT	best available technology
BATF	Bureau of Alcohol, Tobacco, Firearms and Explosives
BBC	Basic Building Code (BOCA; now called National Building Code)
BBDR	biologically based dose-response model
bbl	barrel
BBP	butyl benzyl phthalate
BCF	bioconcentration factor
BCF	bulk continuous fiber
BCM	blood-clotting mechanism effects
BCMC	Board for the Coordination of Model Codes (formed by BOCA and other organizations)
bcs	*Bacillus subtilis*
BCT	best conventional pollutant control technology
BDAT	best demonstrated available technology
BDRP	Biological Defense Research Program (U.S. Navy, Bethesda, MD)
BDS	biohazard detection system
Be	beryllium
Bé	Baumé; arbitrary scale of specific gravities
BEI	biological exposure index
BEK	butyl ethyl ketone
BETEC	Building Environment and Thermal Envelope Council (NIBS)
bfa	body fluids assay
BFD	Boston Fire Department
BFE	bromotrifluoroethylene
BFS	beam foil spectroscopy
BG	bag [as a unit of issue (UI)]
Bh	bohrium

BHA	butylated hydroxyanisole
BHC	benzene hexachloride
BHT	butylated hydroxytoluene
bi-	prefix for "two" (*also* **di-**)
Bi	bismuth
BIA	Bureau of Indian Affairs
BIDS	Biological Integrated Detection System
BIFC	Boise Interagency Fire Center
BIFMA	Business and Institutional Furniture Manufacturers' Association
biol	biological
bis-	prefix meaning "twice" or "again"
Bk	berkelium
B/L	bill of lading
BLD	blood effects
BLEVE	boiling liquid expanding vapor explosion
BLM	Bureau of Land Management
BLS	basic life support
BMC	bulk molding compound
BMC	benchmark concentration
BMD	benchmark dose
BMP	best management practice
bmr	bone marrow
BMR	benchmark response
BNA	Bureau of National Affairs
BOCA	Building Officials and Code Administrators
BOCA-ES	Building Officials and Code Administrators Evaluation Service
BOD	biochemical oxygen demand
BOE	Bureau of Explosives
BOF	basic oxygen furnace
BOLDER	Basic On-Line Disaster Emergency Response
BOM	Bureau of Mines
BOP	basic oxygen process
BOPF	basic oxygen process furnace
BOPP	biaxially oriented polypropylene
BOR	Bureau of Reclamation
bp	boiling point

BP	blood pressure
BPA	blanket purchase agreement
BPT	best practicable (control) technology
Bq	becquerel
Br	bromine
b range	boiling range
brd	bird
BS	British Standards
BSI	British Standards Institution (now called British Standards)
BSO	benzene soluble organics
BSR	Board of Standards Review (ANSI)
BT	bottle [as a unit of issue (UI)]
BTS	Border and Transportation Security (branch of DHS)
Btu	British thermal unit (*also* **BTU**)
BTU	British thermal unit (*also* **Btu**)
BTX	benzene, toluene, and xylene
Bu	butyl
BUBU	big, unconstricting, baggy, and ugly (clothing)
BUR	built-up roofing
BVE	butyl vinyl ether
BW	biological warfare
BW	biological weapon
BWA	biological warfare agent
BWC	biological weapons convention
bwd	wild bird species
BWR	boiling water reactor
BX	box [as a unit of issue (UI)]
Bz	benzoyl (C_6H_5CO-)
BZ	designation for an incapacitating agent

C

c	speed of light
c	calorie
°C	degrees Celsius (centigrade)
C	carbon

C	continuous
C	ceiling (limit)
C_p	specific heat at constant pressure
C_v	specific heat at constant volume
ca	approximately
Ca	calcium
Ca	NIOSH abbreviation denoting a material should be treated as a potential human carcinogen
CA	cellulose acetate
CA	copper azole (wood preservative)
CA	bromobenzylcyanide (agent designation)
CA	California
CA	Chemical Abstracts
CAA	Clean Air Act
CAA	competent authority approval
CAAA	Clean Air Act Amendments
CAB	cellulose acetate butyrate
CABO	Council of American Building Officials
CAD	computer-assisted design
CADK	chemical agent detection kit
CAER	Community Awareness and Emergency Response (CMA program)
CAFE	corporate average fuel economy
CAGE	Commercial and Government Entity (Code)
CAI	computer-assisted instruction
CAIR	Comprehensive Assessment Information Rule (under TSCA)
cal	calorie
calc	calculate
CAM	computer-assisted management
CAM2	(improved) chemical agent monitor (*also* **ICAM**)
CAMEO	Computer-Aided Management of Emergency Operations
CANCEE	Canadian National Committee on Earthquake Engineering
C&EN	*Chemical & Engineering News*
C & F	cost and freight
C & I	cost and insurance
CANUTEC	Canadian Transport Emergency Centre
CAP	cellulose acetate propionate

CAR	carcinogenic effects (*also* **CARC**)
CAR	capability assessment for readiness
CARB	California Air Resources Board
carc	carcinogen
CARC	carcinogenic effects (*also* **CAR**)
CARS	Center for Atomic Radiation Studies (Acton, MA)
CAS	Chemical Abstracts Service
CASRN	Chemical Abstracts Service registry number (standard reference number assigned to chemical substances registered with the Chemical Abstracts Service)
CAT	Crisis Action Team (located at DHS headquarters)
CAT scan	computerized axial tomography scan
Cb	columbium (obsolete name for niobium)
C/B	chemical/biological
CBA	copper boron azole (wood preservative)
CBC	circulating bed combustor
CBD	*Canadian Building Digest*
CBDCOM	Chemical and Biological Defense Command
CBI	confidential business information
CBIRF	Chemical Biological Incident Response Force
CBL	commercial bill of lading
CBM	chlorobromomethane
CBO	certified building official
CBOD	carbonaceous biochemical oxygen demand
CBP	Customs and Border Protection (part of DHS)
CBQRF	Chemical/Biological Quick Response Force
CBR	chemical, biological, and/or radiological
CBRA	Coastal Barrier Resources Act
CBRDT	Chemical/Biological Rapid Deployment Team
CBRN	chemical, biological, radiological, and/or nuclear
CBRNE	chemical, biological, radiological, and/or nuclear emergency
CBRT	Chemical/Biological Response Team
CBW	chemical and biological weapons
CBW	chemical and biological warfare
cc	cubic centimeter
CC	closed cup (test for flash point)
CC	ammoniacal copper citrate (wood preservative)

CCA	chromated copper arsenate (wood preservative)
CCAA	Canadian Clean Air Act
CCBFC	Canadian Commission on Building and Fire Codes
CCC	Commodity Credit Corporation
CCCME	Canadian Commission on Construction Materials Evaluation
CCCS	Council Committee on Chemical Safety (ACS)
CCDEH	California Conference of Directors of Environmental Health
CCFS	Coordinating Committee on Fire Safety (SPI)
CCMC	Canadian Construction Materials Centre
CCN	cloud condensation nuclei
CCNR	Commission Centrale pour la Navigation du Rhin
CCOHS	Canadian Centre for Occupational Health and Safety
CCP	casualty collection point
CCRF	Commissioned Corps Readiness Force (U.S. Public Health Service)
CCT	clean coal technology
CCT	critical care transport
CCTV	closed circuit television
Cd	cadmium
CDA	completely denatured alcohol
CDBG	community development block grants
CDC	Centers for Disease Control and Prevention
CDD	chlorinated dibenzo-p-dioxin
CDDC	copper bis(dimethyldithiocarbamate) (wood preservative)
CDF	chlorinated dibenzofuran
CDG	Carriage of Dangerous Goods (IMO subcommittee)
CDL	commercial driver's license
CDRG	Catastrophic Disaster Response Group
CDT	central daylight time
Ce	cerium
CE	chartered engineer
CEE	International Commission for Certification of Electrical Equipment (now International Electrotechnical Commission)
CEEL	community emergency exposure limits
CEEL-1	Concentration of an airborne substance (gas, vapor, aerosol) below which direct toxic effects are unlikely to lead to discomfort in the general population, but above which discomfort becomes increasingly common

CEEL-2	Concentration below which direct toxic effects are unlikely to lead to disability, but above which disability becomes increasingly common
CEEL-3	Concentration below which death or life-threatening effects are unlikely, but above which death or life-threatening effects become increasingly likely
CEIS	Code Enforcement Information System
CEM	comprehensive emergency management
CEMS	continuous emissions monitoring system
CEN	European Committee for Standardization
CENELEC	European Committee for Electrotechnical Standardization
CEO	chief executive officer
CEP	completed exposure pathway
CEPA	Canadian Environmental Protection Agency
CEPP	Chemical Emergency Preparedness and Prevention (EPA)
CEPPO	Chemical Emergency Preparedness and Prevention Office
CEQ	Council on Environmental Quality
CERCLA	The Comprehensive Environmental Response, Compensation, and Liability Act of 1980 (PL 96-510, 40 CFR 300)
CERT	chemical emergency response team
CERT	community emergency response team
CERT	Computer Emergency Response Team (DHS) (*also called* **US-CERT**)
CET	certified environmental trainer
cf	compare
Cf	californium
CF	causal factor
CFA	Composites Fabricators Association
CFCs	chlorofluorocarbons
CFE	chlorotrifluoroethylene
CFEI	certified fire and explosion investigator
CFFA	Chemical Fabrics & Film Association
CFFDRS	Canadian Forest Fire Danger Rating System
CFI	certified fire inspector
CFL	compact fluorescent lamp
cfm	cubic feet per minute (*also* **CFM**)
CFM	chlorofluoromethanes
CFM	cubic feet per minute (*also* **cfm**)

CFO	chief financial officer
CFPS	certified fire protection specialist
CFR	Code of Federal Regulations
cfs	cubic feet per second
CFSI	Congressional Fire Services Institute
CG	phosgene (agent designation)
CG	Coast Guard
CGA	Canadian Gas Association
CGA	Compressed Gas Association [Chantilly, VA; (703) 788-2700]
CGI	combustible gas indicator
cgs	centimeter-gram-second (metric system)
CGSB	Canadian General Services Board
CHAS	Chemical Health and Safety (division of ACS; *also called* **DCHAS**)
chd	child
ChE	cholinesterase
chem	chemical
chem-bio	chemical and biological
CHEMLINE	on-line chemical database (National Library of Medicine)
CHEMNET	Chemical Industry Mutual Aid Network (CMA) A program established by the CMA to provide mutual aid information and programs to organizations desiring such information.
CHEMRIC	Chemical Monograph Referral Center
CHEMTREC	Chemical Transportation Emergency Center, established and operated by the American Chemistry Council (formerly CMA)
chk	chicken
CHLOREP	Chlorine Emergency Plan (operated by the Chlorine Institute)
CHMM	certified hazardous materials manager
CHO	chemical hygiene officer
CHP	chemical hygiene plan (29 CFR 1910.1450, OSHA Standard)
CHP	certified health physicist
CHRIS	Chemical Hazards Response Information System
CHS	Certification in Homeland Security (levels I–V)
CHST	construction health and safety technologist
Ci	curie
CI	Chlorine Institute
CI	color index
CI	compression ignition

CIA	Central Intelligence Agency
CIAO	Critical Infrastructure Assurance Office (Department of Commerce)
CIB	Current Intelligence Bulletin (NIOSH)
CIC	chloroacetophenone in chloroform
CIDX	Chemical Industry Data Exchange
C.I.F.	cost, insurance, and freight
CIH	certified industrial hygienist
CIIT	Chemical Industry Institute of Toxicology
CINC	Commander-In-Chief
CIP	critical infrastructure protection
cis-	indication that two radicals or groups are positioned on one side of a double bond between two carbon atoms
CIS	consumer information sheets
CIS	Cancer Information Service
CIS	Chemical Information System, Inc.
CISD	critical incident stress debriefing
CISMT	critical incident stress management team
CJCS	chairman of the Joint Chiefs of Staff
CK	cyanogen chloride (a chemical blood agent)
Cl	chlorine
CL	ceiling concentration
CL	ceiling level
CL	chlorine (agent designation)
clr	*Chlamydomonas reinhardi*
CLS	characteristic loss spectroscopy
cm	centimeter
Cm	curium
CMA	Chemical Manufacturers Association (now the ACC)
CMC	carboxymethylcellulose
CMEA	Council for Mutual Economic Assistance
cmpd	compound
CMPF	cyclohexyl methylphosphonafluoridate
CMRA	Chemical Marketing Research Association
CMS	Centers for Medicare and Medicaid Services
CMT	crisis management team
CMV	commercial motor vehicle

CN	cellulose nitrate
CN	can [as a unit of issue (UI)]
CN	chloroacetophenone (agent designation)
CNB	CN in benzene and carbon tetrachloride (agent designation)
CNC	CN in chloroform (agent designation)
CNET	Centre Nationale d'Etudes des Télécommunications
CNG	compressed natural gas
CNOH	cyanic acid (agent designation)
CNS	CN and chloropicrin in chloroform (agent designation)
CNS	central nervous system
Co	cobalt
CO	Colorado
CO_2	carbon dioxide
COC	Cleveland open cup (test for flash point)
COCO	contractor-owned/contractor-operated
COD	chemical oxygen demand
COD	cause of death
COF	certificate of fitness
COFI	Council of Forest Industries (Canada)
COG	council of governments
COH	Center for Occupational Hazards
COH	coefficient of haze
conc	concentration
CONEG	Coalition of Northeastern Governors
CONPLAN	U.S. Government Interagency Domestic Terrorism Concept of Operations Plan
contg	containing
CONUS	continental United States
CONUSA	continental United States Army
COO	chief operating officer
COOP	continuity of operations plans
COPPE	Council on Plastics and Packaging in the Environment
COR	contracting office representative
COR	corrosive effects
COTIF	Convention Relative aux Transports Internationaux Ferroviaires
COTP	captain of the port
cP	centipoise (measure of viscosity)

CP	chemically pure
CP	command post
CPC	chemical protective clothing
CPDA	Chemical Producers and Distributors Association
CPE	chemical protective equipment
CPE	chlorinated polyethylene
CPF	carcinogenic potency factor
CPG	Civil Preparedness Guides (series of FEMA policy documents)
CPG 1-3	*Federal Assistance Handbook: Emergency Management, Direction, and Control Programs* (prepared by FEMA). Provides guidance on administrative and programmatic requirements associated with FEMA funds.
CPG 1-5	*Objectives for Local Emergency Management* (prepared by FEMA). Describes and explains functional objectives that represent a comprehensive and integrated emergency management program. Includes recommended activities for each objective.
CPG 1-8	*Guide for Development of State and Local Emergency Operations Plans* (prepared by FEMA).
CPG 1-8A	*Guide for Review of State and Local Emergency Operations Plans;* standard instrument used to assess EOPs that are developed to satisfy eligibility for funding. Called the *crosswalk checklist.* Prepared by FEMA.
CPG 1-35	*Hazard Identification, Capability Assessment, and Multi-Year Development Plan for local governments* (prepared by FEMA)
CPHP	Centers for Public Health Preparedness (CDC program)
CPI	Consumer Price Index
CPI	chemical process industry
CPR	cardiopulmonary resuscitation
CPS	characters per second
CPS	contour plotting system
CPSC	Consumer Product Safety Commission
CPT	cone penterometer testing
CPVC	chlorinated polyvinyl chloride
Cr	chromium
CR	a riot control chemical (agent designation)
CRC	Chemical Referral Center (CHEMTREC)
CRC	Coordinating Research Council
CRC	contamination reduction corridor
CRC	crisis response cell

CRI cutaneous radiation injury
CRIT DOC NIOSH criteria document
crit press critical pressure
crit temp critical temperature
CRM customer relationship management
CRP child-resistant packaging
CRSP Canadian registered safety professional
CRT cathode ray tube
CRT community response team
crys crystal(s) or crystalline (*also* **cryst**)
cryst crystal(s) or crystalline (*also* **crys**)
CRZ contamination reduction zone
cS centistoke, the unit of kinetic viscosity
Cs cesium
CS a riot control chemical (agent designation)
CS customer service
CSA Canadian Standards Association
CSB United States Chemical Safety and Hazard Investigation Board
CSE Centro Studi ed Esperienze dei Vigili del Fuoco
CSEPP Chemical Stockpile Emergency Preparedness Program
CSF confidential statement of formula
CSHS Center for State Homeland Security
CSI Construction Specifications Institute
CSI critical safety index
CSICC Canadian Steel Industries Construction Council
CSIN Chemical Substances Information Network
CSIRO Commonwealth Scientific and Industrial Research Organization
CSIS Center for Strategic and International Studies
CSM Center for Subsurface Modeling
CSMA Chemical Specialties Manufacturers Association
CSP certified safety specialist
CSP Canadian soft plywood
CST civil support teams, formerly known as RAID teams (National Guard)
CST central standard time
CT Connecticut
CTAC Chemical Transportation Advisory Committee (USCG)

CTBT	Comprehensive Test Ban Treaty
CTBTO	Comprehensive Nuclear Test Ban Treaty Organization
CTFA	Cosmetic Toiletry and Fragrance Association
CTFE	chlorotrifluoroethylene
CTG	control technique guidelines
ctl	cattle
CTNSP	Center for Technology and National Security Policy
CT scan	*See* **CAT scan**
cu	cubic
Cu	copper
cu ft/lb	cubic feet per pound
CUI	Chemical Use Inventory (TSCA)
cu m	cubic meter (*also* **m^3**)
CUM	cumulative effects
CUSA	certified utility safety administrator
CV	chemical vocabulary
CVD	chemical vapor deposition
CVS	cardiovascular effects
CW	chemical warfare
CW	chemical weapons
CWA	Clean Water Act
CWC	Chemical Weapons Convention
CWLM	cumulative working level months
CX	phosgene oxime (agent designation)
cyt	cytogenic analysis
CYT	cytogenic effects
CZC	chromated zinc chloride (wood preservative)
CZM	Coastal Zone Management (Program)
CZMA	Coastal Zone Management Act

D

d	day(s) (*also* **D**)
d	density
d-	dextrorotatory
2,4-D	dichlorophenoxyacetic acid

D	deuterium
D	day(s) (*also* **d**)
D	optical density of smoke
DA	diphenylchloroarsine (agent designation)
DAA	diacetone acrylamide
DAAMS	depot area air monitoring system
DAC	disaster assistance center
DAE	disaster assistance employee (*also called* Stafford Act employee or **SAE**)
DAF	dissolved air flotation
DAMAGES	Disaster Assistance Management Accountability System
D&H	dangerous and hazardous (cargo)
DAP	diallyl phthalate
DARPA	Defense Advanced Research Projects Agency
dB	decibel
DBA	doing business as
DBC	1,4-dichlorobutane
DBMS	database management systems
DBP	dibutyl phthalate
DC	diphenylcyanoarsine (agent designation)
DC	District of Columbia
DCHAL	Division of Chemistry and the Law (ACS)
DCHAS	Division of Chemical Health and Safety (ACS)
dck	duck
DCMAO	Defense Contract Management Area Operations
DCO	defense coordinating officer
DCO	dehydrated castor oil
DDA	Department for Disarmament Affairs (UN)
DDE	dichlorodiphenyl-dichloroethylene
DDNP	diazodinitrophenol
DDP	drug dependence effects
DDT	dichlorodiphenyltrichloroethane
DDTA	derivative differential thermal analysis
DE	Delaware
DEA	diethanolamine
DEA	Drug Enforcement Administration
dec	decomposes (*also* **decomp**)

decomp	decomposes or decomposition (*also* **dec**)
decon	decontamination
DEET	N,N-diethyl-m-toluamide
def	definition
deg	degree
DEG	diethylene glycol
DEHP	di(2-ethylhexyl) phthalate
deliq	deliquescent
DEP	diethyl phthalate
DEP	Department of Environmental Protection (can refer to Australian national organization or individual U.S. state organizations)
deriv	derivative
DES	diethylstilbesterol
DEST	Domestic Emergency Support Team
DF	methylphosphonic difluoride (agent designation)
DFO	disaster field office
DFP	Douglas fir plywood
DFW	Department of Fish and Wildlife
DGP	dangerous goods panel (ICAO)
DHHS	U.S. Department of Health and Human Services
DHS	Department of Homeland Security
di-	prefix for "two" (*also* **bi-**)
Di	didymium
DIA	Defense Intelligence Agency
DIDP	diisodecyl phthalate
dil	dilute
diln	dilution
DIN	Deutsches Institut für Normung
DIOP	diisooctyl phthalate
DISC	Disaster Information Systems Clearinghouse
DISS	diameter index safety system
distln	distillation
DLA	Defense Logistics Agency
dlt	dominant lethal test
dm	decimeter
DM	adamsite (agent designation)
DMA	dimethylamine

DMATs	disaster medical assistance teams (coordinated efforts through FEMA)
DMF	dimethylformamide
dmg	*Drosophila melanogaster*
DMIS	database management information system
DMORTs	disaster mortuary assistant teams (now part of FEMA)
DMS	docket management system
DMS	dimethyl sulfide
DMSO	dimethyl sulfoxide
DMV	Department of Motor Vehicles (state-level)
DNA	deoxyribonucleic acid
DNAPL	dense nonaqueous phase liquid
DNC	dinitrocresol
dnd	DNA damage
DNFSB	Defense Nuclear Facilities Safety Board
dni	DNA inhibition
dnr	DNA repair
DNR	Department of Natural Resources
DNR	do not resuscitate
dns	unscheduled DNA synthesis
DNT	dinitrotoluene
DO	dissolved oxygen
DOA	Department of Agriculture
DOA	dead on arrival
DOB	date of birth
DOC	U.S. Department of Commerce
DOD	U.S. Department of Defense
DODAAC	Department of Defense Activity Address Code
DoDD	Department of Defense directive
DoDI	Department of Defense instruction
DOE	U.S. Department of Energy
DOEd	U.S. Department of Education (*also* **ED**)
DOI	U.S. Department of the Interior
DOJ	U.S. Department of Justice
DOL	U.S. Department of Labor
DOMS	Directorate of Military Support (DOD)
DOP	dioctyl phthalate (*also* di-2-ethylhexyl phthalate)

DOS	U.S. Department of State
DOT	U.S. Department of Transportation
DOT 103	The classification of an insulated or uninsulated nonpressure tank car with an expansion dome of 1%. Can be constructed of carbon steel, aluminum, nickel, or alloy steel. A bottom outlet or washout is allowed, depending on specification.
DOT 104	The classification of an insulated carbon steel, nonpressure tank car with a minimum expansion dome of 2%. Bottom outlet and washout are optional.
DOT 105	The classification of an insulated pressure tank car designed for top loading and unloading. May be constructed of carbon steel or aluminum alloy. No bottom outlet or washout; only one opening in tank.
DOT 111	The classification of an insulated or uninsulated nonpressure tank car without an expansion capacity built into the tank. These tanks have varied fittings according to specification. This tank car is the most common one in service.
DOT 112	The classification of an uninsulated carbon steel pressure tank car designed for top loading and unloading. Bottom outlet and washout are prohibited. Thermal protection is designed to meet specific criteria.
DOT 113	The classification of an insulated vacuum tank car for cryogenic service having an inner container and carbon steel outer shell. The insulation system is designed for protection for 30 days, not protection from fire (thermal).
DOT 114	The classification similar to the DOT 112 class, except bottom outlets and washouts are allowed.
DOT 115	The classification of a tank car with an inner tank, a layer of polyurethane insulation (supporting the inner tank), and an outer tank constructed of carbon steel. Bottom washout and outlets are optional.
DOTC	U.S. Department of Transportation classification
DOT-E	designation of materials exempt from Department of Transportation regulations
DP	diphosgene (agent designation)
DP	degree of polymerization
DPI	dots per inch
dpo	*Drosophila pseudoobscura*
DQO	data quality objective
DR	drum [as a unit of issue (UI)]
DRC	disaster recovery center
DRE	destruction and removal efficiency

DRF	disaster relief fund
DRMO	Defense Reutilization and Marketing Office
DRMS	Defense Reutilization and Marketing Service
DSC	differential scanning colorimetry
DSL	digital subscriber line
DSL	Domestic Substances List (Canadian list similar to TSCA)
DSM	demand-side management
DSP	disodium phosphate
DSS	decision support systems
DTA	differential thermal analysis
DTRA	Defense Threat Reduction Agency
DWEL	drinking water equivalent level
DWI	disaster welfare inquiry
DWS	drinking water standard
dwt	deadweight tonnage
Dy	dysprosium
dyn	dynes

E

E^o	standard reduction potential
E_a	activation energy
E_k	kinetic energy (*also* **KE**)
EA	environmental assessment
EA	each [as a unit of issue (UI)]
EA	Office of Energy Assurance (DOE)
EA 5414	DMAPDMAPP (a chemical nerve agent)
EADS	Environmental Assessment Data Systems
EAF	Environment Assistance Fund
EAK	ethyl amyl ketone
EAS	Emergency Alert System
EAS	Essential Air Service
EASHW	European Agency for Safety and Health at Work
EBITDA	earnings before interest, taxes, depreciation, and amortization
EBS	Emergency Broadcast System
EC	electron capture

EC	European Community
EC	emergency coordinator
EC_{50}	effective concentration of gas or smoke that will produce a response in 50% of the test animals within a specified time.
ECE	Economic Commission for Europe (UN)
ECF	extended care facility
ECG	electrocardiogram
ECS	Emergency Communications Staff
ED	U.S. Department of Education (*also* **DOEd**)
ED	ethyldichloroarsine (a vesicant or blister agent)
ED	effective dose
ED_{10}	effective dose (the lowest dose that should produce a minimal effect)
EDB	ethylene dibromide
EDC	ethylene dichloride
EDD	enforcement decision document
EDF	Environmental Defense Fund
EDI	electronic data interchange
EDT	Eastern Daylight Time
EDTA	ethylene diamine tetraacetic acid
EEC	European Economic Community
EED	estimated exposure dose
EEG	electroencephalogram
EEI	essential elements of information (military report format)
EENET	Emergency Education Network
EF	emission factor
EFV	excess flow valve
e.g.	for example
EHS	environmental health and safety
EHS	extremely hazardous substance
EIA	Electronic Industries Association
EICC	Emergency Information and Coordination Center (FEMA)
EIGA	European Industrial Gases Association
EIMA	Emergency Information and Media Affairs (FEMA)
EINECS	European Inventory of Existing Commercial Chemical Substances
EIR	environmental impact report
EIS	environmental impact statement

EKG	electrocardiogram
EL	exposure level
ELO	environmental liaison officer
ELT	emergency locator transmitter
EM	emergency manager
EM	environmental management
EMAC	Emergency Management Assistance Compact
EMAP	Environmental Monitoring and Assessment Program
emb	embryo
EMF	electromotive force
EMI	electromagnetic interference
EMI	Emergency Management Institute (FEMA)
EMIC	Environmental Mutagen Information Center
EMPA	Emergency Management Planning and Assistance
EMPA	ethyl methylphosphonate
EMPG	Emergency Management Performance Grant
EMR	electron magnetic resonance
EMR-ISAC	Emergency Management and Response-Information Sharing and Analysis Center
EMS	emergency medical services
EMT	emergency medical technician
EMT-B	emergency medical technician-basic
ENBC	enhanced nuclear, biological, and chemical
ENIAC	electronic numerical integrator and computer
ENSO	El Niño-southern oscillation
EO	ethylene oxide
EO	executive order
EOC	emergency operations center
EOL	end of life
EOP	emergency operations plan
EP	extraction procedure
EP	extreme pressure
EP	ethylene propylene
EPA	U.S. Environmental Protection Agency
EPA 402	list of toxic substances [under TSCA Section 402; contains list of extremely hazardous substances (EHS)]
EP&R	Emergency Preparedness and Response (FEMA, under DHS)

EPCRA	Emergency Planning and Community Right-to Know Act of 1986 (*also called* SARA, Title III)
EPDM	ethylene-propylene-diene modified elastomer
EPE	estimated position error
EPIRB	emergency position indicating radio beacon
Epi-X	Epidemic Information Exchange (CDC)
EPM	ethylene-propylene copolymer
EPR	electron paramagnetic resonance
EPR	ethylene propylene rubber
EPS	expanded polystyrene
EPT	ethylene propylene terpolymer
EPTOX	extraction procedure toxicity
eq	equation
eq	gram equivalent weight
equilib	equilibrium
equiv	equivalent
Er	erbium
ER	extra risk
ERB	Economic Resources Board
ERC	energy release component
ERC	emissions reduction credit
ERDC	Engineer Research and Development Center (U.S. Army, Vicksburg, MS)
ERG	*Emergency Response Guidebook*
ERH	electrical resistance heater
ERNS	Emergency Response Notification System (NRC database)
ERP	enterprise resource planning
ERRI	Emergency Response & Research Institute
ERT	Environmental Response Team
ERT	Emergency Response Team
ERT-A	advance element of the Emergency Response Team
Es	einsteinium
ESA	Endangered Species Act
ESA	environmentally sensitive area
ES&H	Office of Environment, Safety, and Health (DOE)
esc	*Escherichia coli*
ESD	electrostatic dissipation

ESF	emergency support function
ESH	environmental safety and health
ESLI	end-of-service-life indicator
ESP	electrostatic precipitator
EST	Eastern standard time
EST	Emergency Support Team (located in FEMA headquarters)
esu	electrostatic units
Et	informal abbreviation for ethyl
ETA	estimated time of arrival
ETFE	ethylene-tetrafluoroethylene
eth	ether
ETIC	Environmental Teratology Information Center
ETO	ethyl alcohol
EtOH	informal abbreviation for ethyl alcohol
Eu	europium
EU	European Union
eug	*Euglena gracilis*
EUSC	Effective U.S. Control Fleet
eV	electron volt
EVA	ethylene vinyl acetate
EVAL	ethylene vinyl alcohol
EVE	ethyl vinyl ether
EVOH	ethylene vinyl alcohol
EVT	emergency vehicle technicians

F

°F	degrees Fahrenheit
F	faraday
F	fluorine
FAA	Federal Aviation Administration
FAR	Federal Aviation Regulations
FAS	free alongside (of ship)
FAST	firefighter assist and safety team [may *also* be called a **rapid intervention team (RIT)**]
FAX	facsimile

fb	fiber
FBC	fluidized bed combustion
FBI	Federal Bureau of Investigation
fbr	fibroblast
FBR	fast breeder reactor
FC	fluorocarbon
f/cc	fibers per cubic centimeter of air
FCC	Federal Communications Commission
FCC	*Food Chemicals Codex*
FCL	full container load
FCO	federal coordinating officer
FD	fire department
FDA	U.S. Food and Drug Administration
FD&C	Food, Drugs, and Cosmetics Act
FDIC	Fire Department Instructor's Conference
FDMS	Federal Docket Management System (EPA)
Fe	iron
FE	fugitive emissions
FEC	facility emergency coordinator
FedCIRC	Federal Computer Incident Response Center
FEL	frank-effect level
FEMA	Federal Emergency Management Agency
FEMA-REP-5	*Guidance for Developing State, Tribal, and Local Radiological Emergency Response Planning and Preparedness for Transportation Accidents*
FEP	fluorinated ethylene propylene
FEPCA	Federal Environmental Pesticide Control Act (enacted as amendments to FIFRA)
FERC	Federal Energy Regulatory Commission
FES	flame emission spectroscopy
FESC	federal emergency support coordinator
FEST	Foreign Emergency Support Team
FETN	Fire and Emergency Training Network
FEV1	forced expiratory volume
FFC	free from chlorine
FFDCA	Federal Food, Drug, and Cosmetic Act
FFPE	firefighter protective ensemble

FGAN	fertilizer grade ammonium nitrate
FGD	flue gas desulfurization
FHML	Federal Hazardous Material Law
FHWA	Federal Highway Administration
FIA	Federal Insurance Administration
FIAT	Field Information Agency, Technical
FID	flame ionization detector
FIFRA	Federal Insecticide, Fungicide, and Rodenticide Act
FIP	federal implementation plan
FIRESCOPE	Firefighting Resources of California Organized for Potential Emergencies
FIRM	flood insurance rate maps (FEMA)
FL	Florida
flam	flammable
flash p	flash point (*also* **Fl. P.** and **FLP**)
FLETC	Federal Law Enforcement Training Center
FLIR	forward looking infrared
Fl. P.	flash point (*also* **flash p** *and* **FLP**)
FLP	flash point (*also* **Fl. P.** *and* **flash p**)
Fm	fermium
FM	titanium tetrachloride (agent designation)
FM	Factory Mutual System
FMA	Flood Mitigation Assistance (FEMA program)
FMC	Federal Maritime Commission
FMCSA	Federal Motor Carriers Safety Administration
FMCSR	Federal Motor Carriers Safety Regulations
FML	flexible membrane liner
FMP	fire management plan
FNS	Food and Nutrition Services (USDA)
FOB	free on board
FOC	FEMA Operations Center
FOG	field operations guide
FOIA	Freedom of Information Act
FONSI	finding of no significant impact
FOP	fire occurrence prediction
FOP	Fraternal Order of Police
FORSCOM	United States Army Forces Command

FOUO	for official use only
fp	freezing point
FP	fine particulate
FPA	Federal Pesticide Act
FPA	Flexible Packaging Association
FPA	Federal Power Act
FPC	Federal Power Commission
FPD	flame photometric detector
FPEIS	Fine Particle Emissions Information System [component of Environmental Assessment Data Systems (EADS)]
FPS	Federal Protective Service
Fr	francium
FR	Federal Register
FR	final ruling
FRA	Federal Railroad Administration
FRA	Federal Register Act
FRC	functional residual capacity
FRERP	Federal Radiological Emergency Response Plan
frg	frog
FRG	Federal Republic of Germany
FRMAC	Federal Radiological Monitoring and Assessment Center (part of NNSA)
FRN	Federal Register Notice
FRN	final rulemaking notice
FRN	FEMA Radio Network
FRP	Federal Response Plan (replaced by the National Response Plan)
FRP	fiberglass-reinforced plastic
FRT	fire retardant treated
FS	sulfur trioxide-chlorosulfonic acid (agent designation)
FS	Forest Service (USDA)
FSN	FEMA Switch Network
FSO	facility security officer
FSS	Federal Supply Service
ft	feet
Ft	Fourier transform
FTA	Free Trade Agreement
FTC	Federal Trade Commission

FT-IR	Fourier transform infrared spectrophotometer
FTMS	Federal Test Method Standards
FTS	Federal Telecommunications Systems
FVC	forced vital capacity
fw	formula weight
FWPCA	Federal Water Pollution Control Act
FY	fiscal year

G

γ	gamma
g	gram (*also* **gm**)
Ga	gallium
GA	tabun (a chemical nerve agent)
GA	Georgia
GAAP	generally accepted accounting principles
GAC	granular activated carbon
gal	gallon
GAO	General Accounting Office
GATT	General Agreement on Tariffs and Trade
GB	sarin (a chemical nerve agent)
GBL	government bill of lading
GC	gas chromatograph
GC	gas chromatography
GC	Office of General Counsel (FEMA)
g/cm^3	grams per cubic centimeter
GC/MS	gas chromatograph/mass spectrophotometer
Gd	gadolinium
GD	soman (a chemical nerve agent)
GDP	gross domestic product
GDR	German Democratic Republic
Ge	germanium
GE	a nerve gas (agent designation)
GEDAPER	A seven-step decision-making process for emergency operations: gather, estimate, determine, assess, plan, evaluate, and review
GEP	good engineering practice

GF	cyclohexyl sarin (a chemical nerve agent)
GHS	Globally Harmonized System (UN system for hazardous materials classification)
GI	gastrointestinal
GIS	geographic information system
GIT	gastrointestinal tract
g/L	grams per liter
glac	glacial
GLC	gas-liquid chromatography
gm	gram (*also* **g**)
GMA	Grocery Manufacturers Association
g/mL	grams per milliliter
GMP	good manufacturing practice
GMT	Greenwich mean time
GMW	gram-molecular weight
GNP	gross national product
GOCO	government-owned/contractor-operated
GOES	geostationary operational environmental satellites
GOGO	government-owned/government-operated
GOP	general operating procedures
GOPO	government-owned/privately-operated
GP	DMAEDMAPP (a chemical nerve agent)
GP	general purpose
GPC	gel permeation chromatography
GPF black	general purpose furnace black
gpg	Guinea pig
gpm	gallons per minute
GPR	ground penetrating radar
GPS	global positioning system
gran	granular or granules
GRAS	generally recognized as safe
grb	gerbil
GRP	glass reinforced plastic
GSA	General Services Administration
GTL	gas to liquid
GWM	groundwater monitoring
GWP	global warming potential

GWPC	Ground Water Protection Council
GWPS	groundwater protection standards
GWPS	groundwater protection strategy

H

h	hour(s) (*also* **H** *and* **hr**)
h	Planck's constant
H	hydrogen
H	mustard; a vesicant or blister agent (*also* **HD)**
H	hour(s) (*also* **h** and **hr**)
HACS	Hazard Assessment Computer System
HAD	heat actuating devices
HAN	*Health Alert Network* (CDC)
HAP	hazardous air pollutants
HARM	*Hazards Analysis Resource Manual*
HASP	health and safety plan
HAZ-1	a subset of HAZARD I developed by the CPSC
HAZARD I	an analysis method and computer program developed by NIST
HazCom	the OSHA Hazard Communication Standard (CFR 29 1910.1200)
hazmat	hazardous materials (*also* **HAZMAT**)
HAZMAT	hazardous materials (*also* **hazmat**)
HAZOP	hazard and operability study
HAZUS	Hazards United States (computer program)
HAZWOPER	Hazardous Waste Operations and Emergency Response (CFR 29 1910.120)
HAZWOPER training	OSHA Hazardous Waste Operations and Emergency Response training
Hb	hemoglobin
HBFC	hydrobromofluorocarbon
HC	hydrocarbon
HC	hexachloroethane (agent designation)
HC	zinc oxide (agent designation)
HCB	hexachlorobenzene
HCB	homemade chemical bombs
HCC	Hazard Characteristic Codes (DOD)
HCCH	hexachlorocyclohexane

HCCPD	hexachlorocyclopentadiene
HCFC	hydrochlorofluorocarbon
HCG	human chorionic gonadatropin
HCP	Hearing Conservation Program
HCS	Hazard Communication Standard (OSHA standard cited in 29 CFR 1910.1200)
HCTS	Hazardous Cargo Transportation Security (subcommittee of CTAC)
HCU	hydrocracking unit
HD	mustard (a vesicant or blister agent); *also* **H**
HDP	high detonation pressure
HDPE	high-density polyethylene
HDT	highest dose tested (in a study)
HDTV	high-definition television
He	helium
HEC	human equivalent concentration
hecto-	prefix meaning "10^2" or "100"
HED	human equivalent dose
hemi-	prefix meaning "half"
HEOD	dieldrin
HEPA	high-efficiency particulate air filter
HEROIC	Hazmat Emergency Response Operations and Information Center
HESIS	Hazard Evaluation System and Information Service (state of California)
HETP	hexaethyl tetraphosphate
hexa-	prefix meaning "six"
Hf	hafnium
HF	high frequency
HFC	hydrofluorocarbon
HFV	hemorrhagic fever virus
H/HD	sulfur mustards
HHDN	aldrin
HHS	Department of Health and Human Services
HI	hazard index
HI	Hawaii
HICA-MYDP	Hazardous Identification Capability Assessment and Multi-Year Development Plan

HIPAA	Health Insurance Portability & Accountability Act
HIPS	high impact polystyrene
HIT	Hazard Information Transmission program
HIV	human immunodeficiency virus
hl	hectoliter (*also* **hL**)
hL	hectoliter (*also* **hl**)
HL	mustard-lewisite mixture
hla	HeLa cell
HLD	homeland defense
HLRW	high-level radioactive waste
HLS	homeland security
HLT	Hurricane Liaison Team (FEMA staff who join with NOAA staff and others during hurricane events)
HLW	high-level waste (radioactive)
hm	hectometer
HM	hazardous material
HM	hazard mitigation
hma	host-mediated assay
HMAC	Hazardous Materials Advisory Council
HMCP	HazMat Contingency Planning Course (designed by FEMA, EPA, and DOT for briefing of SERC and LEPC)
HMEP	Hazardous Materials Emergency Preparedness (grant program and curriculum)
HMF black	high modulus furnace black
HMGP	Hazard Mitigation Grant Program
hmi	*Haemophilus influenzae*
HMI	hazardous materials incident
HMIRS	Hazardous Materials Information Resource System (DOD)
HMIS	Hazardous Materials Identification System
HMIX	Hazardous Materials Information Exchange
HMMP	hazardous materials management plan
hmn	human
HMO	health maintenance organization
HMP	hazard mitigation plan
HMR	Hazardous Materials Regulations
HMRT	hazardous materials response team
HMRU	Hazardous Material Response Unit (FBI; Quantico, VA)

HMTA	Hazardous Materials Transportation Act
HM-TAP	Hazard Mitigation Technical Assistance Program
HMTR	hazardous materials transportation regulations
HMTUSA	Hazardous Materials Transportation and Uniform Safety Act of 1990
HMV	high melt viscosity
HN-1	nitrogen mustard-1 (a vesicant or blister agent)
HN-2	nitrogen mustard-2 (a vesicant or blister agent)
HN-3	nitrogen mustard-3 (a vesicant or blister agent)
Ho	holmium
HOC	halogenated organic carbons
HOS	hours of service
HP	horsepower
HPC black	hard processing channel black
HPLC	high performance liquid chromatography
HPM	hazardous production material
HQ	headquarters
HQDA	Headquarters, Department of the Army
hr	hour
HR	hazard rating
HR	human resources
HRS	Hazardous Ranking System (EPA)
Hs	hassium
HS	Homeland Security (Department of)
HSAB	hard/soft acid/base principle
HSAS	Homeland Security Advisory System
HSC	Homeland Security Council
HSDB	Hazardous Substance Data Bank
HSEES	Hazardous Substances Emergency Events Surveillance
HSL	hazardous substances list
HSO	health and safety officer
HSOC	Homeland Security Operations Center
HSPD	Homeland Security Presidential Directive
HSRT	Homeland Security Response Team
HSt	stearic acid
HSWA	Hazardous and Solid Waste Amendments of 1984 (a group of amendments to RCRA)

ht	height
HT	mustard-T mixture
HTB	high test bleach
htd	heated
htg	heating
HTH	high test hypochlorite
HTH	trademark for a calcium hypochlorite used in bleaching, sterilizing, and in oxidizing swimming pool water.
HTIS	Hazardous Technical Information Service
HTSA	Highway Transportation Safety Administration
HTU	heat transfer unit
HUD	Department of Housing and Urban Development
HVAC	heating, ventilating, and air conditioning
HW	hazardous waste
HWC	Health and Welfare Canada
HWLT	Hazardous Waste Land Treatment Program
HWM	hazardous waste management
HX	general formula for hydrogen halides or the halogen acids
hygr	hygroscopic

I

i-	prefix for “iso”
I	iodine
I	intermittent
IA	Iowa
IA	individual assistance (a category of federal disaster aid to individuals and families; FEMA)
IAEA	International Atomic Energy Agency
IAFC	International Association of Fire Chiefs
IAFF	International Association of Fire Fighters
IAIP	Information Analysis and Infrastructure Protection (Branch of DHS)
ial	intraaural
IAP	incident action plan
IAPD	International Association of Plastics Distributors
IAPMO	International Association of Plumbing and Mechanical Officials

IARC	International Agency for Research on Cancer (World Health Organization)
IATA	International Air Transport Association
IAW	in accordance with
IBC	intermediate bulk container
IBC	International Building Code
IC	incident commander
IC	internal combustion
IC	inspiratory capacity
IC_{50}	incapacitating concentration, median
IC_{50}	inhibition concentration, median
ICAM	improved chemical agent monitor (*also* known as **CAM2**)
ICAO	International Civil Aviation Organization
ICAP	incident communications action plan
ICBO	International Conference of Building Officials
ICC	International Codes Council (est. 1994, made up of BOCA, ICBO, and SBCCI)
ICC	Interstate Commerce Commission
ICCTA	Interstate Commerce Commission Termination Act of 1995
ICE	Immigration and Customs Enforcement (DHS)
ICE	Institution of Chemical Engineers (*also* **IChemE**)
ICE	in case of emergency
IChemE	Institution of Chemical Engineers
ICMA	International City/County Management Association
ICP	incident command post
ICP	inventory control point
ICP	initial compliance period
ICR	information collection request
ICS	incident command system
ICSC	International Chemical Safety Cards
ICT	incident command team
icv	intracervical
ICWM	Institute for Chemical Waste Management
ICWU	International Chemical Workers Union
i.d.	inner diameter
ID	Idaho
-ide	a suffix that indicates a binary compound

IDLH	immediately dangerous to life or health
idr	intradermal
idu	intraduodenal
i.e.	that is
IEA	International Energy Agency
IEC	International Electrotechnical Commission
IED	improvised explosive device
IEEE	Institute of Electrical and Electronics Engineers
IEMIS	Integrated Emergency Management Information System
IEMS	integrated emergency management system
IERL	Industrial Environmental Research Laboratory (EPA)
IETC	Innovative Environmental Technology Conference
IFAI	Industrial Fabrics Association International
IFCS	Intergovernmental Forum on Chemical Safety
IFMIS	integrated financial management information system
IG	Office of Inspector General (FEMA)
IHF	Industrial Health Foundation
ihl	inhalation
IHMM	Institute of Hazardous Materials Management
IL	Illinois
ILO	International Labour Organization (BIT,CH-1211, Geneva,22, Switzerland. U.S. office: 1750 New York Ave., Washington, DC, 20006; (202) 376-2315)
I/M	inspection and maintenance
IMCO	International Maritime Consultative Organization [now called **International Maritime Organization (IMO)**]
IMDG	International Maritime Dangerous Goods Code (International Maritime Organization, #4 Albert Embankment, London SE 175R, UK)
IME	Institute of Makers of Explosives
imm	immersion
IMO	International Maritime Organization
imp	implant
ims	intramuscular
IMS	Integrated Management Information System (OSHA)
IMS	ion mobility spectrometry
IMS	incident management system

IMT	Incident Management Team (designed to operate within the National Incident Management System)
in.	inch
In	indium
IN	Indiana
incomp	incompatible
inf	infant
INN	International Nonproprietary Name
inorg	inorganic
INS	Immigration and Naturalization Service
INS	ion neutralization spectroscopy
insol	insoluble
IOF	interim operating facility
IOM	Institute of Medicine
IP	inhalable particles
IPA	isopropyl alcohol
IPA	isophthalic acid
ipc	intraplacental
IPC	Institute for Interconnecting and Packaging Electronic Circuits
IPCC	Intergovernmental Panel on Climate Change
IPCS	International Programme on Chemical Safety
IPFO	interim principle federal official
ipl	intrapleural
IPM	inhalable particulate matter
IPM	integrated pest management
IPO	initial public offering
IPP	isotactic polypropylene
ipr	intraperitoneal
Ir	iridium
IR	infrared
IRA	Irish Republican Army
IRC	Institute for Research in Construction (Canada)
IRDS	primary irritation dose
IRIS	Integrated Risk Information System (EPA)
IRLC	Ignitable Liquids Reference Collection
IRMS	Information Resources Management Service
irn	intrarenal

IRPTC	International Register of Potentially Toxic Chemicals
IRR	irritant effects
IRRD	issue/release/receipt document
ISBN	International Standard Book Number
ISC	Industrial Source Complex (EPA model)
ISCO	in situ chemical oxidation
ISCOR	in situ chemical oxidation recirculation
ISM	integrated safety management
ISM	International Safety Management (Code)
iso-	a prefix meaning "the same"
ISO	International Organization for Standardization (sometimes incorrectly referred to as "International Standards Organization")
isp	intraspinal
ISP	Internet service provider
ISR	Institute for Standards Research
ISS	ion scattering spectroscopy
IST	incident support team
IT	information technology
ITC	Interagency Testing Committee
ITCO	International Tank Container Organisation (headquartered in Belgium)
ITCZ	intertropical convergence zone
-ite	a suffix indicating the compound contains one less oxygen than it does in its normal state
I-TEF	International Toxicity Equivalence Factor (NATO)
itr	intratracheal
ITS	Information Technology Services Directorate (FEMA)
itt	intratesticular
IU	international units
IUC	International Union of Chemistry
IUPAC	International Union of Pure and Applied Chemistry
IUR	inventory update reporting
IUR	inventory update rule
iut	intrauterine
IV	intravenous (meaning "through the vein")
IVE	isobutyl vinyl ether
ivg	intravaginal

IVHS	intelligent vehicle highway system
ivn	intravenous

J

J	joule
J-4/JCS	Office of the Joint Chiefs of Staff
JBAIDS	Joint Biological Agent Identification and Diagnostic System
JBPDS	Joint Biological Point Detection System
JBREWS	Joint Biological Remote Early Warning System
JCAHO	Joint Commission on Accreditation of Healthcare Organizations
JCAP	Joint Conventional Ammunition Program
J/cm^2	joules per square centimeter
JCPDS	Joint Committee on Powder Diffraction Standards
JCS	Joint Chiefs of Staff
JFHQ-HLS	Joint Forces Headquarters, Homeland Security
JHCS	Joint Hazardous Classification System
JIS	Joint Information System (FEMA)
JIT	just in time
JLOTS	joint logistics over the shore
JOC	Joint Operations Center (an FBI resource at a disaster site)
JON	judgment of need
JOTS	jihadi ops tempo statistics
JP-5	jet fuel grade
JP-8	jet fuel grade
JPIC	Joint Public Information Center
JPL	Jet Propulsion Laboratory
JPO-BIO	Joint Program Office for Biological Defense
JSIPP	Joint Service Installation Pilot Program
JSMG	Joint Service Materiel Group
JTATS	jihadi tactics and targeting statistics
JTF	Joint Task Force
JTF-CS	Joint Task Force-Civil Support
JTRB	Joint Telecommunications Resources Board
JWARN	Joint Warning and Reporting Network

K

k	kilo-
K	degrees kelvin
K	potassium
$\mathbf{K_a}$	acid ionization constant
$\mathbf{K_b}$	base ionization constant
$\mathbf{K_b}$	boiling point ionization constant
$\mathbf{K_c}$	equilibrium constant (*also* $\mathbf{K_{eq}}$)
$\mathbf{K_{eq}}$	equilibrium constant (*also* $\mathbf{K_c}$)
$\mathbf{K_f}$	freezing point depression constant
$\mathbf{K_{sp}}$	solubility product
$\mathbf{K_w}$	water equilibrium constant
KB	kilobyte
KBDI	Keech Byram Drought Index
kc	kilogram calorie
kcal	kilocalorie
KCCO	Kansas City Commodity Office
KDAT	kiln-dried after treatment
kdy	kidney
KE	kinetic energy (*also* $\mathbf{E_k}$)
kg	kilogram
kHz	kilohertz
kilo-	prefix meaning "10^3" or "1,000"
kJ	kilojoule
klp	*Klebsiella pneumoniae*
km	kilometer
kN	kilo-newton
kPa	kilopascal gauge (gauge pressure)
kPa abs	kilopascal absolute (absolute pressure)
Kr	krypton
KS	Kansas
KSC	Kennedy Space Center (United States)
kV	kilovolt
kW	kilowatt
KY	Kentucky

L

l	levorotatory
l	liter (*also* **L**)
L	liter (*also* **l**)
L	lewisite (a vesicant or blister agent)
La	lanthanum
LA	Louisiana
LADD	lifetime average daily dose
LADD	lowest acceptable daily dose
LAER	lowest achievable emission rate
LAH	lithium aluminum hydride
LAL	lightning activity level
LAN	local area network
LAT	live-agent tested
lb/gal	pounds per gallon
lb(s)	pound(s)
LBNL	Lawrence Berkeley National Laboratory
LBP	lead-based paint
LC	lethal concentration
LC	liquid chromatography
LC_{50}	lethal concentration (median)
LC_{Lo}	lowest published lethal concentration
LCL	less-than-carload lot
LCL	lower control limit
LCT_{50}	median lethal dose of a vapor or aerosol
LD	lethal dose
LD_{10}	dose level at which first test subjects died
LD_{50}	lethal dose (median)
LD_{Lo}	lowest published lethal dose
LDPE	low density polyethylene
LDT	lowest dose tested
LEA	local education agency
LECO	local emergency operations center
LED_{10}	lower limit on effective dose
LEF	Life Extension Foundation
LEL	lower explosive limit

LEL lowest effect level (*see* **LOEL**)
LEPC local emergency planning committee
leu leukocyte
LEV low emission vehicle
LFA lead federal agency
LFG landfill gas
LFL lower flammable limit
lfm linear feet per minute
LGR Local Governments Reimbursement Program
LHAMA Labeling of Hazardous Art Materials Act of 1988
Li lithium
LI Langelier Index
LIBOR London Interbank Offered Rate
liq liquid
LKP last known position
LLDPE linear low density polyethylene
LLRW low-level radioactive waste
LLW low-level waste (radioactive)
ln logarithm (natural)
LNAPL light nonaqueous phase liquid
lng lung
LNG liquid natural gas
LOAEL lowest observed adverse effect level
LOC level of concern
LOD limit of detection
LOD line of duty
LODD line of duty death
LOEL lowest observed effect level
log logarithm (common)
LOI limiting oxygen index
LORAN long range navigation (system)
LOX liquid oxygen
LP liquefied petroleum
LPD local planning district (a geographic planning area established by SERC)
LPG liquefied petroleum gas
LQG large quantity generator

Lr	lawrencium
LRFD	load and resistance factor design
LSD	lysergic acid diethylamide
LSZ	life safety zone
LT	long ton (unit of weight that equals 1,016 kg or 2,240 pounds)
LTL	less-than-truckload
Lu	lutetium
LUST	leaking underground storage tank
lvr	liver
lym	lymphocyte

M

m	meter
m	molality
m	minutes
m-	"meta-"
M	molar or molarity (sometimes italicized)
m_l	magnetic quantum number
m^3	cubic meter
M_n	number-average molecular weight of a polymer (*also* **M.N.**)
MA	maleic anhydride
MA	Massachusetts
mAbs	monoclonal antibodies
MAC	multiagency coordination
MAC	maximum allowable concentration
MACA	military assistance to civil authorities
MACO	mutual aid chief officer
MACT	maximum achievable control technology
MAFFS	modular airborne firefighting system
MAK	maximum allowable concentrations (German)
mam	mammal
M&I	management and integration
MARS	U.S. Army Military Affiliate Radio System
MAS	master agreement for services
mass spec	mass spectrometry

MATC	maximum acceptable toxic concentration
MATTS	Mobile Air Transportable Telecommunications System
mb	millibar (*also* **mbar**)
MB	megabyte
mbar	millibar (*also* **mb**)
MBMA	Metal Building Manufacturers Association
mC	milliCurie (*also* **mCi**)
MC	motor carrier
MC-306	A motor carrier tank specification by the DOT. It is designed to carry liquids at low vapor pressures (no more than 3 psig). These nonpressured highway carriers, most commonly made out of aluminum alloy, can be single or multicompartmental (separated by bulkheads with additional circumferential reinforcement provided by baffles). These carriers, popularly called *skin tanks,* typically carry substances with a specific gravity less than 1 (lighter petroleum products like gasoline).
MC-307	A low-pressure tank designed for working pressures of up to 25 psig. Carries products such as poison liquids, mild corrosives, and volatile flammable liquids. This "general chemical trailer" usually will have a horseshoe-shaped cross section.
MC-312	The popular "corrosive tank." Designed for pressures between 35 to 50 psig. Has a smaller capacity than any other of the cargo tanks series due to product density (heavy acids and bases); therefore *also* has support rings around the tank to give additional strength. Most MC-312 tanks are lined.
MC-331	A high-pressure vessel designed for working pressures between 100 and 500 psig. Carries compressed gases and hazardous liquids such as anhydrous ammonia, chlorine, and LPG. An MC-331 has a cylindrical shape, with hemispherical heads.
MC-338	A cryogenic cargo tank used to carry liquefied gases at extremely low temperatures.
MC-406	A vessel similar to the MC-306 series. This vessel, however, is designed to withstand a greater force of movement due to the integrity of the design material and a lower center of gravity.
MC-407	A vessel similar to the MC-307 "general chemical trailer." This vessel, however, is designed to withstand a greater force of movement due to the integrity of the design material and a lower center of gravity.
MC-412	A vessel similar to the MC-312 series "corrosive tank" designed to withstand a greater force of movement due to the structural existence of stiffer outer rings, a thicker shell, and a lower center of gravity.

MC-431	A vessel similar to the high-pressure MC-331; designed to withstand a greater force of movement due to the integrity of the design material and a lower center of gravity.
MCA	Manufacturing Chemists Association
MCAs	monoclonal antibodies
mCi	milliCurie (*also* **mC**)
MCI	mass casualty incident
MCL	maximum contaminant level
MCLG	maximum contaminant level goal
MCS	multiple chemical sensitivity
Md	mendelevium
MD	molecular dynamics
MD	Maryland
MD	methyldichloroarsine (a vesicant or blister agent)
MDD	maximum daily dose
MDI	methylene-p-phenylene isocyanate
MDL	method detection limit
MDMA	3,4-methylene dioxymethamphetamine (Ecstasy)
MDMP	military decision-making process
MDPE	medium density polyethylene
MDT	mountain daylight time
Me	methyl radical (CH_3-)
ME	Maine
MEC	Model Energy Code (CABO)
MEK	methyl ethyl ketone
mEq	milliequivalent
MERS	Mobile Emergency Response System (FEMA)
MeV	million electron-volts
mf	molecular formula
MF	modifying factor
MFN	most favored nation
MFPA	methylfluorophosphonic acid
mg	milligram
Mg	magnesium
MGD	million gallons per day
mg/kg	milligrams per kilogram
mg/m^3	milligrams per cubic meter

μg/m³	micrograms per cubic meter
MGN	multigeneration
MH	maleic hydrazide
MHIDAS	Major Hazard Incident Data Service (UK)
MHW	mean high water
MHz	megahertz
MI	Michigan
MIAK	methyl isoamyl ketone
MIBK	methyl isobutyl ketone
MIKES	mass-analyzed ion kinetic energy spectrometry
mil.	military
mil	one thousandth of an inch
milli-	prefix meaning "one thousandth" (10^{-3})
MILSTAMP	military standard transportation and movement procedures
MILSTRIP	military standard requisition and issue procedures
min	minimum
min	minute(s)
MINICAMS	miniature automatic continuous agent monitoring system
MIOT	Maritime Institute of Technology and Graduate Studies (*also* **MITAGS**)
MIPT	Memorial Institute for the Prevention of Terrorism
misc	miscible
MITAGS	Maritime Institute of Technology and Graduate Studies (*also* **MIOT**)
mixt	mixture
mky	monkey
ml	milliliter (*also* **mL** *and* **ML**)
mL	milliliter (*also* **ml** *and* **ML**)
Ml	milliliter (*also* **ml** *and* **mL**)
ML	maximum likelihood (method) (*see also* **MLE)**
MLD	minimum lethal dose
MLD	mild irritation effects
MLE	maximum likelihood estimate
MLRS	multiple launch rocket system (mobile mass missile launchers such as those used in the Persian Gulf war)
MLW	mean low water
mm	millimeter

mμ	millimicron
μm	micron(s)
MM	molar mass (*also* known as molecular weight)
mma	microsomal mutagenicity assay
MMA	methyl methacrylate
MMAD	mass median aerodynamic diameter
MMG	Medical Management Guidelines
mmo	mutation in microorganisms
mmol	millimole
mmr	mammary gland
MMST	metropolitan medical strike teams
MMWR	*Morbidity and Mortality Weekly Report* (CDC)
Mn	manganese
M.N.	number-average molecular weight of a polymer (*also* $\mathbf{M_n}$)
MN	Minnesota
mnt	micronucleus test
Mo	molybdenum
MO	Missouri
MOA	memorandum of agreement
MOCVD	metal organic chemical vapor deposition
mod	moderately
MODE	the four major transportation methods: rail, highway, air, or water
MODU	mobile offshore drilling unit
MOE	margin of exposure
mol	mole
mol wt	molecular weight
mono-	prefix meaning "one"
MOPP	mission oriented protective posture
MOS	margin of safety
MOST	Ministry of Science and Technology (Korea)
MOU	memorandum of understanding
mp	melting point
MPa	megapascal
MPA	methylphosphonic acid
MPK	methyl propylketone
mppcf	million particles per cubic foot

MQL method quantitation limit
mrc gene conversion and mitotic recombination
MRE meals, ready to eat
MRF materials recovery facility
MRF municipal recycle facility
MRI magnetic resonance imaging
MRL maximum residue limit (pesticide tolerance)
MRP material resource planning
MRS Materials Research Society
MS mass spectrometer
MS mass spectroscopy
MS Mississippi
MS mild steel; carbon-based ferrous alloy (cast iron) with a maximum of about 0.25% carbon
MSA methanesulfonic acid
MSA metropolitan statistical area
msc mutation in somatic mammalian cells
MSCA military support to civil authorities
MS-DOS Microsoft Disc Operating System
MSDS material safety data sheet
MSG monosodium glutamate
MSHA Mine Safety and Health Administration
MSK muscular-skeletal effects
MSL mean sea level
MSP monosodium phosphate
MSP Maritime Security Program
MSST maximum safe storage temperature
MST mountain standard time
MSW municipal solid waste
Mt meitnerium
MT Montana
MT Mitigation Directorate (FEMA)
M/T metric ton; unit of weight equal to 1,000 kg or 2,204.6 lb (*also* **t**)
MTB Materials Transportation Bureau (Department of Transportation)
MTBE methyl tertiary butyl ether
MT black medium thermal black
MTD maximum tolerated dose

MTMC	Military Traffic Management Command
mul	multiple routes
mumem	mucous membranes
mus	mouse
MUT	mutagen
MVA	motor vehicle accident (emergency room usage)
MVE	methyl vinyl ether
MVSS	Motor Vehicle Safety Standards
mw	molecular weight (*also* **Mw**)
Mw	molecular weight (*also* **mw**)
MW	megawatt
MWC	municipal waste combustor
MWEAC	Mount Weather Emergency Assistance Center
MWEOC	Mount Weather Emergency Operations Center (FEMA asset in Virginia)

N

n	refractive index
n	principal quantum number
n-	"normal" (used in chemical formulas)
N	newton(s)
N	nitrogen
N	normality
N	Avogadro's number
N-	a symbol used in some chemical names indicating that the next section of the name refers to a chemical group attached to a nitrogen atom
N_2	nitrogen (chemical formula)
N_2O	nitrous oxide
Na	sodium
NA	not applicable
NA	North American
NAAQS	National Ambient Air Quality Standards
NAC	National Agricultural Chemists
NAC	Nebraska Avenue Complex (location of DHS headquarters)
NACA	National Agricultural Chemicals Association

NACCHO	National Association of County and City Health Officials
NACE	National Association of Corrosion Engineers
NACEPT	National Advisory Council for Environmental Policy and Technology
NAERG	*North American Emergency Response Guidebook*
NAFI	National Association of Fire Investigators
NAFTA	North American Free Trade Agreement
NAHB	National Association of Home Builders
NAICS	North American Industry Classification System
NaK	sodium potassium alloy
NAMAS	National Measurement & Accreditation Service
nano-	prefix meaning "10^{-9}"
NAPA	National Asphalt Pavement Association
NAPL	nonaqueous-phase liquid
NAPM	National Association Purchasing Management
NARA	National Agrichemical Retailers Association
NARM	naturally occurring and accelerator-produced radioactive materials
NAS	National Academy of Sciences
NASA	National Aeronautics and Space Administration
NASAR	National Association for Search and Rescue
NATO	North Atlantic Treaty Organisation
NAVSAC	Navigation Safety Advisory Council
NAWAS	National Warning System
Nb	niobium
NBAR	nonbinding allocations of responsibility
NBC	National Building Code (BOCA)
NBC	National Building Code (AIA)
NBC	National Building Code of Canada
NBC	nuclear, biological, and chemical
NBCC	nuclear, biological, chemical, and conventional
NBE-CPI	Norma Basica de la Edificación-Conditiones de Proteccion contra Incendio en los Edificios
NBI	National Bridge Inventory
NBR	nitrile-butadiene rubber
NBS	National Bureau of Standards [now the National Institute for Standards and Technology (NIST)]
NC	nitrocellulose

NC	North Carolina
NCAR	National Center for Atmospheric Research
NCB	National Codification Bureau
NCC	National Coordinating Center
NCFS	National Center for Forensic Science
NCI	National Cancer Institute
NCP	National Contingency Plan (EPA)
NCP	National Oil and Hazardous Substances Pollution Contingency Plan (EPA)
NCPOA	National Chronic Pain Outreach Association
NCRIC	National Chemical Response and Information Center
NCRP	National Council on Radiation Protection and Measurement
NCS	National Communications System
NCSP	National Communications Support Plan
NCTC	National Counterterrorism Center
NCTR	National Center for Toxicological Research
Nd	neodmium
ND	North Dakota
ND	not determined
ND	"new drugs"
NDMOC	National Disaster Medical Operations Center
NDMS	National Disaster Medical System (DHS)
NDPO	National Domestic Preparedness Office (FBI)
NDRF	National Defense Reserve Fleet.
Ne	neon
NE	Nebraska
NE	sulfur with small amounts of silica gel
NEBOSH	National Examination Board for Occupational Safety and Health (British)
NEC	National Electrical Code (published by NFPA)
NECC	National Emergency Coordination Center (FEMA)
NEHA	National Environmental Health Association
NEHRP	National Earthquake Hazards Reduction Program
NEIS	National Earthquake Information Service (USGS)
NEMA	National Electrical Manufacturers Association
NEMA	National Emergency Management Association
NEMIS	National Emergency Management Information System (FEMA)

NEMP	National Emergency Management Plan
NEMS	National Emergency Response System (Canada)
neo-	prefix meaning "new"
neo-	prefix indicating a hydrocarbon where a carbon is bonded directly to four other carbons
NEPA	National Environmental Policy Act
NERR	National Emergency Resource Registry (DHS)
NESHAP	National Emissions Standards for Hazardous Air Pollutants
NEST	Nuclear Emergency Support Team
NETC	National Emergency Training Center
NETL	National Energy Technology Laboratory (DOE)
NEW	net explosive weight
NEXRAD	Next Generation Weather Radar Program
NF	National Formulary grade of chemical
NFA	National Fire Academy
NFC	National Fire Code (published by NFPA)
NFCL	National Fire Code (Canada)
NFDA	National Funeral Directors Association
NFDRS	National Fire Danger Rating System
NFIC	National Fire Information Council
NFIF	National Flood Insurance Fund
NFIP	National Flood Insurance Program (overseen by FEMA)
NFIRS	National Fire Incident Reporting System
NFPA	National Fire Protection Association
NFPA 704	National Fire Protection Association's standard for hazard warning for stationary containers
NFPCA	National Fire Prevention and Control Administration (later became the U.S. Fire Administration)
NFSA	National Fire Sprinkler Association
ng	nanogram (10^{-9} grams)
NGA	National Governors Association
NGB	National Guard Bureau
NGS	National Geodetic Survey (United States)
NH	New Hampshire
NHMIE	National Hazardous Materials Information Exchange
Ni	nickel
NIAID	National Institute of Allergy and Infectious Diseases

NIBS	National Institute of Building Sciences
NICC	National Interagency Coordination Center
NIEHS	National Institute for Environmental Health Sciences
NIFCC	National Interagency Fire Coordination Center (U.S. Forest Service)
NIH	National Institutes of Health
NIH	"not invented here"
NIIMS	National Interagency Incident Management System
NIIN	National Item Identification Number
NIJ	National Institute of Justice
NIMBY	"not in my back yard"
NIMH	National Institute of Mental Health
NIMS	National Incident Management System (DHS)
NIOSH	National Institute for Occupational Safety and Health
NIRT	Nuclear Incident Response Team
NISA	National Invasive Species Act of 1996
NIST	National Institute of Standards and Technology [formerly National Bureau of Standards NBS)]
NITL	National Industrial Transportation League
nitro-	prefix indicating the presence of the -NO_2 radical
NH	New Hampshire
NJ	New Jersey
NJIT	New Jersey Institute of Technology
NKB	Nordiska Kommittén för Byggbestämmelser
NLM	National Library of Medicine
NLSI	National Lightning Safety Institute
nm	nanometer
NM	New Mexico
NM	dimethylpolysulfide (agent designation)
NMAB	National Materials Advisory Board
NMFS	National Marine Fisheries Service
NMFTA	National Motor Freight Traffic Association
NMHC	nonmethane hydrocarbons
NMIM	National Mobile Inventory Model
NMOC	nonmethane organic component
NMOG	nonmethane organic gases
NMR	nuclear magnetic resonance

NMRI	Naval Medical Research Institute
NMU	National Maritime Union
NMVOC	nonmethane volatile organic chemicals
NNRTs	national nursing response teams (coordinated through FEMA)
NNSA	National Nuclear Security Administration (DOE)
No	nobelium
NO	nitric oxide (chemical formula)
NO	nitric oxide (designation)
NO_x	nitrogen oxides
NOAA	National Oceanic and Atmospheric Administration
NOAEL	no-observed-adverse-effect level
NOEL	no-observed-effect level
NOES	National Occupational Exposure Survey
NOHSCP	National Oil and Hazardous Substances Contingency Plan
noi	not otherwise indexed
NOI	notice of interest
noibn	not otherwise indexed by name
non-	prefix meaning "nine"
NOR	not otherwise regulated
NORAD	North American Aerospace Defense Command
NORM	naturally occurring radioactive material
n.o.s.	not otherwise specified
NOS	not otherwise specified
Np	neptunium
NPACI	National Partnership for Advanced Computational Infrastructure
NP&CA	National Paint and Coatings Association (*also* **NPCA**)
NPCA	National Paint and Coatings Association (*also* **NP&CA**)
NPD	nitrogen-phosphorus detector
NPDES	National Pollutant Discharge Elimination System (EPA)
NPG	*NIOSH Pocket Guide to Chemical Hazards*
NPIRS	National Pesticide Information Retrieval System
NPK mixtures	fertilizers containing nitrogen, phosphorus, and potassium
NPL	National Priority List (EPA sites for chemical waste)
NPPTL	National Personal Protective Technology Laboratory
NPR	National Public Radio
NPRA	National Petrochemical & Refiners Association

NPRM	notice of proposed rulemaking
NPRTs	National Pharmacy Response Teams (FEMA program)
NPS	National Park Service
NPS	nonpoint source (pollution)
NPT	national pipe thread
NPTN	National Pesticide Telecommunications Network
NPTS	National Plan for Telecommunications Support
NR	natural rubber
NRC	National Recycling Coalition
NRC	National Response Center
NRC	nonreusable container
NRC	Nuclear Regulatory Commission
NRCA	National Roofing Contractors Association
NRCC	National Research Council Canada
NRCS	Natural Resources Conservation Service
NRDC	National Resources Defense Council
NRDC	National Resources Development Corporation
NRL	Naval Research Laboratory (Washington, D.C.)
NRP	National Response Plan (replaces the FRP)
NRS	National Response System
NRS	nuclear reaction spectroscopy
NRT	National Response Team
NRT-1	*Emergency Planning Guide* (issued by NRT)
NRT-1a	"Criteria for Review of Hazardous Materials Emergency Plans"
NS	Office of National Security Affairs (FEMA)
NSA	National Security Agency
NSAID	nonsteroidal anti-inflammatory drugs
NSC	National Safety Council
NSC	National Service Center
NSDWR	National Secondary Drinking Water Regulations (EPA)
NSEC	National System for Emergency Coordination
NSEP	National Security Emergency Preparedness
NSF	National Sanitation Foundation (now called NSF International)
NSF	National Science Foundation
NSF	National Strike Force
NSN	National Stock Number (DOD)

NSN	National Supply Number
NSPS	New Source Performance Standards
NSR	nitrile silicone rubber
NSR	New Source Review
NSTA	National Science Teachers Association
NTA	nitrilotriacetic acid
NTAC	National Threat Assessment Center (U.S. Secret Service)
NTDB	National Trade Data Bank
NTE	neurotoxic esterase
NTI	National Toxics Inventory
NTIA	National Telecommunications and Information Administration
NTIS	National Technical Information Service
NTP	National Toxicology Program
NTPS	National Transportation Planning System
NTSB	National Transportation Safety Board
NTTC	National Tank Truck Carriers Inc.
Nureg 0654/FEMA-Rep-1	"Criteria for Preparation and Evaluation of Radiological Emergency Response Plans and Preparedness in Support of Nuclear Power Plants"
NV	Nevada
NVLAP	National Voluntary Laboratory Accreditation Program
NVOAD	National Voluntary Organizations Active in Disasters (includes the American Red Cross and Salvation Army)
NVOCC	nonvessel operating common carrier
NWCG	National Wildfire Coordinating Group
NWF	National Wildlife Federation
NWS	National Weather Service
NY	New York

O

o-	ortho
O	oxygen
O_2	formula for molecular oxygen
O_3	ozone
OAG	Office of the Attorney General
OC	capsaicin

OC	open cup (test for flash point)
OC	oxygen consumed
OC	operations chief
OCAW	Oil, Chemical, and Atomic Workers Union
OCDETF	Organized Crime Drug Enforcement Task Force
OCIS	OSHA Computerized Information System
OCMI	officer in charge of marine inspection
OCONUS	outside the continental United States (international)
OCR	optical character recognition
OCTI	Office Central des Transports Internationaux par Chemins de Fer
ocu	ocular
od	outer diameter
ODC	ozone depleting chemical
ODP	Office of Domestic Preparedness (DOJ)
ODP	ozone-depleting potential
ODS	ozone-depleting substance
OEC	Office of Enforcement and Compliance Assurance (EPA)
OECD	Organization for Economic Cooperation and Development
OEL	occupational exposure limit
OEM	original equipment manufacturer
OEP	Office of Emergency Preparedness (U.S. Public Health Service)
OET	Office of Emergency Transportation
OFDA	Office of U.S. Foreign Disaster Assistance
OFM	Office of Financial Management (FEMA)
ofs	other fish
OH	Ohio
OHI	Occupational Health Institute
OHMTADS	Oil and Hazardous Materials/Technical Assistance Data System
OHS	Office of Homeland Security
OHST	occupational health and safety technologist
OIA	Office of International Affairs (part of DHS)
OIAA	Office of Information Analysis and Access (EPA)
OIG	Office of Inspector General
OK	Oklahoma
-ol	a suffix indicating one or more hydroxyl (-OH) groups are present in an organic compound
OLA	Office of Legislative Affairs

OM	outcome measurement
OMB	Office of Management and Budget
omi	other microorganisms
oms	other mutation test systems
ONP	Office of National Preparedness (FEMA)
OP	Office of Policy and Regional Operations (FEMA)
OPA	Oil Pollution Act of 1990
OPCW	Organization for the Prohibition of Chemical Weapons (UN)
open	open irritation test
OPIC	overseas private investment corporation
OPIDN	organophosphate-induced delayed neuropathy
OPM	Office of Personnel Management
OPM	organization and procedure manual
OPP	Office of Pesticide Programs (EPA)
OPP	oriented polypropylene
OPS	oriented polystyrene
OPS	Office of Pipeline Safety
OPSEC	operational security
OR	Oregon
OR	Oak Ridge
OR	odds ratio
OREIS	Operation Respond Emergency Information System
org	organic
orl	oral
ORM	other regulated materials
ORM-A	U.S. Department of Transportation (DOT) designation for "other regulated materials." The "A" designation is for materials that have an anesthetic, irritating, noxious, toxic, or other similar property that can cause an extreme annoyance or discomfort to passengers or crew if a leak occurs during transportation.
ORM-B	DOT designation for "other regulated materials." The "B" designation is for materials that are capable of causing significant damage to an airplane from leakage during transportation. They are corrosive to aluminum only.
ORM-C	DOT designation for "other regulated materials." The "C" designation is for materials that have characteristics that make them unsuitable for shipment unless properly identified.

ORM-D	DOT designation for "other regulated materials." The "D" designation is for materials that are consumer commodities that present a limited hazard during transportation.
ORM-E	DOT designation for "other regulated materials." The "E" designation is for materials that are not included in any other hazard class, but are subject to DOT regulations. Includes hazardous wastes.
ORNL	Oak Ridge National Laboratory
ORO	Oak Ridge Operations (DOE)
ORP	oxidation reduction potential
Os	osmium
OS	Operations Support Directorate (FEMA)
OSB	oriented strand (or stranded) board
OSC	on-scene coordinator
OSC	on-scene commander
-ose	suffix indicating a carbohydrate compound, usually a sugar
OSHA	Occupational Safety and Health Administration
OSH Act	Occupational Safety and Health Act
OSHP	Office of Safety and Health Protection (ORNL)
OSHRC	Occupational Safety and Health Review Commission
OSLDP	Office for State & Local Domestic Preparedness [(DOJ; now called the Office for Domestic Preparedness (ODP)]
OSM	Office of Surface Mining
OSS	Office of Strategic Services
OST	Office of Science and Technology (DOE)
OST	Office of the Secretary of Transportation
OSTP	Office of Science Technology Policy
OSU-DRC	Ohio State University Disaster Research Center
OTA	Office of Technology Assessment
OTC	over-the-counter
OTFDC	One- & Two-Family Dwelling Code
oth	other cell types
otr	oncogenic transformation
OUO	official use only (information)
OTV	odor threshold value
OVA	organic vapor analyzer
ovr	ovary
oz	ounce

P

p-	meaning "para"
p-	meaning "primary"
P°	standard pressure
P	phosphorus
Pa	protactinium
Pa	Pascal
PA	polyamide (nylon)
PA	phthalic anhydride
PA	public affairs
PA	Public Assistance (FEMA's federal disaster assistance to governments)
PA	Pennsylvania
PAAS	Public Assistance automated system
PAC	Public Assistance coordinator
PAHs	polynuclear aromatic hydrocarbons
PA-ID	Public Assistance applicant identification number
2-PAM chloride	pralidoxine (2-pyridine aldoxime methyl) chloride
PAN	polyacrylonitrile
PAN	peroxyacetylnitrate
PAO	public affairs officer
PAO	Public Assistance officer (FEMA)
PAPR	powered air-purifying respirators
par	parental
Pa·s	pascal-second (viscosity)
PAS	photoacoustic spectroscopy
pat.	patent
Pb	lead
PB	polybutylene (polybutene-1)
PB	polybutadiene
PBA	Plastic Bag Association
PBA	Professional Bowlers Association
PBI	polybenzimidazole
PBPK	physiologically based pharmacokinetic model
PBS	Public Broadcasting System
PBS	Public Building Service (GSA)

PBT	polybutylene terephthalate
PBX	Private Branch Exchange
PC	personal computer
PC	polycarbonate
PCA	patient-controlled analgesia
PCA	Portland Cement Association
PCB	polychlorinated biphenyl
PCDD	polychlorinated dibenzo-p-dioxin
PCDD/F	dioxins and furans
PCDF	polychlorinated dibenzofuran
PCE	perchloroethylene
PCE	tetrachloroethylene (*also* perchlorethylene)
PCE	pyrometric cone equivalent
PCI	Precast/Prestressed Concrete Institute
PCNB	pentachloronitrobenzene
PCP	pentachlorophenate
PCP	phencyclidine; a veterinary anesthetic that causes euphoria and hallucinations in humans
PCTFE	polychlorotrifloroethylene
pcu	pound centigrade unit
Pd	palladium
PD	phenyldichloroarsine (a vesicant or blister agent)
PDA	preliminary damage assessments
PDB	p-dichlorobenzene
PDMS	plasma desorption mass spectrometry
PDS	Professional Development Series (FEMA)
PDT	Pacific daylight time
PE	polyethylene
PE	pentaerythritol
PE	professional engineer
PEEK	polyetheretherketone
PEG	polyethylene glycol
PEI	polyetherimide
PEI	Petroleum Equipment Institute
PEL	permissible exposure limit (OSHA)
PEN	polyethylene naphthalate
penta	pentachlorophenol

PEO STRI	program executive office for simulation, training, and instrumentation
PES	polyethersulfone
PES	photoelectron spectroscopy
PES	potential energy surface
PET	peroxide explosive tester
PET	polyethylene terephthalate (*also* **PETE**)
PETE	polyethylene terephthalate (*also* **PET**)
PETG	polyethylene terephthalate glycol
PETN	pentaerythritol tetranitrate
petr	petroleum
PEX	cross-linked polyethylene
PF	phenol formaldehyde
PFA	perfluoroalkoxy
PFA	Polyurethane Foam Association
PFC	perfluorated carbon
PFO	principal federal official
PFOA	perfluorooctanoic acid
Pf resins	phenol-formaldehyde resins
PFT	permanent full-time (employee)
pg	picogram (one trillionth of a gram; 10^{-12} g)
PG	polyethylene glycol
pgn	pigeon
pH	The negative logarithm of the hydronium ion concentration, which is the indication of the acidity or alkalinity of a substance in water
PHA	process hazard analysis
PHC	principal hazardous constituent
PHCP	prehospital care provider
PHIB	perfluoroisobutylene
PHMSA	Pipeline and Hazardous Materials Safety Administration (DOT)
PHS	U.S. Public Health Service (DHHS)
PI	plasticity index
PI	polyimide
PIA	Plastics Institute of America
PIAT	public information assistance team
PIB	polyisobutylene

pic	phage inhibition capacity
PIC	products of incomplete combustion (*also* **PICs**)
pico-	prefix meaning "10^{-12}"
PICs	products of incomplete combustion (*also* **PIC**)
PID	procurement item description
PID	photoionization detector
PIDX	Petroleum Industry Data Exchange (API)
PIH	poison inhalation hazard
PIH	poisonous by inhalation
PIN	personal identification number
PIN	Pesticide Information Network
PIO	public information officer
PIR	polyisocyanurate
PIRG	Public Interest Research Group
PIV	post indicator valve
PIW	project identification worksheet
pixel	picture element
pK	represents the extent of dissociation of a weak acid
pK	peak concentration
pkg	package
PLA	polylactic acid
PLB	personal locator beacon
PLSS	Public Land Survey System (United States)
Pm	promethium
PM	particulate matter (*also* micron particulate matter)
PM2.5	particulate matter (smaller than 2.5 μm in diameter)
PM10	particulate matter (nominally 10 μm and less)
PM15	particulate matter (nominally 15 μm and less)
PMA	Pacific Maritime Association
PMA	Pharmaceutical Manufacturers' Association
PMCC	Pensky-Martens closed cup (flash point tester)
PMMA	polymethyl methacrylate
PMN	premanufacture notification (under TSCA)
pmol	picomole
PMP	polymethylpentene
PMR	proportionate mortality ratio

PMRA	Pest Management Regulatory Agency (Canada)
PN	part number
PN	positive notification
PNA	polynuclear aromatic hydrocarbons
PNOC	particulates not otherwise classified (ACGIH)
PNOR	particulates not otherwise regulated (OSHA)
PNP	private nonprofit
PNS	peripheral nervous system effects
Po	polonium
PO	project officer
PO_x	general designation for the oxides of phosphorus
POC	point of contact
POC	project officer coordinator
POD	probability of detection
POE	point of exposure
POGO	privately-owned/government-operated
POHCs	principal organic hazardous constituents
POL	petroleum, oil, and lubricants
poly-	prefix meaning "many"
POM	particulate organic matter
POM	polycyclic organic matter
POM	polyoxymethylene
POP	performance-oriented packaging
POP	persistent organic pollutant
POTUS	President of the United States
POTWs	publicly owned/operated treatment works
PP	polypropylene
PPA	Pollution Prevention Act
PP&E	property, plant, and equipment
ppb	parts per billion
PPC	Prevention Preparedness Council
PPDI	p-phenylene diisocyanate
PPE	personal protective equipment
PPG	polypropylene glycol
pph	parts per hundred
PPI	Plastics Pipe Institute

PPIC	Pesticide Programs Information Center
PPIS	Pesticide Product Information System
PPIS	Pollution Prevention Incentives for States
ppm	parts per million
PPO	polyphenylene oxide
PPS	polyphenylene sulfide
PP-SCBA	positive-pressure self-contained breathing apparatus
ppt	parts per trillion
ppt	precipitate
ppth	parts per thousand
PPV	positive pressure ventilation
P/QA	performance/quality assurance
PQL	practical quantitation limit
Pr	praseodymium
PR	pair [as a unit of issue (UI)]
PR	Puerto Rico
PRCS	permit required confined space
precip	precipitate
PRF	Plastics Recycling Foundation
PROACT	Protective and Responsive Options for Airport Counterterrorism
Prop 65	Proposition 65 (California Safe Drinking Water and Toxic Enforcement Act of 1986)
PROTECT	Program for Response Options and Technology Enhancements for Chemical/Biological Terrorism
PRP(s)	potentially responsible party (or parties)
PS	designation for chloropicrin
PS	polystyrene
PS	point source
PSC	polar stratospheric cloud
PSD	Prevention of Significant Deterioration
psi	pounds per square inch
PSI	pollutant standards index (now called the air quality index)
PSI	Proliferation Security Initiative
psia	pounds per square inch absolute
psig	pounds per square inch gauge; psia minus local atmospheric pressure
PSM	Process Safety Management

PST	Pacific standard time
PSTN	Pesticide Safety Team Network
Pt	platinum
PT	Preparedness, Training, and Exercises Directorate (FEMA)
PTE	preparedness, training, and exercises
PTFE	polytetrafluoroethylene
PTMEG	polytetramethylene ether glycol (*also referred to as* **PTMO** *or* **PTMG**)
PTMG	polytetramethylene ether glycol (*also referred to as* **PTMO** *or* **PTMEG**)
PTMO	polytetramethylene ether glycol (*also referred to as* **PTMG** *or* **PTMEG**)
PTT	polytrimethylene terephthalate
Pu	plutonium
PUC	public utility commission
PUL	pulmonary system effects
PUR	polyurethane
PURPA	Public Utilities Regulatory and Policy Act
PVA	polyvinyl alcohol (*see also* **PVOH**)
PVA	polyvinyl acetate (*see also* **PVAc**)
PVAc	polyvinyl acetate (*see also* **PVA**)
PVAL	polyvinyl alcohol
PVB	polyvinyl butyral
PVC	polyvinyl chloride
PVCs	premature ventricular contractions
PVD	physical vapor deposition
PVDC	polyvinyl dichloride
PVDC	polyvinylidene chloride
PVDFR	polyvinyl difluoride
PVE	polyvinyl ether
PVF	polyvinyl fluoride
PVI	polyvinylisobutyl ether
PVK	polyvinyl carbazole
PVM	polyvinyl methyl ether
PVM/MA	polyvinyl methyl ether/maleic anhydride
PVOH	polyvinyl alcohol (*see also* **PVA**)
PVP	polyvinyl pyrrolidone

PVSA	Passenger Vessel Services Act
PVT	pressure, volume, and temperature
PW	public works
PWS	public water supply
PWSS	public water supply system
PZEV	partial zero-emission vehicle
PZVC	prolonged zero-visibility conditions

Q

Q	sesquimustard (a vesicant or blister agent)
Q	reaction quotient
q	heat
QA	quality assurance
QAP	quality assurance program
QA/QC	quality assurance/quality control
QC	quality control
QL	quantification limit
QR	quick response
QRV	quick release valve
qt	quart
QT	quality testing
QT	quench and temper (*also* quenched *and* tempered)
QUP	quantity unit pack

R

R'	the designation for an additional organic group or alkyl radical in a general formula
R	roentgen
R	gas constant
R-	the designation for an organic group or alkyl radical
Ra	radium
RA	remedial action
RACES	Radio Amateur Civil Emergency Service
RACM	reasonably available control measures

RACM	regulated asbestos-containing material
RACT	reasonably available control technology
rad	radiation absorbed dose
RADAR	radio detecting and ranging
RADCON	radiological control team
RAID Teams	Rapid Assessment and Initial Detection Teams [now known as Civil Support Teams (CST)]
R&D	research and development
RAP	Radiological Assistance Program (part of NIRT; provides first response capability)
RARA	Resource Conservation and Recovery Act
RAWS	remote automatic weather station
Rb	rubidium
RBC	red blood cells
RC	residual capacity
RCA	riot control agent
RCMA	Roof Coatings Manufacturers Association
RCO	regional compliance officer
RCP	Regional Oil and Hazardous Substances Pollution Contingency Plan
RCRA	Resource Conservation and Recovery Act of 1976
RCRIS	Resource Conservation and Recovery Information System (EPA)
RD	regional director
RDA	recommended dietary allowances
RDD	radiological dispersal device
RDD	regional deposited dose
RDDR	regional deposited dose ratio
RDECOM	Research, Development, and Engineering Command (Army Materiel Command)
RDF	refuse-derived fuel
rDNA	recombinant DNA
RDV	reference dose values
RDX	cyclonite (agent designation)
Re	rhenium
REACT	Radio Emergency Associated Communications Teams
READY	radio, equipment, air, duties, yes
REC	regional emergency coordinator
REE	rare earth elements

ref	reference
refr	refractive
REL	recommended exposure limit
rem	roentgen equivalent man
REM	rapid eye movement
REMP	Regional Emergency Management Plan
REMS	RCRA Enforcement Management System
REO	regional environmental officer
REP	roentgen equivalent physical
REP	Radiological Emergency Preparedness (FEMA)
REPI	Renewable Energy Production Incentive
RfC	reference concentration
RfD	reference dose
RFD	reference dose value
RFID	radio frequency identification
RFNA	red fuming nitric acid
RFP	request for proposal
RGDR	regional gas dose ratio
RGL	Regulatory & Guidance Library
Rh	rhodium
RH	relative humidity
rhomb	rhombic
RHYTHM	registered trademark for the Du Pont Company's Safe Distribution Program: Remember How You Treat Hazardous Materials
RI	Rhode Island
RIA	resource identification and analysis
RIC	Radon Information Center
RICO	Racketeer Influenced and Corrupt Organizations Act
RID	dangerous goods by rail (European regulations; Règlements Concernant le Transport International Ferroviaire des Marchandises Dangereuses)
RIM	reaction injection molding
RIS	resonance ionization spectroscopy
RISC	Regulatory Information Service Center
RIT	rapid intervention team [*may also be called a* **firefighter assist and search team (FAST)**]
RITA	Research and Innovative Technology Administration

RMA	Rubber Manufacturers Association
RMCL	recommended maximum contaminant level
RMP	Resource Management Plan
RMP	risk management plan (or program)
RMPP	risk management and prevention plan
Rn	radon
RNA	ribonucleic acid
RNA	rapid needs assessment team
rns	rinsed with water
ROAM	Rule of Air Management
ROC	regional operations center
ROD	report of discrepancy
ROD	record of decision
ROG	reactive organic gases
RO/RO SHIP	freight ship or ferry with facilities for vehicles to drive on and off ("roll-on/roll-off")
ROU	Radio Officers' Union
RP	red phosphorous (agent designation)
RP	reinforced plastic
RPAR	rebuttable presumption against registration
RPCH	rural primary care hospital
rpm	revolutions per minute
RPM	remedial project manager
RPVC	rigid polyvinyl chloride
RQ	reportable quantity
RR	relative risk
RR	risk ratio
RR	response and recovery
RR	Response and Recovery Directorate (FEMA)
RRF	Ready Reserve Force
RRIS	Rapid Response Information System (FEMA)
RRP	regional response plan
RRT	regional response teams
RSCAAL	remote sensing chemical agent alarm
RSD	risk-specific dose
RSI	roofing/siding/insulation

RSPA	Research and Special Programs Administration, DOT (HM-181; since reorganized within DOT)
RSS	remote storage sites
RTECS	Registry of Toxic Effects of Chemical Substances
RTF	response task forces
RTG	radioisotope thermoelectric generator
RTK	right-to-know
Ru	ruthenium
RV	residual volume
RVF	Rift Valley fever

S

s	second
s-	prefix for "secondary"
S	sulfur
SA	arsine (a chemical blood agent)
SAA	Standards Association of Australia
SAB	Science Advisory Board (EPA)
SAC	special agency in charge
SADT	self-accelerating decomposition temperature
SAE	Society of Automotive Engineers
SAE	Stafford Act employee [*also* known as disaster assistance employees (DAE)]
SAF black	super abrasion furnace (carbon) black
SAME	Society of American Military Engineers
SAMPE	Society for the Advancement of Material and Process Engineering
SAN	styrene acrylonitrile (copolymer)
S&T	Science and Technology Directorate (DHS)
SANE	sulfur and nitrogen emissions
SAR	start action request
SAR	search and rescue
SAR	supplied-air respirators
SARA	Superfund Amendments and Reauthorization Act of 1986 (Title III is *also* known as EPCRA)
SARS	severe acute respiratory syndrome
SAS	sodium aluminum sulfate

SATP	standard ambient temperature and pressure
SAW	surface acoustic wave
Sb	antimony
SB	styrene butadiene (a copolymer)
SBA	secondary butyl alcohol
SBA	Small Business Administration (provides disaster assistance along with FEMA)
SBC	styrene-butadiene copolymers
SBC	Standard Building Code (SBCCI)
SBCCI	Southern Building Code Congress International
SBCCOM	Soldier and Biological Chemical Command (U.S. Army)
SBG	standard battery grade
SBR	styrene-butadiene rubber
SBS	styrene butadiene styrene
SBS	sick building syndrome
SBX	inorganic boron (wood preservative)
Sc	scandium
SC	special considerations
SC	South Carolina
SCBA	self-contained breathing apparatus
SCC	Setaflash closed (cup) tester
SCC	Shipping Coordinating Committee (U.S. Department of State)
SCC	Standards Council of Canada
SCE	standard calomel electrode
SCFM	standard cubic feet per minute
SCM	shipping container marking
SCO	state coordinating officer
SCP	Standards Completion Program
scu	subcutaneous
SCUBA	self-contained underwater breathing apparatus
SD	South Dakota
SDA	specially denatured alcohol
SDAT	state damage assessment team(s)
SDI	Steel Deck Institute
SDI	Strategic Defense Initiative
SDO	standards development organization
SDWA	Safe Drinking Water Act

SDWIS	Safe Drinking Water Information System
Se	selenium
SE	synchronous excitation (fluorescence spectroscopy)
SEAM	surface, environment, and mining
SEAOC	Structural Engineers Association of California
SEAS	strategic environmental assessment system
SEB	Staphylococcal enterotoxin B
SEBS	styrene-ethylene-butadiene-styrene
sec	second
sec-	prefix for "secondary"
SECDEF	Secretary of Defense
SECNAV	Secretary of the Navy
SEED	Safety Evaluation of Existing Dams (U.S. Bureau of Reclamation)
SEM	standard error of the mean
SEP	supplemental environmental project
SER	steam enhanced remediation
SERC	state emergency response commission
SERI	Solar Energy Research Institute
SES	secondary emissions standard
SESHA	Semiconductor Environmental Safety and Health Association
SETAC	Society for Environmental Toxicology and Chemistry
SEV	severe irritation effects
SFAR	Special Federal Aviation Regulations
SFE	supercritical fluid extraction
SFIP	standard flood insurance policy
SFPE	Society of Fire Protection Engineers
sg	specific gravity
SGF-2	fog oil
SGR	steam gas recycle
SHED	sealed housing for evaporative determinations
SHG	second harmonic generation
SHMO	state hazard mitigation officer
Si	silicon
SI	International System of Units (Système Internationale de Unites; SI)
SIC	Standard Industrial Classification
SIC Code	Standard Industrial Classification Code

SICEA	Steel Industry Compliance Extension Act
SIMS	secondary ion mass spectrometry
SIOC	Strategic Information and Operations Center (an FBI resource)
SIP	state implementation plan
SIP	Streamlined Inspection Program (USCG)
SIRS	satellite infrared spectrometer
SIS	styrene-isoprene-styrene
SITA	Système Internationale Transport Aeronautique
SITREP	situation report
SIU	Seafarers International Union
SJI	Steel Joist Institute
SLA	service level agreement
SLAR	single layer antireflection coating
SLPS	State and Local Programs and Support Directorate (FEMA)
SLR	side-looking radar
Sm	samarium
SMACNA	Sheet Metal and Air Conditioning Contractors' National Association
SMART	Sensitive Membrane Antigen Rapid Test (trademarked test for biological agents)
SMC	sheet molding compound
SME	subject matter expert
SMMA	styrene methyl methacrylate
SMMA	standard mitigation measures agreement
SMOA	Superfund memorandum of agreement
SMR	standardized mortality ratio
SMSA	standard metropolitan statistical area [*also called* **metropolitan statistical area (MSA)**]
Sn	tin
SNG	synthetic natural gas
SNL	Sandia National Laboratories
SNPRM	supplemental notice of proposed rulemaking (EPA)
SNS	Strategic National Stockpile
SNUR	significant new use rule (EPA)
SO_2	sulfur dioxide
SOC	Special Operations Command
SOCMA	Synthetic Organic Chemical Manufacturers Association

SOCMI	synthetic organic chemical manufacturers industry
SOC(s)	synthetic organic chemical(s)
SOD	soil oxidant demand
SOEH	Society for Occupational and Environmental Health
SOG	standard operating guideline
sol	soluble
SOLAS	International Convention for the Safety of Life at Sea
soln	solution
SONAR	sound navigation and ranging
SOP	standard operating procedures
SOW	scope of work
SOW	statement of work
SOx	general designation for the oxides of sulfur
SPAO	state Public Assistance officer
SPC	statistical process control
SPCC	Spill Prevention, Control, and Countermeasure rule (EPA)
SPCC plan	Spill Prevention, Control, and Countermeasure plan
SPCP	spill prevention, containment, and countermeasures
SPE	secondary particulate emissions
SPE	Society of Plastics Engineers
sp gr	specific gravity
SPI	Society of the Plastics Industry
SPI	special packing instruction
SPI	Strategic Planning Initiative
SPM	*Shore Protection Manual*
SPS	syndiotactic polystyrene
spt	sputtering
sp vol	specific volume
SPWG	special work group
sq	square
SQ3R	survey, question, read, recite, and review (*also* **SQRRR**)
SQG	small quantity generator (of hazardous waste)
SQRRR	survey, question, read, recite, and review (*also* **SQ3R**)
Sr	strontium
SRD	simple radiological device
SRF	state-administered Water Pollution Control Revolving Funds (EPA grants)

SRF black	semi-reinforcing furnace (carbon) black
SRI	Southwest Research Institute
S.S.	steamship (*also* **SS**)
SS	steamship (*also* **S.S.**)
SSC	scientific support coordinators
SSI	sensitive security information
SSPC	Steel Structures Painting Council
SSS	side-scan sonar
S/T	short tons (2,000 lbs)
START	simple triage and rapid transport
STATEX	statutory exclusion (FEMA)
STB	Surface Transportation Board (DOT)
STC	single trip container
STCC	standard transportation commodity code
STCW	International Convention on Standards of Training, Certification, and Watchkeeping for Seafarers, 1978
std	standard
STD	sexually transmitted disease
STEL	short-term exposure limit
STEM	scanning transmission electron microscope
STEV	short-term exposure value
STL	small toxic laboratory
STMA	Standard Treatment Measures Agreement (FEMA)
STN	Scientific and Technical Information Network
STP	standard temperature and pressure
STPP	sodium tripolyphosphate
STR	subcontract technical representative
subl	sublimes
SUP	standard unit of processing
SUS	Saybolt universal second (unit measure of viscosity for heated oils)
Sv	sievert (SI unit of dose equivalent; 1 Sv = 100 rem)
SV	sampling visit
SV	significant violator
SVC	Society of Vacuum Coaters
SVD	swine vesicular disease
SW	slow wave

SWAP	Source Water Assessment Program
SWAT	special (or strategic) weapons assault team (former usage)
SWAT	special weapons and tactics (current usage)
SWC	settlement with conditions
SWDA	Solid Waste Disposal Act
SWE	single wavelength excitation (fluorescence spectroscopy)
SWIE	Southern Waste Information Exchange
SWIR	shortwave infrared
SWMU	solid waste management unit
SWPA	source water protection area
SWQPPP	source water quality protection partnership petitions
SWTR	Surface Water Treatment Rule
SXAPS	soft X-ray appearance potential spectroscopy
sym	symmetrical
SYSOP	systems operator

T

t	tera-
t-	tertiary
T	O-mustard (a vesicant or blister agent)
T	tritium
$T_{1/2}$	half-life
T2	transverse relaxation time
T_{Lm}	medium tolerance unit
T_m	melting point of a polymer in °C
Ta	tantalum
TA	technical approach
TAC	technical assistance contractor
TAG	technical assistance grant
TAM	turnaround annual maintenance
TAMS	toxic air monitoring system
T&E	threatened and endangered (species)
TAP	triaryl phosphate
TAPDS	Toxic Air Pollutant Data System
TAPPI	Technical Association of the Pulp and Paper Industry

TAS	technical assistance specialist
TATP	triacetone triperoxide [*also called tricyclic acetone peroxide (TCAP)*]
Tb	terbium
TBD	to be determined
TBP	tributyl phosphate
TBT	tributyltin
TBV	to be verified
Tc	technetium
TC	toxic concentration
TC	Transport Canada
TC_{Lo}	lowest published toxic concentration
TCA	Truckload Carriers Association
TCAP	tricyclic acetone peroxide, or *tricyclo; also called triacetone triperoxide (TATP), peroxyacetone,* or *acetone peroxide*
TCC	Tagliabue closed cup (test for flash point)
TCDD	2,3,7,8-tetrachlorodibenzo-p-dioxin
TCDF	tetrachlorodibenzofurans
TC/DOT	Transport Canada and/or the U.S. Department of Transportation
TCDS	Type Certificate Data Sheets (FAA)
TCE	trichloroethylene
TCF	total chlorine free
TCIM	Threat Countermeasures and Incident Management Directorate
TCLP	toxicity characteristic leaching procedure
TCM	transportation control measures
TCMD	transportation control movement document
TCP	telecommunications priorities
TCP	trichloropropane
TCP	tricresyl phosphate
TCRI	toxic chemical release inventory
TCV	total containment vessel
TD	toxic dose
TD_{Lo}	lowest published toxic dose
TDCC	Transportation Data Coordinating Committee
TDFS	time-dependent fluorescence shifts
TDG	Transportation of Dangerous Goods (Canadian regulations)
TDI	toluene diisocyanate

TDS	total dissolved solids
TDY	temporary duty
Te	tellurium
tech	technical
TECP	totally encapsulating chemical protective suit
TEG	tetraethylene glycol
TEGD	technical enforcement guidance document
TEL	tetraethyl lead
TEM	transmission electron microscopy
temp	temperature
TENS	transcutaneous electrical nerve stimulation
TEP	triethyl phosphate
ter	teratogen
TERC	Tribal Emergency Response Commission
tera-	prefix meaning "10^{12}"
tert-	prefix for "tertiary"
tetra-	prefix for "four"
TEU	Technical Escort Unit (U.S. Army)
TEU	20-ft equivalent unit (containers)
TFBA	Task Force for *Bacillus anthracis*
TFD	terrestrial field dissipation
TFE	tetrafluoroethylene
TFR	temporary flight restrictions
TFX	toxic effects
Tg	glass transition temperature
TGA	thermogravimetric analysis
TGA	technical-grade active ingredient (*also* **TGAI**)
TGAI	technical-grade active ingredient (*also* **TGA**)
Th	thorium
TH	temporary housing
THC	total hydrocarbons
THF	tetrahydrofuran
thia-	prefix indicating presence of sulfur in a compound
thio-	prefix indicating presence of sulfur in a compound, usually substituted for oxygen
THLPSSC	Technical Hazardous Liquid Pipeline Safety Standards Committee
THM	trihalomethane

THO	temporary housing officer
THR	toxic and hazard review
Ti	titanium
TI	Transportation Institute
TIB	toxic industrial biologicals
TIC	Technical Information Center (NASA)
TIC	toxic industrial chemicals
TIH	toxic inhalation hazard (same as **PIH**)
TIM	toxic industrial material
TIR	toxic industrial radiological materials
TIR	thermal infrared
TIRS	thermal infrared scanner
TIS	Tolerance Index System (EPA)
TISE	take it somewhere else
Tl	thallium
TLC	total lung capacity
TLC	thin-layer chromatography
TLC	territory logistics centers
TLm	aquatic toxicity (*also* **AQCX**)
TLV	total lung volume (lung volume at maximal inspiration)
TLV	threshold limit value
TLV-C	threshold limit value-ceiling
TLV-STEL	threshold limit value–short-term exposure limit
TLV-TWA	threshold limit value–time-weighted average
Tm	thulium
TM	trademark
TMA	trimethylamine
TMA	trimellitic anhydride
TMCP	tri-m-cresyl phosphate
TMDL	total maximum daily limit
TMDL	total maximum daily load
TML	trimethyl lead
TMRC	theoretical maximum residue contribution
TMU	ton multiunit tank
TN	Tennessee
TNB	trinitrobenzene

TNT	trinitrotoluene
TO	technical order
TOA	trace organic analysis
TOC	Tagliabue open cup (test for flash point)
TOC	total organic carbon
TOC	total organic compounds
TOCP	tri-o-cresyl phosphate
TODI	3, 3'-dimethyl-4, 4'-biphenylene diisocyanate
TOF	time of flight
TOF	trioctylphosphite
TOMPs	toxic organic micropollutants
TOMS	total ozone mapping spectrometer
torr	unit of pressure equal to 1 mm of mercury
TOX	tetradichloroxylene
TP	thermoplastic
TPA	terephthalic acid
TPCC	Trade Promotion Coordinating Committee
TPCP	tri-p-cresyl phosphate
TPE	thermoplastic elastomer
TPH	total petroleum hydrocarbons
TPI	thermoplastic polyimide
TPO	thermoplastic polyolefin
TPO rubber	thermoplastic polyolefin rubber
TPP	triphenyl phosphate
TPQ	threshold planning quantity
TPSSC	Technical Pipeline Safety Standards Committee
TPTH	triphenyltinhydroxide
TPU	thermoplastic polyurethane
TPV	thermoplastic vulcanizate
TPY	tons per year
TQM	total quality management
TR	technical report
TRACEM	thermal, radiological, asphyxiation, chemical, etiological, and mechanical
TRANSCAER	Transportation Community Awareness and Emergency Response
TRB	Transportation Research Board
TRC	thermodynamics research laboratory

TREAS	Department of the Treasury
TREPR	time-resolved electron paramagnetic resonance
tri-	prefix meaning "three"
TRI	Toxic Release Inventory (database)
TRIP	Toxic Release Inventory Program
TRIPS	Travel, Reporting, and Information Planning System
TRIS	Toxic Chemical Release Inventory System
TRO	temporary restraining order
TRQ	threshold reportable quantity
TRS	total reduced sulfur
TRU	transuranic waste (radioactive)
TS	thermoset
TSA	Transportation Security Administration
TSA	toluene sulfonic acid
TSAC	Towing Safety Advisory Committee
TSCA	Toxic Substances Control Act (40 CFR 700–799)
TSCAPP	Toxic Substances Control Act, Plant and Production Database
TSCC	Toxic Substances Coordinating Committee
TSD	treatment, storage, and disposal
TSDF	treatment, storage, and disposal facility
TSI	thermal system insulation
TSO	Technical Standard Orders (FAA)
TSP	Telecommunications Service Priority
TSP	total suspended particulates
TSP	trisodium phosphate
TSS	total suspended solids (nonfilterable)
TSWG	Technical Support Working Group
TTHM	total trihalomethane
TTMA	Truck Trailer Manufacturers Association
TTO	total toxic organics
TTY	teletype (*also called* a *teletypewriter*)
TUR	toxic use reduction
TV	tidal volume
TVA	Tennessee Valley Authority
TVOC	total volatile organic compounds
TWA	time-weighted average

TWGFEX	Technical Working Group for Fire and Explosions
TWS	transient water system
TX	Texas
TXDS	toxic dose
TZ	treatment zone

U

U	uranium
U/A	urinalysis
UAC	Uniform Administrative Code
UAQI	Uniform Air Quality Index
UARG	Utility Air Regulatory Group
UARS	upper atmosphere research satellite
UBC	Uniform Building Code (ICBO)
UCC	ultra clean coal
UCL	upper control limit
UCR	usual, customary, and reasonable
UCS	uniform color space
UCS	unified command suite
UCS	Uniform Communications Standard
UDI	under the direct influence
UDMH	unsymmetrical dimethyl hydrazine
UEL	upper explosive limit
UF	urea formaldehyde
UF	uncertainty factor
UFAC	Upholstered Furniture Action Council
UFC	Uniform Fire Code (Western Fire Chiefs Association and NFPA)
UFFI	urea-formaldehyde foam insulation
UFL	upper flammable limit
UHF	ultrahigh frequency
UHMWPE	ultra high molecular weight polyethylene
UHV	ultrahigh vacuum (UV)
UIC	Underground Injection Control (Program)
UIC	Union Internationale des Chemins de Fer (International Union of Railways)

UK	United Kingdom
UL	Underwriters Laboratory
ULC	Underwriters' Laboratories of Canada
ULC	Underwriters Laboratory Classification
ULCC	ultra large crude carriers (tankers larger than 300,000 dwt)
ULDPE	ultra low density polyethylene
UMC	Uniform Mechanical Code
UN	United Nations
UNCED	United Nations Conference on Environment and Development
UNECE	United Nations Economic Commission for Europe
UNEP	United Nations Environment Program
UNESCO	United Nations Educational, Scientific and Cultural Organization
UNIDR	United Nations Institute for Disarmament Research
UN/ISO	United Nations International Standards Organization
UN/NA numbers	United Nations/North American (U.S. DOT or Transport Canada) numbers
unr	unreported
uns-	unsymmetrical
unsym-	unsymmetrical
UP	unsaturated polyester
UPAC	International Union of Pure and Applied Chemistry
UPC	Uniform Plumbing Code
UPC	Uniform Product Code
UPC	Universal Product Code
UPIN	unique physician identification number
UPS	uninterruptible power supply
UPS	ultraviolet photoemission spectroscopy
URAC	Utilization Review Accreditation Commission
URO	utilization review organization
U.S.	United States
USACE	United States Army Corps of Engineers
USAF	United States Air Force
USAID	U.S. Agency for International Development
USAMRIID	United States Army Medical Research Institute of Infectious Diseases
USAN	United States Adopted Name (Council)
US&R	urban search and rescue

USBR	U.S. Bureau of Reclamation
USC	Unified Soil Classification (System)
USC	United States Code
USCA	United States Code Annotated
USCE	United States Army Corps of Engineers
US-CERT	United States Computer Emergency Response Team (DHS)
USCG	United States Coast Guard
USDA	United States Department of Agriculture
USDC	United States Department of Commerce
USDI	United States Department of the Interior
USDW	underground source of drinking water
USEPA	United States Environmental Protection Agency
USFA	United States Fire Administration
USFS	United States Forest Service
USFWS	United States Fish and Wildlife Service
USGS	United States Geological Survey
USN	United States Navy
USNC	United States National Committee
USP	United States Pharmacopeia
USPHS	United States Public Health Service
USP-NF	*United States Pharmacopeia-National Formulary*
USPS	United States Postal Service
USQ	unreviewed safety question
USQD	unreviewed safety question determination
USQD	unreviewed safety question document
USSS	United States Secret Service
UST	underground storage tank
USTRANSCOM	United States Transportation Command
UT	Utah
UTI	urinary tract infection
uv	ultraviolet (*also* **UV**)
UV	ultraviolet (*also* **uv**)
UVB	ultraviolet radiation band
UV/Vis	ultraviolet/visible spectrophotometry

V

V	vanadium
V	volts
V_T	tidal volume (volume of air inhaled/exhaled during normal breathing)
VA	Veterans Affairs
VA	Virginia
VAB	value-added bank
vac	vacuum
vad	vapor-air density
VAD	value-added distributor
val	value
VAL	volunteer agency liaison
VAN	value-added network
vap	vapor
vap d	vapor density
vap press	vapor pressure
var	variety
VAR	value-added reseller
VAT	value-added tax
VB	valence bond
VBIED	vehicle borne improvised explosive devices
VB theory	valence bond theory
VC	vital capacity
VC	vinyl chloride
VC	vinylidene chloride
VCE	polyvinyl chloride-ethylene
VCEMA	polyvinyl chloride-ethylene-methyl acrylate
VCM	vinyl chloride monomer
VCMA	polyvinyl chloride-methyl acrylate
VCR	video cassette recorder
VCVAC	polyvinyl chloride-vinyl acrylate
VCVDC	polyvinyl chloride-vinylidene chloride
VDT	video display terminal
VE	a nerve gas (agent designation)
VE	visual emissions

VEO	visible emission observation
VFD	volunteer fire department
VFR	visual flight rules
VG	a nerve gas (agent designation)
V-gas	a nerve gas (agent designation)
VHA	Veterans Health Administration (Department of Veterans Affairs)
VHAP	volatile hazardous air pollutant
VHF	viral hemorrhagic fever
VHF	very high frequency
VHMWPE	very high molecular weight polyethylene
VHS	vertical and horizontal spread (model)
VI	viscosity index
VI	Virgin Islands
VICS	Voluntary Interindustry Communications Standard
VISA	Voluntary Intermodal Sealift Agreement
visc	viscosity
VIVM	vendor independent messaging interface
VKT	vehicle kilometers traveled
VLCC	very large crude carriers (tankers between 200,000 and 300,000 dwt)
VM	a chemical nerve agent (agent designation)
VMATs	veterinary medical assistance teams (coordinated through FEMA)
VMT	vehicle miles traveled
VNIR	visual and near infrared
VOAD	volunteer organizations active in disasters
VOC	volatile organic compound
vol	volume
VOLAG	voluntary agency
VOM	volt-ohm meter
VOS	volatile organic substances
VP	vapor pressure
VPC	vapor phase chromatography
vs.	versus
VSD	virtually safe dose
VSEPR	valence shell electron pair repulsion theory
vsol	very soluble
VSS	volatile suspended solids

VT	Vermont
VUV	vacuum ultraviolet
Vx	a chemical nerve agent (agent designation)
VX	a chemical nerve agent (agent designation)

W

w	weight
W	tungsten
W	weeks
W	work
WA	Washington
WB	wet bulb
WBC	white blood cell count
WBC	white blood cells
WCO	World Customs Organization
WEDI	Workgroup for Electronic Data Interchange
WERL	Water Engineering Research Laboratory
WES	Waterways Experiment Station (U.S. Army Corps of Engineers)
WET	whole effluent toxicity (test)
WFNA	white fuming nitric acid
WG	work group
WH	Warnock Hersey (professional services)
WHMIS	Workplace Hazardous Materials Information System
WHO	World Health Organization
WHPS	Warnock Hersey Professional Services, Ltd.
WHWT	water and hazardous waste team
WI	Wisconsin
WICEM	World Industry Conference on Environmental Management
WIMPs	weakly interacting massive particles
WIMS	Weather Information Management System
WIP	work in progress
WISER	Wireless Information System for Emergency Responders (NLM, DHHS)
WL	working level
WLA/TMDL	waste load allocation/total maximum daily load

WLM	working level month
WMD	weapons of mass destruction
WMD chem/bio	weapons of mass destruction, chemical/biological
WMD-CST	Weapons of Mass Destruction Civil Support Teams (National Guard; originally called RAID teams)
WMO	World Meteorological Organization
WNS	Warehouse Information Network Standard
WOBO	World Organization of Building Officials
WOE	weight-of-evidence (for carcinogenicity)
WOHRC	Women's Occupational Health Resource Center
WP	wettable powder
WP	white phosphorus
WPCF	Water Pollution Control Federation
WQA	Water Quality Act
WQM	water quality monitor
WQS	water quality standards
WQSDB	National Water Quality Standards Database (EPA)
WRAP	Waste Reduction Assessments Program
WRC	Water Resources Council
WRDA	Water Resources Development Act
WREAFS	Waste Reduction Evaluations at Federal Sites Program
WRI	World Resources Institute
WRIS	Wildland Resources Information System
WRITE	Waste Reduction Innovative Technology Evaluation Program (EPA)
WRSIC	Water Resources Scientific Information Center
WSF	water soluble fraction
WSRA	Wild and Scenic Rivers Act
WSS	work smart standards
WSTB	Water Science and Technology Board
WSTP	wastewater sewage treatment plant
wt	weight
WTE	waste-to-energy
wt/gal	weight per gallon
WV	West Virginia
WWEMA	Waste and Wastewater Equipment Manufacturers Association
WWF	World Wildlife Fund

WWPI Western Wood Preservers Institute
WWTP wastewater treatment plant
WWTU wastewater treatment unit
WWW World Wide Web
WY Wyoming
WYSIWYG "What you *see* is what you get."

X

Xe xenon
XEPS extruded expanded polystyrene
XLPE cross-linked polyethylene
XRF X-ray fluorescence spectroscopy

Y

y year(s)
Y yttrium
Yb ytterbium
-yl suffix indicating a molecular fragment or group

Z

Z atomic number
ZEV zero emissions vehicle
Z list OSHA list of Toxic and Hazardous Substances (29 CFR 1910.1000, tables Z-1, Z-2, and Z-3; worker right-to-know)
Zn zinc
Zr zirconium
ZRL zero risk level
Z table *see* **Z list**